D04414682

A Colour Handbook

Skin Diseases
of the
Dog and Cat
SECOND EDITION

Tim Nuttall
BSc, BVSc, PhD, CertVD, CBiol, MSB, MRCVS
Senior Lecturer in Veterinary Dermatology,
University of Liverpool Small Animal Teaching Hospital, Leahurst Campus, Neston, UK

Richard G. Harvey
BVSc, PhD, FBiol, DVD, DipECVD, MRCVS
The Veterinary Centre, Coventry, UK

Patrick J. McKeever
DVM, MS, DACVD
Professor Emeritus
McKeever Dermatology Clinics, Eden Prairie, Minnesota, USA

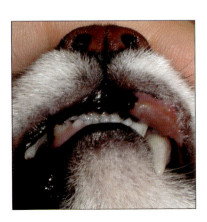

MANSON PUBLISHING/THE VETERINARY PRESS

Second impression 2011

Copyright © 2009 Manson Publishing Ltd

ISBN: 978-1-84076-115-3

All rights reserved. No part of this publication may be reproduced, stored in a retrieval system or transmitted in any form or by any means without the written permission of the copyright holder or in accordance with the provisions of the Copyright Act 1956 (as amended), or under the terms of any licence permitting limited copying issued by the Copyright Licensing Agency, 33–34 Alfred Place, London WC1E 7DP, UK.

Any person who does any unauthorized act in relation to this publication may be liable to criminal prosecution and civil claims for damages.

A CIP catalogue record for this book is available from the British Library.

For full details of all Manson Publishing Ltd titles please write to:
Manson Publishing Ltd, 73 Corringham Road, London NW11 7DL, UK.
Tel: +44(0)20 8905 5150
Fax: +44(0)20 8201 9233
Email: manson@mansonpublishing.com
Website: www.mansonpublishing.com

Commissioning editor: Jill Northcott
Project manager: Ayala Kingsley
Editor: Peter Beynon
Cover and book design: Ayala Kingsley
Layout: DiacriTech, Chennai, India
Colour reproduction: Tenon & Polert Colour Scanning Ltd, Hong Kong
Printed by: New Era Printing Co Ltd, Hong Kong

CONTENTS

ALPHABETICAL INDEX OF DISEASES

Drug names

Generic name	Trade name
acetic acid and aloe	AloCetic Ear Rinse
adrenocorticotropic hormone	Synacthen
chlorine dioxide	Earigant Liquid
ciclosporin/cyclosporine	Neoral, Atopica
fluocinolone acetonide in 60% dimethylsulfoxide	Synotic
hydrocortisone aceponate	Cortavance
imiquimod cream	Aldara
isotretinoin	Accutane
mitotane (o,p′-DDD)	Lysodren
moxidectin/imidacloprid	Advocate
parachlorometaxylenol (PCMX)	Epi-Otic Advanced
pentoxifylline	Trental
phytosphingosine	Douxo Seborrhea Spot-on, Douxo Micellar Solution, Chlorhexidine PS shampoo
propylene glycol, malic acid, benzoic acid, and salicylic acid	Multicleanse Solution, Oti-Clens, Dermisol
recombinant feline interferon omega	Virbagen
selamectin	Stronghold, Revolution
staphage lysate	Staphage Lysate

PREFACE

Veterinary dermatology has had an exponential growth in information since publication of the first edition of *A Color Handbook of Skin Diseases of the Dog and Cat* in 1998. This has necessitated a complete revision of all the chapters and the inclusion of twenty-one new diseases. In addition, one hundred and thirty-one new illustrations of dermatologic diseases have been added. The authors have tried to provide the relevant information concerning the diagnosis and treatment of dermatologic diseases in such a format that it is easily accessible by the busy practitioner.

ACKNOWLEDGEMENTS

The authors would like to acknowledge the support given by their families through the sacrifices they have made to allow us time to complete this book. We are also grateful for the wonders of modern technology, without which this book would not have come to fruition. Finally, we would like to thank the referring veterinarians who have trusted their dermatologic cases to us so that we could accumulate the knowledge and experience necessary to undertake the writing of this book.

Tim Nuttall, Richard Harvey, Patrick McKeever

INTRODUCTION

A practical approach to the diagnosis of dermatologic cases

A dermatologic case can be viewed as a jigsaw puzzle, with history, clinical findings, and diagnostic procedures as the major pieces. As with a puzzle, one piece by itself will generally not let you know what the picture is but, if you combine the pieces, the picture becomes clear. Likewise, a clinician will generally need the information in the history, the clinical findings, and the results of diagnostic procedures to see the picture or arrive at a definitive diagnosis.

APPROACH, HISTORY, AND SIGNALMENT

Initially, it is important to determine what are the client's concerns. In many chronic cases these concerns may be different from, or not relate to, the primary disease but reflect concerns due to secondary manifestations. Also, it is important to determine what are the client's expectations. These may well be unrealistic, since many cases cannot be cured, just controlled.

Signalment and particulars about the animal's diet and environmental surroundings are obtained next, as these may give clues to contagion, zoonotic potential, and idiosyncratic managemental factors. Information pertaining to other body organs (appetite, thirst, exercise capability, etc.) is also important, because the dermatologic lesions may reflect systemic disease and/or concurrent diseases may limit investigation and treatment options and radically alter the prognosis.

Attention should then be focused on the skin by enquiring about the initial appearance and location of the lesions, any subsequent changes, and the time frame of any progression. Finally, one can ask what the response has been to at-home or veterinary prescribed therapies.

PHYSICAL EXAMINATION

The skin and all body organs should be examined in a systematic manner. It is important to record the findings so that progress can be monitored objectively rather than subjectively. This methodology will also ensure that information is available should another clinician be asked to evaluate the case. It is especially important to note the distribution of lesions, along with the types of lesions, and whether they are primary or secondary. It is therefore important to be able accurately to identify commonly encountered skin lesions and recognize their significance.

DIFFERENTIAL DIAGNOSIS

Using information obtained from the history and physical examination, a list of differential diagnoses or rule-outs is developed. Findings obtained from the history and physical examination are compared with key features of the diseases in the list of differential diagnoses so that they can be prioritized.

DIAGNOSTIC PLAN

Consideration of the prioritized differential diagnosis list will allow formulation of a diagnostic plan, which will either yield a definitive diagnosis or allow diseases to be ruled out. This plan should be reviewed with the animal's owner and the reasons for the plan, the likelihood of success, and the cost of the various diagnostic procedures explained to the client. Communication is essential, as many cases take a considerable amount of time to work up and may incur considerable expense. It is important to ensure that owners understand and accept this. Scheduling extra consultation time can be very useful.

THERAPY

After explaining the various treatment options, their expected success rate, cost, and possible side-effects, a treatment plan is developed that is acceptable to the client. If appropriate, follow-up examinations are scheduled to assess progress and/or adjust medication doses.

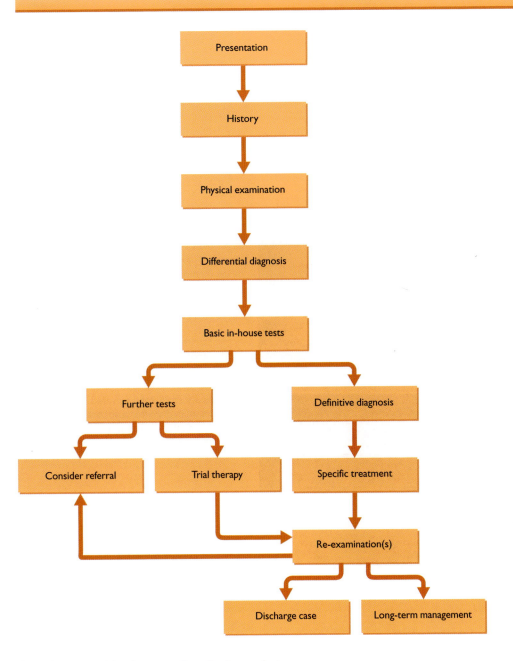

Algorithm summarizing the approach to the dermatologic case.

Terminology used in the description of dermatologic lesions

PRIMARY LESIONS

Primary lesions are directly associated with the disease process. They are not pathognomonic, but give a valuable clue as to the type of disease process occurring.

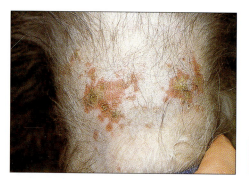

Macules are flat areas of discoloration up to 1 cm (0.4 in) in diameter, whereas *patches* are larger than 1 cm in diameter. Changes can involve increased blood flow (erythema), extravasated blood (hemorrhagic petechiae and ecchymoses), or pigment changes. Erythema can be distinguished from hemorrgage by blanching on digital pressure or using a glass slide (diascopy).

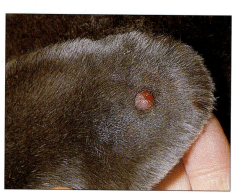

Papules are small, solid, elevated lesions up to 1 cm (0.4 in) in diameter associated with cell infiltration and/or proliferation, in this case a mast cell tumor.

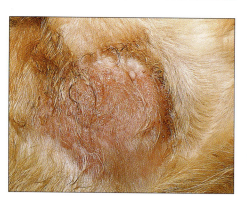

A **plaque** is a flat, solid, elevated lesion of more than 1 cm (0.4 in) in diameter, again associated with cell infiltration and/or proliferation. The lesions illustrated are eosinophilic plaques on a cat.

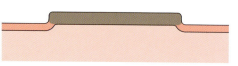

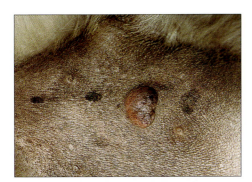

A **nodule** is a solid elevation of the skin greater than 1 cm (0.4 in) in diameter, again associated with cell infiltration and/or proliferation. The nodule illustrated is a mast cell tumor on the abdomen of a dog. A *tumor* is a large nodule, although not necessarily neoplastic.

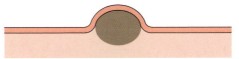

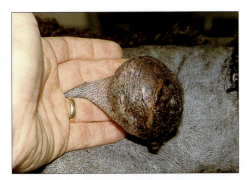

A **tumor** is a large growth. A lipoma on the flank of a dog is illustrated.

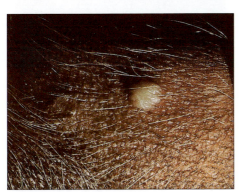

A **pustule** is a small circumscribed skin elevation containing purulent material. This consists of degenerate inflammatory cells (most commonly neutrophils) with or without microorganisms or other cells (e.g. acanthocytes in pemphigus foliaceus). Pustules and vesicles rapidly rupture in dogs and cats, leaving epidermal collarettes and crusts (see below).

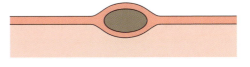

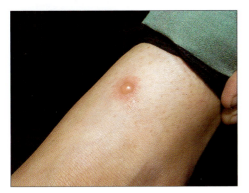

A **vesicle** is a circumscribed elevation of the skin up to 1 cm (0.4 in) in diameter filled with serum. The illustrated vesicle occurred on this veterinary nurse's arm within minutes of a flea bite. A bulla is a vesicular lesion greater than 1 cm (0.4 in) in diameter.

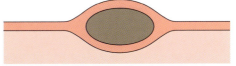

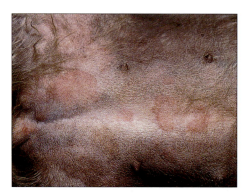

A **wheal** is an irregular elevated edematous skin area that often changes in size and shape. The wheals in this case were acute, transient, and of unknown etiology.

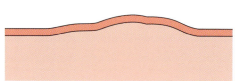

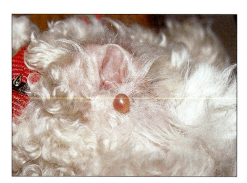

A **cyst** is an enclosed cavity with a membranous lining that contains liquid or semi-solid matter. The illustration is of a cystic basal cell tumor on the head of a dog.

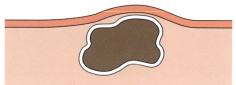

SECONDARY LESIONS

Secondary lesions are a result of trauma, time, and degree of insult to the skin. Often, primary lesions evolve into secondary lesions. Thus papules become pustules, which become focal encrustations, often hyperpigmented. Secondary lesions are much less specific than primary lesions.

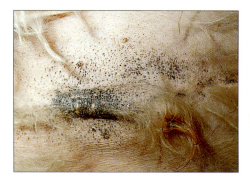

Comedones are the result of sebaceous and epidermal debris blocking a follicle. They may be seen in many diseases, but are often very prominent in cases of hyperadrenocorticism, as in this instance.

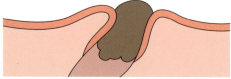

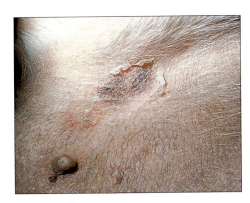

Scale results from accumulations of superficial epidermal cells that are dead and cast off from the skin. In this case there is an epidermal collarette surrounding a postinflammatory patch of hyperpigmentation. This presentation is frequently seen in cases of superficial pyoderma and other pustular diseases.

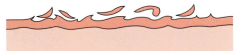

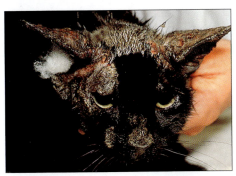

Crust is composed of cells and dried exudates. It may be serous, sanguineous, purulent, or mixed. This cat has pemphigus foliaceus.

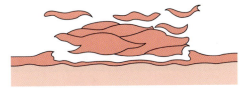

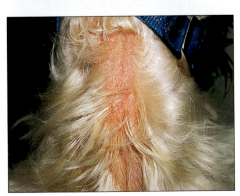

Erythema is reddening of the skin due to increased blood flow (see under macules p.10). The pattern of erythema may be diffuse to generalized (e.g. atopic dermatitis) or macular–papular (e.g. pyoderma or ectoparasites). In this Springer Spaniel the erythema is due to *Malassezia pachydermatis* infection.

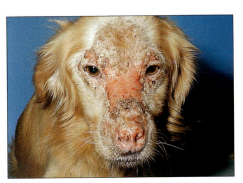

An **erosion** occurs following loss of the superficial part of the epidermis (i.e. down to but not including the basement membrane), as on the face of this dog with discoid lupus erythematosus. Erosions heal without scar formation.

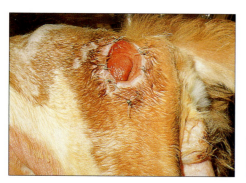

An **ulcer** is deeper than an erosion. They occur following loss of the epidermis and basement membrane and exposure of the deeper tissues of the dermis. Lesions may scar, as in this decubital ulcer overlying the bony prominence of the hip.

A **sinus** or **fistula** is a draining lesion. This dog has panniculitis and there are draining fistulas on the flank. The term sinus is usually reserved for an epithelialized tract that connects a body cavity and the skin surface.

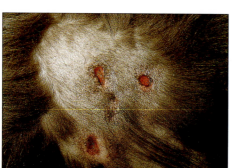

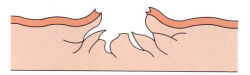

An **excoriation** results from self-trauma. In some cases, often in cats, the damage can be extensive, as in this Persian cat with food allergy.

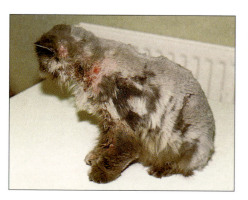

A **scar** results from the abnormal fibrous tissue that replaces normal tissue after an injury, such as a burn as in this case.

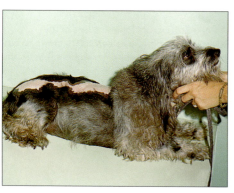

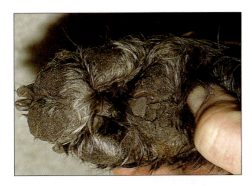

A **fissure** forms when thickened, usually lichenified or heavily crusted, skin splits. The illustration shows the foot of a dog with necrolytic migratory erythema.

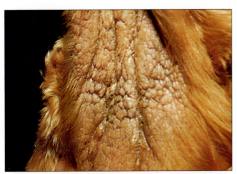

Lichenification occurs following chronic inflammation, as in this case of *M. pachydermatis* infection. There is thickening of the skin associated with accentuation of normal skin markings. Histopathologically, lichenification consists of thickening of the epidermis (acanthosis) and the stratum corneum (hyperkeratosis).

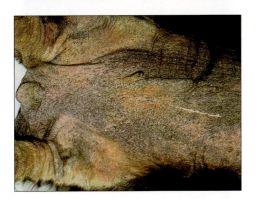

Hyperpigmentation, an increase in cutaneous pigmentation, usually occurs after chronic inflammation, as with this West Highland White Terrier with atopic dermatitis. Hyperpigmentation may also be seen in cutaneous changes associated with an endocrinopathy.

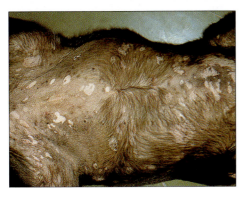

Hypopigmentation, a decrease in cutaneous pigmentation, occasionally follows inflammation, as in this case where it occurred after a superficial pyoderma. It is more commonly associated with immune-mediated inflammatory dermatoses. Vitiligo, a rare non-inflammatory, though possibly immune-mediated condition, is characterized by symmetrical hypopigmentation. There are also a number of hereditary conditions associated with complete or partial loss of pigmentation (e.g. albinism).

Pruritic dermatoses

General approach
- Rule out ectoparasites, particularly fleas
- Do not assume that the diagnosis is an allergy
- Remember that superficial pyoderma is pruritic
- Remember that immune-mediated diseases, keratinization disorders, and many other dermatoses are occasionally pruritic

Diseases that may be refractory to steroid therapy
- Sarcoptic mange, *Pelodera strongyloides* dermatitis, and other ectoparasites
- *Malassezia* dermatitis and pyoderma
- Allergic or irritant contact dermatitis
- Cutaneous adverse food reactions
- Epitheliotropic lymphoma

Diseases that may result in zoonoses
- Sarcoptic mange
- Cheyletiellosis
- Flea allergic dermatitis
- Syringomyelia

Common diseases
- Canine atopic dermatitis
- Cutaneous adverse food reactions (food or dietary allergy or intolerance)
- Flea bite hypersensitivity (flea allergy dermatitis)
- Sarcoptic mange (scabies, sarcoptic acariosis)
- Pyotraumatic dermatitis
- Superficial pyoderma
- *Malassezia* dermatitis

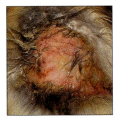 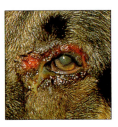 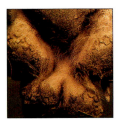 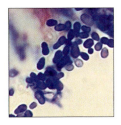

Pyotraumatic dermatitis

DEFINITION
Pyotraumatic dermatitis (acute moist dermatitis, hot spot) is a localized area of acute inflammation and exudation in skin that is traumatized by licking, scratching, or rubbing.

ETIOLOGY AND PATHOGENESIS
There is no single etiology, but rather multiple factors that predispose to the development of pyotraumatic dermatitis. Some of these factors include: acute focal inflammation resulting from allergic conditions such as atopic dermatitis, allergic contact dermatitis, and flea bite and other parasite hypersensitivities; skin maceration due to continued wetting or accumulation of moisture under a thick coat; trauma due to abrasions, foreign bodies in the coat, or irritation from clipper blades; and a primary irritant contacting the skin. Serum exudation from the inflammatory process creates a favorable climate for bacterial overgrowth and surface pyoderma.

CLINICAL FEATURES
Lesions are noted more frequently during hot, humid weather. Animals are presented because they are persistently licking or scratching a particular area, which can vary in size and is generally sharply demarcated. The areas most commonly involved are the dorsal and dorso-lateral lumbosacral region and the periaural region[1]. Affected skin is erythematous, moist, and, in the majority of cases, exudative (**1–3**). The typical lesion will evidence alopecia or thinning of the hair. However, hair may still cover the lesion if it is detected early or if it is in a location that is difficult to lick or scratch. Excoriations are occasionally present due to licking or scratching. The surrounding skin should be checked carefully for satellite lesions including superficial folliculitis and, less commonly, deep pyoderma with draining sinus tracts.

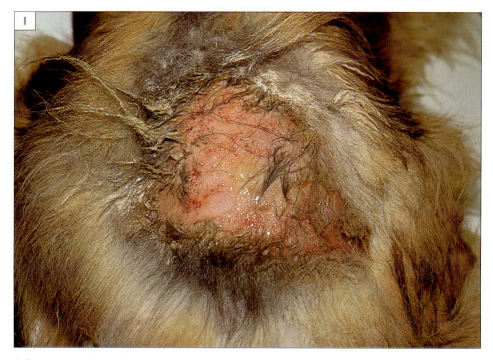

1 Pyotraumatic dermatitis. A well-demarcated moist, erythematous, alopecic patch on the dorsal lumbosacral region of a Collie cross.

DIFFERENTIAL DIAGNOSES

- Calcinosis cutis
- Superficial burn
- Irritant contact dermatitis
- Flea bite hypersensitivity
- Atopic dermatitis
- Cutaneous adverse food reaction
- Deep folliculitis and furunculosis

DIAGNOSIS

Diagnosis is generally made on the clinical appearance of lesions and a history of predisposing factors. Impression smears may be appropriate for determination of the number and type of bacteria, and a skin biopsy would be appropriate if calcinosis cutis was suspected.

MANAGEMENT

Sedation may be necessary for initial treatment if the lesions are painful or the animal is fractious. Any remaining hair should be clipped from affected areas and the lesions cleaned with a shampoo containing chlorhexidine or ethyl lactate and thoroughly rinsed with clean water. Other antimicrobial washes (see Superficial pyoderma, p. 146) may be appropriate. The lesion can then be treated with a drying solution of 2% aluminum acetate (Domeboro solution) for 3–5 minutes to decrease exudation. After cleaning and drying, an antibiotic–steroid cream or ointment can be applied. Application of the drying solution and antibiotic–corticosteroid preparation can be continued at home by the owner 2–3 times a day. A novel, topical diester glucocorticoid spray (hydrocortisone aceponate) is highly effective, with minimal adverse effects when applied once daily. If the lesion is extensive or severe, systemic corticosteroids at antiinflammatory doses can be used for 3–7 days, or as necessary, to reduce the inflammation and shorten the time necessary for resolution of the lesion. Most lesions resolve in 3–7 days, but they may recur if predisposing factors are not corrected.

Some individuals of certain breeds, particularly Labrador Retrievers and St. Bernards[2], may be affected by deeper infection and may require systemic antibacterial therapy (see Deep pyoderma, p. 166).

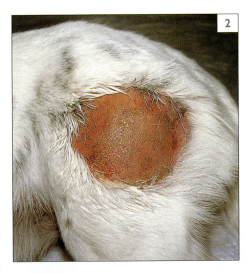

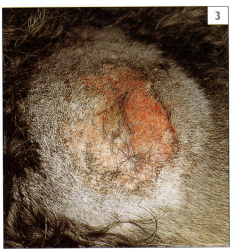

2, 3 Pyotraumatic dermatitis.

KEY POINTS

- Do not underestimate the capacity of this disease to cause problems.
- Treat aggressively and make regular re-examinations.

Canine atopic dermatitis

DEFINITION

Atopic dermatitis (atopy, atopic disease) is characterized as a genetically predisposed tendency to develop IgE antibodies to environmental allergens, resulting in a characteristic inflammatory and pruritic skin disease.

ETIOLOGY AND PATHOGENESIS
Immunology

The pathogenesis of atopic dermatitis is complex and new concepts on the etiology of the disease are still emerging. It is currently felt that epidermal contact with the allergen results in Langerhans cell uptake processing, then presentation of the allergen to T lymphocytes[1]. It has been documented in humans and postulated in the dog that there is an abnormality in the ratio between T helper 1 (TH_1) cells (which promote delayed hypersensitivity, macrophage activation, production of opsonizing and complement fixing antibodies, and antibody-dependent cell mediated cytotoxicity) and T helper 2 (TH_2) cells (which promote the development of mast cells and eosinophils, down-regulate the production of IgG_1, but stimulate the synthesis of IgE and IgA). The increase in TH_2 cells results in B-cell overproduction of IgE. In addition, there are other changes in cell-mediated immunity[1]. These cellular irregularities, along with the release of other mediators of inflammation from mast cells and basophils due to coupling of allergen with antigen-specific IgE, result in a cascade of substances promoting inflammation and pruritus.

Heritability

Because of the clinical observation that atopic dermatitis occurs more frequently in certain breeds of dogs and in certain familial lines, it is presumed that there is a genetic predisposition for the disease. In a study using Beagle dogs, the capacity to produce high levels of IgE was determined to be genetically inherited in a dominant manner[2]. However, the high levels of IgE could only be produced if the animals were sensitized with antigens repeatedly between one and four weeks of age. A recent study evaluated 144 West Highland White Terrier puppies from 33 litters. A high prevalence of atopic dogs was noted in certain litters, but clear evidence of consistent heritability could not be demonstrated[3]. Heritability of 0.47 has, however, been demonstrated in British guide dogs, which are largely Labrador/Golden Retriever crosses[4].

Epidermal barrier defect

The stratum corneum is composed of desquamating corneocytes surrounded by intercellular lipids that are thought to play a role in normal skin barrier function and provide protective function for the host. There is ample evidence of defective skin barrier function in atopic humans. In particular, recent studies have identified a loss-of-function filaggrin mutation in 25% of atopic patients, especially early-onset, high-IgE, and severe cases. There is some evidence that there may be defects of fatty acid metabolism in the skin of atopic dogs[5,6]. Another study demonstrated that the length and thickness of the stratum corneum lipid deposits were lower in non-lesional atopic canine skin than in normal canine skin. In addition, it was determined that the intercellular lipid lamellae exhibited many structural defects in the stratum corneum of dogs with atopic dermatitis[7]. Therefore, there is evidence for an epidermal barrier defect in the skin of dogs with atopic dermatitis.

Role of staphylococci in the pathogenesis or perpetuation of lesions

Cutaneous infections with *Staphylococcus* species are a common finding. Studies have shown that corneocytes of atopic dogs have a greater adherence for *Staphylococcus intermedius* and numbers of this organism are increased in the skin of symptomatic atopic dogs[8]. Some studies suggest that the inflamed skin allows for transepidermal penetration of staphylococcal antigens[9]. In addition, serum levels of anti-staphylococcal IgE were found to be higher in dogs with recurrent superficial pyoderma secondary to atopic dermatitis[10]. Therefore, it is possible that there could be an immediate-type hypersensitivity reaction to staphylococcal antigens that could contribute to the inflammatory process. Staphylococcal toxins may also contribute to the inflammation as well as serving as allergens[11]. There is some evidence that dogs with atopic dermatitis have abnormal cell-mediated immune responses, which could possibly contribute to the development of infection[12]. A recent study found that *S. intermedius* organisms produce superantigens, which are potent inducers of T-cell proliferation and inflammation in human atopic dermatitis and rodent models[13].

Role of *Malassezia* in the pathogenesis and perpetuation of lesions

A prominent feature of secondary *Malassezia* dermatitis is pruritus, which can be severe in some animals. Surface counts of this organism in dogs with atopic dermatitis are higher than or equal to those in normal dogs. Dogs with atopic dermatitis exhibit higher levels of serum IgE against *Malassezia* antigens than non-atopic dogs or dogs with *Malassezia* dermatitis but without atopic dermatitis[14]. Specific intradermal tests, T-cell proliferation, and passive transfer of hypersensitivity for *Malassezia* have also been demonstrated[15]. Therefore, there could be an immediate-type hypersensitivity to this organism, resulting in inflammation. In addition, yeast also contain or secrete a variety of substances that can initiate the complement cascade and trigger an inflammatory response[16].

Threshold phenomenon
Threshold for pruritus

With this concept a certain level of pruritic stimulus may be tolerated without manifestation of clinical signs. However, if there is an increase in stimuli from one or more sources such as bacteria, yeast, or ectoparasites, the threshold will be exceeded and pruritus will result.

Threshold for development of clinical signs of atopic dermatitis

With this concept a certain amount of allergen load may be tolerated. However, if the allergen load is increased, the threshold will be exceeded and clinical disease will develop. An example of this would be an animal who has a hypersensitivity to house dust mites, but does not itch during the winter, and who also has a hypersensitivity to ragweed, which will push it over the threshold and result in clinical disease during the time of year when there are high ragweed pollen counts. Concurrent food or parasite hypersensitivities are other examples of situations that may result in the threshold being exceeded.

CLINICAL FEATURES

The clinical features of canine atopic dermatitis are extremely variable, with no single physical or historical finding that definitively diagnoses the disease.

The true incidence of canine atopic dermatitis is unknown and probably varies by geographical region and the given population within that region. In one survey the incidence within 53 private veterinary practices in the US was 8.7%[17].

Generally, clinical signs of atopic dermatitis are first seen when animals are between one and three years of age. However, the disease has been noted in very young (approximately 12 weeks of age) and very old (approximately 16 years of age) animals.

The breed predisposition to atopic dermatitis will vary with the local gene pool, but in the US, UK, and Europe, a number of breeds are recognized to be particularly at risk. These include the Beauceron, Boston Terrier, Boxer, Cairn Terrier, Chinese Shar Pei, Cocker Spaniel, Dalmatian, English Bulldog, English Setter, Fox Terrier, Golden Retriever, Labrador Retriever, Lhasa Apso, Miniature Schnauzer, Pug, Scottish Terrier, Sealyham Terrier, West Highland White Terrier, Wire Haired Fox Terrier, and Yorkshire Terrier[18].

If sensitivities develop to pollens, the clinical signs are likely to be seasonal (i.e. spring and/or autumn depending on the pollens). However, many animals exhibit perennial disease, a reflection of the importance of allergy to indoor allergens such as house dust mites. There is also a group of animals with perennial signs that become much worse in a particular season. An example of this would be a dog with a house dust mite sensitivity, who develops severe clinical signs during the pollen season. It has been noted that worsening of a particular animal's condition may occur during late fall or early winter when a forced air heating system is put into use, resulting in a greater circulation of dust and molds. Forced air or central heating can also dry the skin and coat.

The degree of pruritus evidenced may vary from very mild to intense and may be generalized or, more commonly, localized. If localized, it may be specific to one or more of the following areas: ears, periocular, muzzle, ventral neck, antecubital, axilla, groin, flank, feet (especially the interdigital webs), and under the tail.

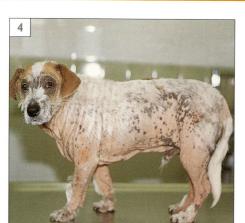

Primary lesions

Some animals with atopic dermatitis will have no primary lesions and only evidence pruritus. Erythema, when present, is thought to be the primary lesion and it may be generalized (**4, 5**) or specific to one or more of the following areas: ears (particularly the ventral or concave pinna) (**6**), periocular (**7**), muzzle, ventral neck (**8**), antecubital, axilla (**9**), groin (**10**), flank, feet (especially the interdigital webs) (**11**), and under the tail (**12**). In most cases the erythema will be diffuse rather than macular–papular, although this is often complicated by self-trauma and excoriation.

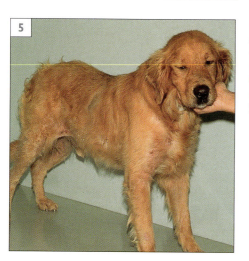

4–7 Atopic dermatitis. Extensive erythema and alopecia on the ventral trunk and proximal limbs of a Jack Russell Terrier (**4**); erythroderma (generalized erythema, scale, and alopecia) in a Retriever (**5**); erythematous otitis externa in a Boxer (**6**); facial excoriations in a German Shepherd Dog (**7**).

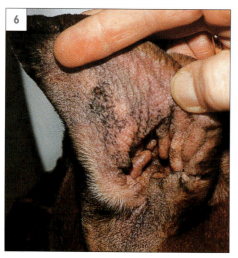

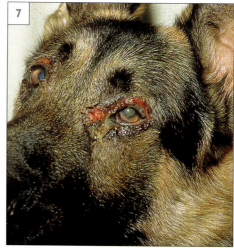

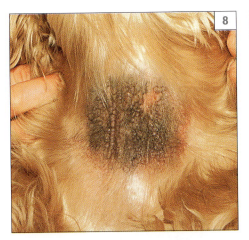

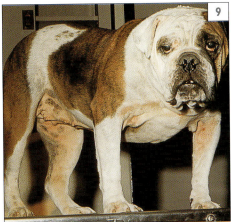

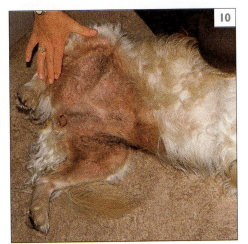

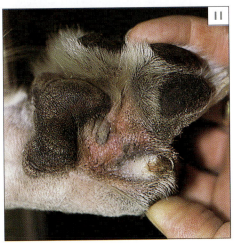

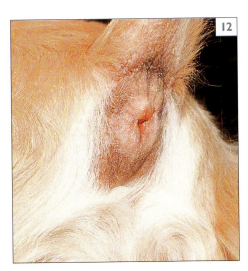

8–12 Atopic dermatitis. Focal hyperpigmentation and erythema on the ventral neck of a Cocker Spaniel due to secondary *Malassezia pachydermatis* infection (**8**); erythema in the axillae, groins, and medial aspects of the proximal limbs in an English Bulldog (**9**); erythematous papules and localized erythematous alopecia in the groin of a Labrador Retriever (**10**); plantar interdigital erythema in a West Highland White Terrier (**11**); perineal erythema in a Cocker Spaniel (**12**).

Secondary changes, complications, and additional features

Hyperpigmentation

This may occur in any area where there has been inflammation or irritation to the skin. Focal areas are often noted at the sites of resolving staphylococcal lesions.

Lichenification

A thickening and exaggeration of skin markings. This may develop in any location where there is chronic inflammation or irritation to the skin. Constant licking by the animal may contribute significantly to its development. It is most frequently noted in the ears (particularly on the concave aspect of the pinnae and in the vertical canal), periocular, ventral neck (especially in Cocker and Springer Spaniels) (**8**), axilla, flank folds, lips, and under the tail.

Seborrhea

This may be generalized and often contributes to a significant and objectionable odor about the animal. It may be localized and, if so, the ears, ventral neck (especially in Cocker and Springer Spaniels), webs of the toes, axilla, and groin are frequently involved.

Scaling

Increased scaling may occur due to either an increased turnover time of the epidermis or due to a dyskeratosis.

Alopecia

Inflammation of the skin can occasionally result in a synchronization of hair to the telogen phase, resulting in either a diffuse thinning of the coat or complete hair loss. More commonly, focal areas of alopecia may occur at the sites of secondary staphylococcal infection or from scratching, biting, or licking at the skin.

Secondary staphylococcal infection

Lesions start as small erythematous papules, which may or may not develop into pustules. The lesion may enlarge slightly, and crust formation can occur. More frequently, it expands in a circumferential manner with a scaling and sometimes erythematous border (epidermal collarettes). If a lesion develops in a haired area, a tuft of hair corresponding in size to the lesion will fall out; this is particularly noticeable in short-coated breeds, where it results in a patchy, multifocal alopecia. Lesions are generally about 1 cm in diameter, but they may enlarge to 6–7 cm in diameter. Initially, erythema is seen in the center of lesions, but this may fade with time and often the affected area becomes hyperpigmented. With time, new hair may be seen starting to regrow in the center of lesions. In some animals, pruritus will only occur when the pruritic threshold has been exceeded due to the infection. Lesions may be seen on any area of the body, but they are very common in the axilla, ventral abdomen, and under the tail.

Secondary *Malassezia* infection

There are no specific lesions associated with secondary *Malassezia* infection, although there may be an increase in intensity of erythema and pruritus, which in some cases is very significant. The organism tends to be associated with areas of seborrhea such as the ear, ventral neck, and skin of the foot webs. Lesions can be greasy, malodorous, alopecic, lichenified, erythematous, and/or hyperpigmented.

Secondary otitis

Chronic or recurrent otitis is seen in 80% of atopic dogs and may be the only or most prominent clinical sign in up to 20% of cases. Protracted inflammation will often lead to hyperplasia of the tissues on the inside of the pinnae and the ear canals. It also predisposes to sebaceous and ceruminous hyperplasia, resulting in excess wax accumulation that predisposes to further infection.

Interdigital papules, nodules, furunculosis, or cysts

Inflammation in the skin between the toes results in the walls of the hair follicles becoming hyperplastic and hyperkeratotic. A follicle may become plugged and balloon out as sebaceous and apocrine gland secretions continue to be secreted into it. Finally it ruptures into the dermis, resulting in a foreign body reaction to sebum, keratin, and hair. If there are bacteria in the hair follicles, they may add an infectious component to the lesion. Clinically the lesions are seen as papules or nodules, which may break open and drain a serosanguineous fluid. In many cases these lesions will develop spontaneously and then disappear. Single or multiple feet may be affected.

Alopecia and scaling of ear margins

In a minority of cases, alopecia and scaling will affect the margins of the pinna and the animal will have a pinna pedal reflex mimicking sarcoptic mange. This finding can occur in any breed, but is most frequently noted in German Shepherd Dogs and Cocker and Springer Spaniels.

Perianal dermatitis

This is often misdiagnosed as either intestinal parasitism or anal sacculitis. Lesions occur in the skin under the tail as well as in the skin of the peri-anal area. Erythema may be the only finding in some cases, but in others the skin of the affected areas becomes very hyperplastic. Animals will either drag their rectal areas across the floor or spin in circles on the rectal area as they try to relieve the pruritus.

Obsessive compulsive behavior

Some animals, especially those of the Bichon Frise breed, become obsessive–compulsive towards an area of minimal erythema and will lick, bite, or scratch a particular area of skin incessantly until it is excoriated and bleeding.

DIFFERENTIAL DIAGNOSES

- Flea bite hypersensitivity
- Sarcoptic mange
- Cutaneous adverse reaction to food
- *Malassezia* dermatitis
- Staphylococcal pyoderma
- Cheyletiellosis
- *Otodectes cynotis* infestation
- Pediculosis
- Allergic or irritant contact dermatitis
- *Pelodera strongyloides* dermatitis
- Cutaneous lymphoma
- Harvest mite (chiggers or berry bugs) infestation
- Ancylostomiasis (hookworm dermatitis)
- Dermatophytosis
- Psychogenic dermatitis (obsessive–compulsive disorder)

Some of these differential diagnoses, especially cutaneous infections and adverse food reactions, may be concurrent with atopic dermatitis.

DIAGNOSIS

Various set criteria for the diagnosis of canine atopic dermatitis have been proposed[19,20]. However, it has been shown that these criteria would be incorrect in one out of every five cases[16]. Nevertheless, the diagnosis of canine atopic dermatitis is based on characteristic histor-ical and clinical findings with the exclusion of other pruritic conditions. There is no one specific diagnostic test that is infallible in ruling atopic dermatitis in or out.

Skin scrapings

These are necessary to rule out parasites. If sarcoptic mange is suspected, appropriate therapy should be instituted to rule it out, as it may be difficult to demonstrate the mite on skin scrap-ings. Anti-*Sarcoptes* IgG serology is also useful, although titers can last for up to six months post infestation and false-positive tests can be seen in dogs strongly reactive to *Dermatophagoides* species house dust mites. Serology can be nega-tive for the first 2–4 weeks of infestation.

Impression smears
Seborrheic skin

A clean scalpel blade can be used to collect sebor-rheic debris, which can be smeared on a slide, stained with Gram's stain or a modified Wright's stain (e.g. Diff-Quik), and examined for the pres-ence of yeast and bacteria. Clear acetate tape may also be used by pressing the sticky side to the skin lesion and then staining with a modified Wright's stain and affixing the tape to a glass slide for examination.

Pustules on or under edges of circular scaling lesions

The bevel of a needle or the tip of a scalpel blade can be used to collect material from a pustule or from under scale at the leading edge of a lesion. This can then be smeared on a slide and stained with Gram's stain or a modified Wright's stain (e.g. Diff-Quik) and examined for the presence of bacteria.

Ears

If wax or exudate is present in the ears, it should be collected on a swab or curette, smeared on a slide, stained as previously described, and examined to determine the presence of bacteria or yeast and their morphology.

Moist lesions

A glass slide can be pressed against the lesion and then stained as previously described and exam-ined for the presence of bacteria or yeast.

Diet trials
If the condition is non-seasonal, an appropriate diet trial should be instituted for 6–10 weeks to rule out food hypersensitivity (see Cutaneous adverse food reaction, p. 31).

Skin biopsy
Histiopathologic findings are not specific for atopic dermatitis, but they would be definitive to rule out cutaneous lymphoma.

Dermatophyte culture
If lesions are present that are suspicious for dermatophytes, hair and scale should be cultured on dermatophyte test medium or Sabouraud's medium for a definitive diagnosis.

Intradermal skin testing
If properly performed, intradermal skin testing will result in positive results that concur with the history in approximately 85% of cases (**13**). To prevent inaccurate test results, short-acting steroids such as prednisone, prednisolone, and methylprednisolone should be discontinued three weeks prior to testing, and repository injectable steroids should be discontinued 6–8 weeks prior to testing. Antihistamines should be discontinued 7–10 days before testing. Control of pruritus pending testing may be achieved by bathing the animal every 1–3 days using emollient moisturizing shampoos, oatmeal and paroxamine-based shampoo, or, alternatively, a simple cleansing shampoo followed by application of a conditioner containing paroxamine. Lotions or sprays containing 1% hydrocortisone or 0.0584% hydrocortisone aceponate may be applied to pruritic inflamed skin twice daily as long as it is not applied to the skin site used for testing. Performance and interpretation require experience in order to obtain the best results. If the procedure is not performed routinely, or if the clinician has not had appropriate training, referral is recommended.

Serologic allergy testing
Serum allergen-specific measurement (RAST, ELISA, and liquid-phase immunoenzymatic assay) can be performed to determine if there are increased concentrations of allergen-specific IgE present. The major problem with these tests is lack of specificity. Almost all normal dogs, and all dogs with skin disease, reacted to at least one and, sometimes, many substances in one study[21]. In another pilot study, results from aliquots of the same serum sample, sent in with different identifying information and tested by the same laboratories on different dates, varied unacceptably among replicate tests[22]. However, in some situations, serologic testing may be helpful in the selection of allergens for immunotherapy.

MANAGEMENT
Treatment of atopic dermatitis must be tailored to the specific signs and secondary changes or complications present in an individual animal. Owners need to be aware that lifelong management is the norm and it is not possible to predict initially which animal will respond to a particular therapy. They also need to understand that clinical manifestations frequently change, resulting in the need to adjust the therapy. Also, it is necessary for the owner to appreciate the time and financial commitment needed for the management of the atopic dog.

Systemic therapy
Antihistamines
Less severe cases of atopic dermatitis may be controlled with antihistamines or antihistamines plus topicals. A crude and certainly not infallible guideline to determine if antihistamines could possibly be effective, is whether or not the animal is sleeping through the night. If the animal is

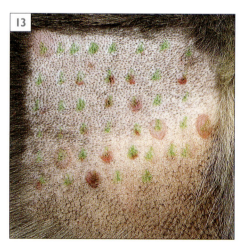

13 Positive intradermal skin test. The green dots are text highlighter and positive reactions are seen as darkly colored (edematous) swellings.

sleeping through the night without waking up to lick or scratch, there is a greater chance that their use may be beneficial.

A recent evidence-based assessment[23] concluded that there is fair evidence for medium efficacy for a combination of chlorpheniramine and hydroxyzine (1–4 mg and 25–100 mg, respectively, p/o q24h). There is little evidence that other antihistamines are effective, but therapeutic trials using drugs from different classes for two weeks each in sequence may be helpful in individual cases. Chlorpheniramine (0.4 mg/kg p/o q8h), diphenhydramine (2–4 mg/kg p/o q8h), and hydroxyzine (2 mg/kg p/o q8h) are the three drugs used most frequently for these trials. Clemastine fumerate (0.05 mg/kg p/o q8h) and ketotifen (2–4 mg/kg p/o q8h) may also be effective, but the cost will be higher. Terfenadine, astemizole, and lortadine have not proved beneficial for the treatment of pruritus in dogs due to allergic reactions[22]. There is a synergistic effect between essential fatty acids and antihistamines. Adverse effects are uncommon but include sedation and gastrointestinal upsets. The second-generation drugs can induce potentially fatal cardiac arrhythmias.

Glucocorticoids

Methylprednisolone (0.4–0.8 mg/kg) is the preferred agent for the control of erythema and pruritus. Prednisolone and prednisone may also be used (0.5–1.0 mg/kg), but they are more likely to cause polyuria/polydipsia and polyphagia in some dogs. Induction doses should be given twice daily for 8 days or until remission, then once daily in the morning for 8 days, and then on alternate mornings.

The dose is then decreased by 20% every 8 days to determine the least amount that will keep the animal comfortable. The dose is then decreased by 20% every eight days to determine the least amount that will keep the animal comfortable. Antihistamines or essential fatty acid supplementation may also be administered in an attempt to further reduce the dose. The client should be forewarned that the minimal dose may change if the animal contracts a secondary infection, is exposed to fleas or to a hotter and more humid environment, or encounters a higher dose of the antigen. Failure promptly to re-establish control of pruritus in a case that was previously well controlled should prompt suspicion of secondary infection with *S. intermedius* or *M. pachydermatis*, flea or sarcoptic mange infestation, or development of calcinosis cutis. Ever-increasing doses of glucocorticoid should not be permitted without re-examination.

The rapid action of glucorticoids makes them ideal to use in short bursts. Topical products or prednisone (0.5–1.0 mg/kg p/o q24h for 3–5 days) or methylprednisolone (0.4–0.8 mg/kg p/o q24h for 3–5 days) are very effective when used at the owners' discretion to control short-term exacerbation in dogs otherwise controlled on non-steroidal therapy or during food trials. Adverse effects are rarely seen with this protocol.

Methylprednisolone acetate (0.25–1.0 mg/kg i/m) or betamethasone (0.08–0.4 mg/kg i/m) injections are generally not recommended because of the prolonged pituitary adrenal suppression. However, occasional use of these injectable steroids may be warranted if the dermatitis is extremely severe, if only 1–3 injections are needed per year to control a seasonal allergy, or if the client finds it impossible to administer oral medications to the animal.

Adverse affects of systemic glucocorticoids, including polyuria, polydipsia, polyphagia, and mood changes (including aggression), are common. The onset of iatrogenic hyperadrenocorticism is dose and duration dependent, but varies between individual dogs. Regular monitoring and checks for occult infections of the skin, oral cavity, and urinary tract are appropriate for dogs on long-term therapy.

Ciclosporin

Ciclosporin (cyclosporine) is a polypeptide isolated from the fungus *Tolypocladium inflatum*. Its main use is as an immunosuppressive drug to prevent rejection following organ transplants. Ciclosporin has been found to inhibit mast and eosinophil cell function, inhibit T lymphocyte function (especially lymphocyte activation and cytokine production), inhibit the lymphocyte activating function of antigen-presenting Langerhans cells as well as decreasing their numbers in the skin, inhibit keratinocyte cytokine production, and inhibit mast cell-dependent cellular infiltration at sites of inflammation[23]. Ciclosporin marketed for humans is supplied as soft gel capsules containing either 25 or 100 mg of drug per capsule or as a liquid containing 100 mg/ml. Ciclosporin marketed to veterinarians comes in four strengths of soft gel capsules: 10 mg, 25 mg, 50 mg, and 100 mg. The recommended dose for dogs is 5 mg/kg p/o q24h[24]. The drug does not cause immediate improvement in pruritus and erythema, but significant improvement should be seen within three weeks, continuing slowly until six weeks[24]. Once disease is controlled the frequency of dosing can be changed to every other day or, if still controlled, to twice weekly. A rough guideline would be that approximately 30% of cases can be maintained on alternate day dosing and another 15–20% can be maintained with every third day dosing[25]. Alternatively, the dose may be reduced to 2.5 mg/kg q24h[26]. Satisfactory control of lesions will occur in approximately 60–80% of the cases treated with ciclosporin[25,27]. Emesis is a major side-effect of this treatment and is reported to occur in 14–40% of cases[28]. In some cases an animal will tolerate the drug after a few days; in other cases, giving the drug after a meal will be beneficial. The problem may also be reduced by giving a partial dose of the drug after a meal for three days, then increasing the dose every three days until the recommended dose is reached. Metoclopramide (0.2–0.4 mg/kg p/o), sucralfate (0.5–1.0 g/dog p/o), ranitidine (1 mg/kg p/o), or cimetidine (5–10 mg/kg p/o) given thirty minutes prior to dosing may also decrease the frequency of emesis. Some animals will not tolerate the drug and it has to be discontinued. Other less common side-effects are diarrhea, gingival hyperplasia, papilloma-type lesions of the epidermis, hirsuitism, and a psoriasiform–lichenoid-like dermatitis with coccoid bacteria [29,30]. In rare instances, pinnal erythema, lameness, and muscle pain may be observed. Ciclosporin is metabolized by the liver, so extreme caution should be used if the animal to be treated has liver disease, as very high blood levels will develop. If the drug is to be used in these situations, blood level assays should be performed and the dose adjusted accordingly. In animals without liver disease blood levels are fairly consistent, so monitoring is not necessary[31]. A year-long study in Beagles treated with ciclosporin at up to nine times the recommended dose did not evidence any hepatotoxic, nephrotoxic, or myelotoxic effects[32]. However, creatinine levels should be monitored in treated dogs with renal failure and co-administration with potentially nephrotoxic drugs is contraindicated. Drugs that inhibit cytochrome P450 microsomal enzyme activity (e.g. ketoconazole, itraconazole, fluconazole, erythromycin, and allopurinol), if given concurrently, will result in very high blood levels of ciclosporin and potentiate possible toxicity or other side-effects[33]. Conversely, anticonvulsants and trimethoprim–sulfonamides that increase P450 metabolism may reduce plasma levels of ciclosporin. This drug is expensive and cost may preclude its use in larger dogs.

Phytopica

Phytopica™ is a preparation derived from *Rehmanannia glutinosa, Paedonia lactiflora,* and *Glycyrrhiza uralensis. In vitro* studies and rodent models have demonstrated a number of immunomodulating effects including expression of the immunosuppressive cytokines, inhibition of histamine, pro-inflammatory cytokine release, and antioxidant and antibacterial activity. In a recent randomized, double blind, placebo controlled trial of 120 dogs, a dose of 200 mg/kg q24h administered in food led to a 20% reduction in clinical signs in up to 59% of dogs, and a 50% reduction in up to 36%. Response was typically evident within four weeks. Adverse effects were limited to mild gastrointestinal disturbances, although a few dogs refused to eat the medicated food as it has a strong licorice flavor.

Antibacterial agents

To control secondary staphylococcal infections animals should be treated for three weeks with one of the following: cefalexin (cephalexin) (25 mg/kg p/o q12h), cefpodoxime proxetil (5–10 mg/kg p/o q24h), oxacillin or dicloxacillin (20 mg/kg p/o q12h), clindamycin (11 mg/kg p/o q12h), lincomycin (22 mg/kg q12h), clavulanic acid-potentiated amoxicillin (25 mg/kg p/o q12h), or enrofloxacin (5 mg/kg p/o q24h). (See Superficial pyoderma, p. 146, for additional antibacterial agents that would be appropriate.)

Antifungal agents

To control secondary *Malassezia* infection, treat with ketoconazole (10 mg/kg p/o q12h) for 10–14 days. Alternatively, itraconazole could be used at a dose of 5 mg/kg p/o q24h, but this would be more expensive. Topical therapy (see below) is also effective.

Essential fatty acids (EFAs)

Supplements containing omega-3 and/or omega-6 fatty acids may be useful in cases where the pruritus is minimal, or as adjunct therapy in more severe cases. The response to fatty acid supplements is dose related (i.e. the more that is given, the better the effect) and there is a time lag of up to 12 weeks before maximal response is seen. It is unclear whether EFAs act primarily on the skin barrier or inflammatory cascade. Foods enriched with EFAs and other micronutrients may also be beneficial. Clinical trials have shown that Royal Canin Skin Support and Eukanuba Dermatosis FP ameliorate the clinical signs of atopic dermatitis, although the improvement is generally <50%.

Allergen specific immunotherapy (ASIT)

Hyposensitization has been reported to provide benefits to 50–80% of dogs with atopic dermatitis[18]. In addition, approximately 75% of atopic dogs can be controlled without the use of systemic glucocorticoids when hyposensitization is combined with other non-steroidal treatments[18]. In one (US) author's (PJM) experience, 60–65% of atopic dogs can be maintained on hyposensitization alone, another 15–20% can be maintained with hyposensitization plus non-steroidal treatments, while 20–25% do not benefit from hyposensitization; in another (European) author's (TJN) experience, 75% of treated dogs derive a greater than 50% improvement from treatment, although the success rate may be lower for less experienced clinicians. It may take animals as long as 6–12 months to respond to immunotherapy and, therefore, critical clinical evaluation should not take place until a year of therapy has been completed. Other concurrent therapy, including glucocorticoids if necessary, is appropriate pending its full effects. The percentage of dogs with an excellent response to hyposensitization appears to be greater when therapy is based on intradermal rather than serologic testing[18,34] and when hyposensitization is based on strong intradermal reactions in a 2–6-year-old animal. Chronically affected older animals with long-standing disease appear to have a poorer response. Adverse effects are uncommon. Injection site reactions and anaphylactic shock are very rare. Some dermatologists give the first 5–6 doses in the veterinary hospital and observe the animal for 20–30 minutes post injection. Increased pruritus after an injection indicates that the dose is too high. Mild reactions can generally be prevented by pretreating with antihistamines two hours prior to the injection. Intervals between injections can be individualized to the needs of the animal. Retesting may reveal new sensitivities in dogs who were tested when they were <12 months of age, dogs who have a poor response to ASIT, or dogs who respond well initially and then relapse. When new sensitivities are found, reformulation of ASIT may be beneficial.

Topical therapy

Topical therapy is beneficial, although it can be time consuming. As it is likely that percutaneous exposure to allergens plays a role in pathogenesis, bathing to remove allergens from the skin is likely to be helpful.

Shampoos

If a secondary bacterial infection is present, shampoos containing benzoyl peroxide should be used every 4–7 days depending on the severity of the lesions. Shampoos containing chlorhexidine or ethyl lactate are not as irritating as those containing benzoyl peroxide and may be more appropriate for animals that have severely inflamed skin. If yeasts are found on impression smears or skin scrapings, shampoos containing miconazole or ketoconazole should be used. Scaling should be treated with shampoos containing tar and salicylic acid, unless it is due to xeroderma. Shampoos containing phytosphingosine are especially beneficial for those cases with seborrhea and odor associated with seborrhea. Monosaccharides can inhibit microbial adherence to keratinocytes, and they may inhibit inflammatory cytokine production.

Conditioners and humectants

The use of skin and coat conditioners and humectants after bathing has been found to be beneficial in preventing drying of the skin (xeroderma) and reducing irritation of the animal's dermatitis. Emollient moisturizing shampoos are indicated in these cases. A conditioner containing oatmeal and paroxamine has been found to be particularly beneficial.

Glucocorticoids

Topical glucocorticoid treatment is beneficial as an adjunctive treatment to antihistamines, and the combination will limit the necessity for systemic glucocorticoids in many cases. Focal areas of mild inflammation may be treated with either sprays or lotions containing 1% hydrocortisone twice daily. Areas of severe inflammation and lichenification can be treated with betamethasone valerate cream 0.1% twice daily. This cream is especially beneficial in treating erythema and pruritus of the web skin between the toes and the skin under the tail and around the rectum. Betamethasone valerate is a potent steroid and systemic absorption can occur, causing adrenocortical suppression. Clients should also be instructed to wear gloves when betamethasone valerate is applied, as it can cause a thinning of the skin with continued contact. Triamcinolone spray 0.015% applied twice daily may be very beneficial for treating focal areas as well as larger areas of inflammation. A topical spray formulation of the diester glucocorticoid hydrocortisone aceponate has recently become available. Diester glucocorticoids have potent local anti-inflammatory effects, but they are metabolized in the skin thus minimizing systemic adverse effects and cutaneous atrophy. Results from randomized, placebo controlled trials indicate that once daily hydrocortisone aceponate is highly effective and well tolerated in canine atopic dermatitis. It may be possible to reduce the frequency of application once the clinical signs are in remission to every other day or twice weekly. Glucocorticoid-containing eye and ear drops can be useful for managing inflammation in the ear canals.

Therapy for special situations
Interdigital papules and nodules
These lesions (as described above [Clinical features]) can often be the primary manifestation of disease in a dog. Tacrolimus ointment 0.1% applied to the dorsal and ventral web skin between the toes twice daily will often prove to be a very effective treatment. It may take 6–8 weeks for lesions to resolve and continuous treatment is necessary to prevent the formation of new lesions. Concurrent systemic glucocorticoids and antibacterials may be used for the first 14 days to hasten resolution of lesions.

Periocular dermatitis
This will evidence itself as varying degrees of erythema, alopecia, and lichenification about the eyes. A conjunctivitis may be present and the animals will scratch at their eyes or rub them along furniture or the floor. It may occur as the only sign or in conjunction with other features of atopic dermatitis. Ophthalmic preparations containing dexamethasone 0.1% applied to the eyes and the skin around the eyes 3–4 times a day are often very beneficial. 0.2% ciclosporin ointment applied twice daily to remission and then tapering the frequency is also effective.

Obsessive–compulsive behavior
Animals with atopic dermatitis and obsessive–compulsive behavior (as described in Clinical features above) often have a poor response to the usual treatments for atopy. Some may do better if clomipramine is given (1–3 mg/kg p/o q24h).

Reoccurring staphylococcal infections
Generally, the initial antibacterial therapy will result in resolution of the lesions. However, even though other treatments for atopy keep the animal comfortable, predisposing factors may still be present and the staphylococcal infection may return. Managing the underlying inflammation will prevent recurrence in most animals, but some that are very prone to repeated infection will benefit from an alternative to constant antibacterial treatment. In these cases the animal is given the standard dose of an antibacterial (e.g. cefalexin or dicloxacillin) twice daily on 2–3 consecutive days per week (e.g. 'weekend therapy') after initial resolution of the infection with standard dosing. An alternative to this is for the animal to receive standard treatment for one week, then no antibacterial treatment for two weeks.

Secondary otitis
(See Chapter 10: Otitis externa, p. 254.)

KEY POINTS
- Clients must be made to understand that this is a disease that is not cured but just controlled with periodic or continuous use of medications.
- Bilateral otitis externa occurs in 55–80% of atopic dogs.
- Recurrent superficial pyoderma and *Malassezia* infection are common in atopic dogs.
- The pruritus is usually steroid responsive.

Cutaneous adverse food reaction (food or dietary allergy or intolerance)

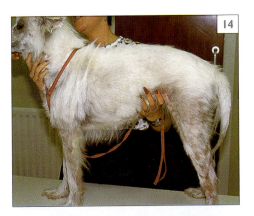

ETIOLOGY AND PATHOGENESIS

Cutaneous adverse food reaction (CAFR) is an uncommon dermatosis caused by an abnormal response to an ingested food or additive. The etiology of most cases of dietary intolerance is not determined, but it may involve either food intolerance or food hypersensitivity. Food intolerance is any clinically abnormal response to the ingestion of a food that does not have an immunologic component (e.g. food poisoning, food idiosyncrasy, metabolic reactions, and dietary indiscretions)[1]. Food hypersensitivity or allergy is an abnormal response that is immunologically mediated.

Most dogs tend to react to more that one food; in one study of 25 dogs, the average was 2.4[2]. Beef, chicken, dairy products, maize, wheat, soy, and eggs all seem to be common allergens in canine CAFR[1–3]. The range of allergens seems similar in cats, although fewer cases have been studied[4,5].

The incidence of adverse reaction to food is controversial and difficult to determine, as it may coexist with atopic dermatitis. About 10–15% of all cases of allergic dermatosis are attributable to adverse reactions to food[1], although the incidence is higher in some reports[6–8]. A range of IgE binding proteins, including IgG and phosphoglucomutase, have been identified in cattle and sheep extracts[9].

Up to 52% of dogs present at less than one year of age[1,3], although there is no sex or breed predisposition.

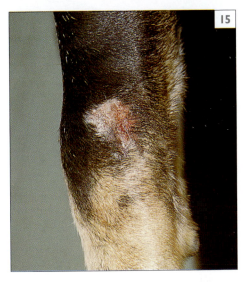

CLINICAL FEATURES

The clinical signs are usually very similar to those of atopic dermatitis (**14–16**). Pruritus is the most prominent feature in the majority of cases; it is usually non-seasonal, although dogs with a seasonal exacerbation may have concurrent atopic dermatitis or flea allergic dermatitis, or there may

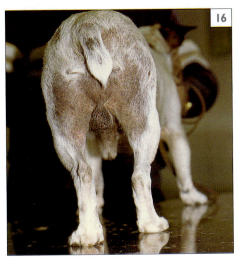

14–16 Dietary intolerance. A Samoyed with extensive alopecia, scale, and crust (**14**); a Rottweiler with a focal lesion on the forelimb (**15**); a Jack Russell Terrier with symmetrical alopecia secondary to pruritus (**16**).

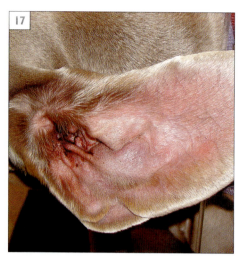

17 *Malassezia* otitis externa in a Weimeraner with a cutaneous adverse food reaction.

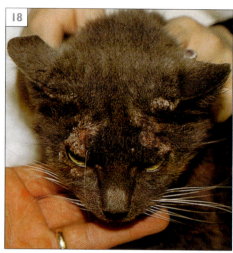

18 Dietary intolerance. Extensive alopecia, scale, and crust on the head of a domestic shorthair cat (the crusting is due to self-trauma).

only be seasonal exposure to certain foods. Primary lesions such as erythema and papules may be noted, but most lesions (e.g. erythema, papules, pustules, scale, crust, hyperpigmentation, lichenification, and alopecia) result from self-trauma and secondary infection[2,3,5,10,11]. The location of any dermatologic lesions can be quite varied. Unilateral or bilateral otitis externa (17) is common, and may occur in the absence of other signs of skin disease.

CAFRs can also cause gastrointestinal tract (GIT) signs including soft feces, flatulence, intermittent diarrhea, and colitis. In one study, 60% of dogs also had some form of GIT signs, usually manifested by an increased number of bowel movements (greater than or equal to six per day)[10]. It has also been reported to trigger recurrent pyoderma[12] and nail disorders[13].

Pruritus, crusting, and excoriations of the head and neck are the most common clinical findings of adverse reaction to food in cats (18). Other presentations include localized or generalized scale or crusts, miliary dermatitis, symmetric or localized areas of alopecia, eosinophilic granulomas, eosinophilic plaque, pinnal erythema, feline acne, and otitis externa[4,5,8,14].

DIFFERENTIAL DIAGNOSES
Dogs
- Atopic dermatitis
- Flea allergic dermatitis
- Other ectoparasites
- Drug eruption
- Superficial staphylococcal folliculitis
- *Malassezia* dermatitis
- Contact dermatitis
- Defects in keratinization
- Epitheliotropic lymphoma (mycosis fungoides)

Cats
- Flea allergic dermatitis
- Other ectoparasites
- Dermatophytosis
- Atopic dermatitis
- Idiopathic miliary dermatitis
- Idiopathic eosinophilic granuloma complex
- Psychogenic alopecia
- Pyoderma
- Drug eruption
- Feline acne

DIAGNOSIS

Definitive diagnosis is based on feeding a restricted diet composed of unique ingredients to which the animal has never, or only very rarely, been exposed. It is therefore critically important to obtain a full dietary history including data on commercial diets, scraps or leftovers, biscuits or chews, flavored medicines, and any vitamin or mineral supplements.

Diet trials may be based on home cooked diets (see *Table 1*) or commercially prepared dried or tinned (canned) foods[5]. Limited studies have demonstrated that commercial diets are inferior to home cooked diets, but the latter could be

---

Table 1 Home cooked diets

Vegetarian test diet for dogs

1.4 kg (3 lb) carrots

1.4 kg (3 lb) peas

1.4 kg (3 lb) green beans

1.4 kg (3 lb) fresh or tinned tomatoes

285 g (10 oz) broccoli

450 g (1 lb) greens (cabbage, kale, spinach)

2 kg (4 lb 6 oz) white rice (or equivalent amounts of turnip, maize, potato, sweet potato, quinoa, sago, tapioca, etc.)

Cook the rice and vegetables in water according to the instructions on the packaging and without seasoning. Separate the rice and vegetables into eighteen 0.6 liter (20 fl oz) containers and place in the freezer. Thaw when required, mix one portion of vegetables with the cooked rice, and feed half to three-quarters of a cup of the vegetable–rice mixture for each 4.5 kg (10 lb) body weight. For very large dogs, you may have to feed extra rice. To prevent diarrhea, slowly switch to the vegetarian diet over 8–10 days. The dog's stools may be softer on the vegetarian diet. Compared with most commercial foods, this diet is low in protein and some dogs may lose weight.

Meat and rice diet for dogs

2.5 kg (10 cups) cooked rice

450 g (1 lb) cooked meat (e.g. turkey, rabbit, venison, duck, etc.)

1$\frac{1}{3}$ tsp calcium carbonate

1 tsp dicalcium phosphate

5 tbsp vegetable oil

1 tsp salt substitute (potassium chloride)

Non-flavored, additive-free multivitamin/mineral supplement (follow recommended dose)

Bake or boil the meat. Cook the rice according to directions and add salt substitute to the water. Grind or finely chop the meat and set aside. Pulverize the calcium carbonate, dicalcium phosphate, and vitamin/mineral supplement. Mix the oil, minerals, and supplements with the rice and then add the meat. Mix well, cover, and refrigerate. Some dermatologists recommend starting with 10 g/kg meat and 20 g/kg carbohydrate, and then adjusting according to response and palatability.

Meat and rice diet for cats

100 g (3.5 oz) rice and 100 g (3.5 oz) chicken or other meat (poached in water, which is added back as gravy) is adequate. Some cats refuse to eat carbohydrates, however, and may find meat-only diets more palatable. It can also be worth adding the oil and the vitamin and mineral supplements as above, and many feline specialists advise adding 150 mg taurine.

nutritionally imbalanced, are labor intensive and expensive, may cause gastrointestinal upsets and weight loss, may result in poor compliance, and the dogs may not go back to commercial foods[5]. Single protein, single carbohydrate, complete dried and tinned food diets are often marketed as 'hypoallergenic', although they are only hypo-allergenic for animals that do not react to any of the ingredients. They are easy to prepare, nutri-tionally balanced, and usually palatable, although the exact ingredients may be unknown (color-ings, flavorings, preservatives, and other fats) and it may not be possible to find a commercial diet that contains a novel ingredient. IgE binding studies with canine serum have shown that cattle and sheep extracts cross-react[9], and in humans there is extensive cross-reaction between proteins derived from related fish, birds, and mammals. The only true hypoallergenic diets are those in which the proteins have been hydrolysed to reduce their molecular weight to <10 kDa, theo-retically rendering them non-immunogenic. Recent studies have demonstrated good effi-cacy[11,15], but they are more expensive and may be less palatable than single protein diets.

The length of a diet trial necessary to confirm an adverse reaction to food is controversial, but most authorities now recommend at least six weeks. However, one prospective study of 51 dogs found that 23.5% required 6–7 weeks and 17.6% required 8–10 weeks[3]. Some authors, furthermore, recommended 12-week diet trials in cats. It may also be necessary to keep cats indoors to prevent them feeding on wild animals or in other homes, and to muzzle or leash dogs that scavenge.

Any animal that improves with a restricted diet should be challenged with its original diet, which should include all treats, scraps, biscuits, chews, and dietary supplements. If a CAFR is involved, there will be an increase in pruritus within seven to ten days of the dietary challenge. If there is no increase in pruritus following the dietary challenge, then a CAFR can be ruled out and the apparent improvement was probably due to some other effect. If there is recrudescence of pruritus with the dietary challenge, then the restricted diet should be reinstituted and there should once again be resolution of pruritus. If a diagnosis of CAFR is made, it is helpful to be able to identify the specific foods to which the animal is reacting using a series of sequential food challenges.

Failure to recognize and treat secondary infec-tions and ectoparasites during a dietary trial is a common cause of problems. Another major reason for poor compliance during a dietary trial is continued pruritus. One possible solution is to allow the use of short courses of glucocorticoids (0.5–1.0 mg/kg p/o q24h for 3–5 days) as necessary during the trial.

The use of serology or IDT (intradermal testing) in the diagnosis of CAFR is controversial. Currently, there is no evidence that these tests are reliable for the following reasons:

- Two percent of all ingested food antigen is absorbed and presented to the immune system.
- Cross-reactions between dietary and environmental allergens have been demonstrated, particularly carbohydrate determinants.
- Both the above lead to the formation of circulating allergen specific IgE and IgG, and IgA-containing mucosal secretions in healthy dogs.
- As previously stated, not all adverse food reactions in dogs are immunologically mediated.

Bearing these points in mind, there is still no substitute for undertaking a properly conducted dietary trial using either a novel protein or hydrol-ysed diet to rule out CAFR in dogs or cats[1,16].

MANAGEMENT
Feed a complete and balanced, highly digestible, limited antigen diet that does not contain the offending ingredients (as identified in the chal-lenge studies).

KEY POINTS
- Dietary intolerance is uncommon.
- Recurrent otitis externa and recurrent superficial pyoderma may be associated with dietary intolerance.
- Diagnosis relies on a properly conducted food trial and challenge.

Allergic and irritant contact dermatitis

ETIOLOGY AND PATHOGENESIS

Allergic (ACD) and irritant (ICD) contact dermatitis are two very similar conditions mediated by direct contact with environmental substances and, therefore, they affect sparsely haired, predominantly ventral skin[1]. ACD is a type 4 (cell-mediated) hypersensitivity reaction to small, low molecular weight chemicals (haptens) that bind to host proteins. Haptenated proteins are phagocytosed, processed, and presented by antigen presenting cells, especially epidermal Langerhan's cells, to T cells bearing the appropriate T cell receptors. These recirculate to the skin and, on subsequent exposure to the hapten, trigger a cell-mediated immune response[2]. ICD, in contrast, is directly triggered by noxious compounds[2]. The effector stages and inflammation in ACD and ICD share similar immunologic pathways, resulting in almost identical clinical signs and histopathology[1,2].

CLINICAL FEATURES

The refractory period for allergic contact dermatitis is reported to be rarely less than two years, so one would not expect it to appear in very young animals[1]. However, the inquisitive nature of puppies and, perhaps, their juvenile pelage, might predispose them to exposure to irritants and, therefore, ICD. German Shepherd Dogs comprised 50% of the dogs in one series of confirmed ACD cases[3]. ACD requires multiple exposures, whereas ICD will occur on first exposure[2]. ACD usually affects individual animals, but ICD can affect all in-contact animals[2]. Most cases of ACD and ICD are perennial, although it does depend on the timing of exposure, and seasonal examples will be met, typically to vegetative allergens/irritants[1,2,4,5].

Acute and severe ACD/ICD may result in erythema, edema, vesicles, and even erosion or ulceration (**19, 20**)[1–3,5,6]. Primary lesions include erythematous macules, papules, and occasionally vesicles. Secondary lesions (e.g. excoriation, alopecia, lichenification, and hyperpigmentation)

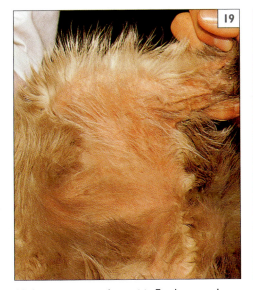

19 Irritant contact dermatitis. Erythema and alopecia following exposure to irritant oil.

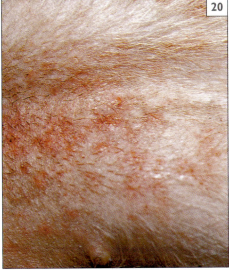

20 Allergic contact dermatitis. Primary lesions (erythematous papules) on the ventral midline of a Labrador Retriever.

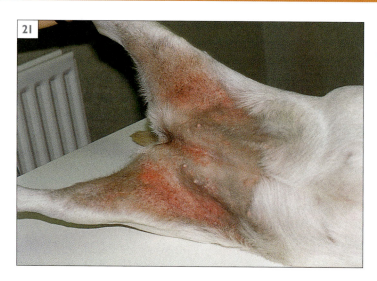

21 Well-demarcated erythema and alopecia in the groin and ventral abdomen of a Labrador Retriever.

tend to mask these primary lesions. There is usually a well-defined margin between affected and normal skin (**21**). Pruritus is variable, but may be intense[1–3,6].

The distribution of the lesions reflects the exposed contact areas and, therefore, hairless dogs and cats are at more risk[7]. Clinical signs are usually confined to sparsely haired skin, but prolonged contact will result in extension to adjacent areas and, with time, the chin, ventral pinna, ventral neck, medial limbs, and the entire ventrum will be affected[1,5]. Generalized reactions may be seen in cases of reactions to shampoos[1,5]. Chronic otitis externa may result from sensitivity to topical neomycin or other potential irritants and sensitizers[5,8,9]. Other potential substances include metals, plastics, fibers, leather, dyes, oils, and cleaning fluids[1–3,5–7].

DIFFERENTIAL DIAGNOSES
- Atopic dermatitis
- Cutaneous adverse food reaction
- Sarcoptic mange
- Demodicosis
- Harvest mite or chigger infestation
- Superficial pyoderma
- *Malassezia pachydermatis* dermatitis
- *Pelodera strongyloides* dermatitis
- Hookworm dermatitis

DIAGNOSIS
A tentative diagnosis can be based on history, clinical signs, and eliminating the differential diagnoses[2]. Histopathology from primary lesions or acute cases may reveal intraepidermal spongiosis or vesiculation and keratinocyte necrosis, but most biopsies are non-specific[1,2,10]. Exclusion trials and closed patch testing may be necessary if definitive diagnosis is deemed necessary for management.

If the environment is suitable, exclusion trials are useful tests. These can include: avoiding carpets, grass or concrete (wet concrete is a common irritant); plain cotton bedding; cleaning with water only; glass or ceramic food and water bowls; avoiding rubber or plastic toys; and avoiding topical medications. If the dermatitis goes into remission, provocative exposure may allow identification of the allergen/irritant. Closed patch testing may be indicated if exclusion trials are unrewarding, but this is a specialist procedure and referral is advised[1,2,7,9]. Briefly, the animal is hospitalized, the thoracic wall close-clipped, and samples from a standard panel of chemicals (such as The European Standard Battery of Allergens [**Note:** these are not standardized for animals]) are placed into Finn chambers (small nickel cups), which are taped to the clipped skin. In addition, samples from the household (e.g. carpet fibers or vegetation) can be

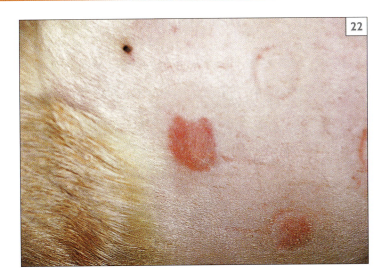

22 Positive closed patch test read after 48 hours. Circular impressions of the Finn chambers are apparent, and the edematous, erythematous patches are readily visible.

placed into adjacent chambers. An Elizabethan collar and foot bandages are used to prevent the animal removing the Finn chambers. The sites are inspected at 48 hours, with any erythematous and indurated sites classed as positive (**22**). Punch biopsies can be taken from positive sites to confirm the reaction[10]. Small-scale patch tests (e.g. for suspect shampoos and topical medications) can be set up by applying the fluid absorbed onto cotton swabs held in place by adhesive dressings such as Opsite® and a body bandage as above.

MANAGEMENT

If the allergen or irritant can be identified, and if exposure can be restricted, then the prognosis is good. Failure to identify the cause or prevent access results in reliance on symptomatic therapy, usually with systemic glucocorticoids. Topical therapy can be appropriate with localized lesions. In some individuals, complete control may be very hard to achieve without the side-effects of glucocorticoid therapy becoming apparent. Ciclosporin (cyclosporine) or topical tacrolimus (not licenced for animals) can be effective and better tolerated. Pentoxifylline (10 mg/kg p/o q12h) ameliorated lesions in three dogs sensitized to plants of the Commelinaceae family[11]. Barrier creams and/or prompt washing can be used if some exposure is unavoidable.

KEY POINTS

- Allergic contact dermatitis is rare.
- The pruritus may be refractory to steroid therapy.
- Focal lesions may result from reactions to topical medications, food bowls, or toys.
- Generalized lesions may result from shampoos.

Flea bite hypersensitivity
(flea allergic dermatitis)

ETIOLOGY AND PATHOGENESIS
Flea bite hypersensitivity (FBH) or flea allergic dermatitis (FAD) develops following introduction of flea salivary proteins into the epidermis and dermis[1]. Hypersensitivity to these proteins initiates immediate, late phase, and chronic inflammatory reactions[2]. Flea bites may be irritating, but it is considered that clinical signs in affected animals are associated with FBH/FAD rather than flea bite dermatitis[3]. In dogs, early and regular flea exposure may prevent or delay FBH/FAD. Intermittent exposure seems to be the most potent inducer of clinical sensitivity[3]. Fleas are vectors for *Bartonella* (cat scratch fever),

Rickettsia felis, *Haemoplasma* (feline infectious anemia), and *Dipylidium caninum*[4]. The vast majority of infestations are associated with the cat flea (*Ctenocephalides felis felis*). A variety of other fleas have been found on dogs and cats. Species identification can help to determine the epidemiology and aid control in difficult infestations.

CLINICAL FEATURES
Dogs
Dogs exhibit more predictable clinical signs than cats. There is no breed incidence, except that atopic dogs may be predisposed. Dogs aged 1–3 years are most commonly affected[3]. Pruritus is usually present, although variable. Lesions are mostly over the caudal back, flanks, tail, and perineum (**23**, **24**) and, less commonly, the limbs, ventral or rostral trunk, and head. Clinical signs include symmetrical to irregular alopecia, erythema, papules, crusts, excoriation, hyperpigmentation, and lichenification. The severity of the lesions is related to the degree and duration of pruritus. Acute pyotraumatic dermatitis ('hot spots') and superficial bacterial folliculitis are also commonly reported.

Cats
Cats rarely manifest overt pruritus or primary lesions. Feline FBH/FAD is a common cause of a number of clinical presentations including miliary dermatitis (a macular papular, crusting dermatitis) (**25**), symmetrical self-induced alopecia (**26**, **27**), and lesions of the eosinophilic granuloma complex (eosinophilic plaque, eosinophilic granuloma, linear granuloma, and indolent ulcers) (**28**, **29**).

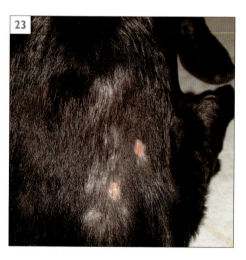

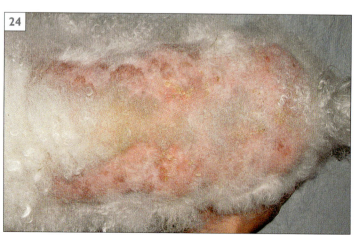

23, 24 Symmetrical self-trauma, alopecia, erosions, and crusts in two dogs with FBH/FAD.

25 Miliary dermatitis in a cat with FBH/FAD.

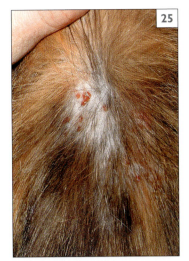

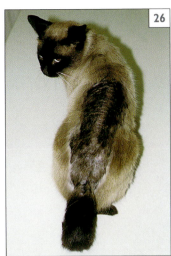

26, 27, 28, 29 Flea bite hypersensitivity. Alopecia and hyperpigmentation due to acromelanism along the dorsal midline of a dark-pointed Siamese cat (**26**); extensive alopecia involving the entire caudal trunk and hindlimbs of a cat (**27**); linear (collagenolytic) granuloma on the medial aspect of the hindlimb of a cat (**28**); cluster of eosinophilic plaques on the caudal aspect of the hindlimb of a cat (**29**).

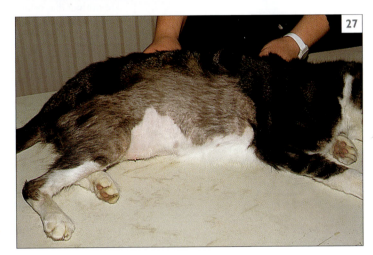

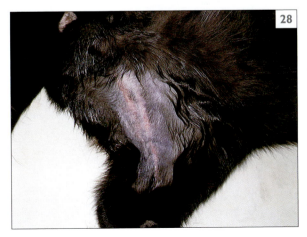

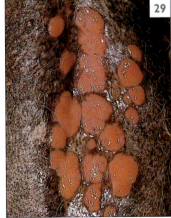

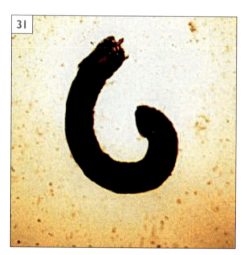

DIFFERENTIAL DIAGNOSES
- Pediculosis
- Sarcoptic mange
- Cheyletiellosis
- Ectopic *Otodectes cynotis* infestation
- *Neotrombicula* infestation
- *Lynxacarus radovsky* infestation
- Superficial staphylococcal pyoderma (usually a secondary problem)
- Dermatophytosis
- Atopic dermatitis
- Cutaneous adverse food reaction
- Pemphigus foliaceus
- Drug eruption
- Idiopathic eosinophilic granuloma complex
- Pyschogenic alopecia

DIAGNOSIS
Definitive diagnosis of FBH/FAD requires compatible clinical signs, the presence of fleas or flea feces on the animal and, strictly speaking, a positive flea-specific intradermal or serology test. In practice, negative allergen tests should not be used to rule out FBH/FAD, particularly in cats. Reports of positive tests to flea extracts vary from 2% to 77%[5], which probably reflects the proportion of atopic, flea allergic, and concurrent cases seen at different centers. Recent studies have shown that intradermal tests using the purified flea salivary antigen were more accurate than those using whole body extracts, and that intradermal tests with either extract were superior to an FcεRIα based ELISA using the purified flea salivary antigen[6,7].

It can also be difficult to demonstrate fleas. Flea feces are often the only sign of infestation (**30–32**), but they may not be found in severely pruritic overgrooming animals. It can be easier to detect fleas and/or feces on clinically normal in-contact animals. The presence of *Dipylidium* is diagnostic and contagion is highly suggestive of fleas or other parasites. Lesions in humans are small, pruritic, erythematous papular lesions, typically on the lower limbs. Sensitized humans may develop large bullous lesions, ulceration, and secondary infection[8].

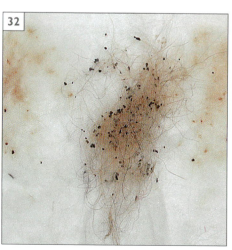

30–32 Flea feces demonstrated in coat combings (**30**), tape-strip cytology ×40 (**31** [photo courtesy P Forsythe]), and red staining on wet cotton wool (**32**).

MANAGEMENT

Adult fleas are obligate ectoparasites that lay eggs in the coat. These readily fall into the immediate local environment, where all the immature stages from egg through to pupa develop[3,9]. Although buildings are the preferred breeding environment, fleas may breed outside in warm climates. In reality, however, outdoor flea burdens are small and contact with other animals or contaminated environments is much more likely to be a source of infestation[3,10].

The principal problem in trying to control domestic flea populations is the resistant pupa[9]. Pupae can lie dormant for several months and yield viable adults after all other eggs, larvae, and adults are killed. Repeated environmental treatments may therefore be necessary. It is important to treat all potential environments (including sheds, cars, etc.) and in-contact animals. This may require tactful conversations about flea control with neighbors, family, and friends.

Variation in insecticide susceptibility between laboratory and field strains of fleas has been shown[11]. This suggests that fleas can develop extensive cross-resistance to insecticides. The clinical implications are unclear, but it could obviously affect the success of a flea control program[10].

In theory, systemic (e.g. nitenpyram, selamectin), slow-kill (e.g. fipronil, imidacloprid), or insect growth regulators (IGRs) (e.g. lufenuron, pyriproxifen) that either require or do not necessarily prevent feeding should be less effective in flea allergic animals. However, it is now thought that it is the overall burden of fleas that contributes to FBH/FAD, and that population control is more important than preventing individual bites.

Environmental treatment

Vacuum cleaning will help remove adult fleas from the flooring, reduce the numbers of eggs and larvae within the carpet, elevate the carpet pile thus enhancing penetration of the insecticide, and stimulate emergence of pupated adults[9].

Environmental products are usually aerosol sprays consisting of a permethrin/pyrethroid combined with an IGR such as methoprene, pyriproxifen, or cyromazine. The insecticide provides a rapid kill of larvae and adults that can be effective for up to 2–3 months. IGRs prevent normal development of the eggs, larvae, and pupae, with residual activity for up to 12 months.

Foggers, available for some products, are easier to apply, but they often miss protected sites under furniture and do not penetrate carpets and rugs very well. Great care must be taken when using environmental treatments in homes with small rodents, birds, and fish. Fleas are susceptible to sunlight, but shaded outdoor areas can be treated with insecticides and/or the parasitic nematode *Steinernema carpocapsa*.

On-animal adulticides

Proprietary shampoos and washes are not particularly effective, as they are rinsed off and have little residual activity. Flea collars are convenient, particularly in cats, but used alone often fail to provide adequate flea control, may trigger contact reactions, are toxic if ingested, and may cause strangulation if fitted incorrectly.

Topical permethrin/pyrethroid spot-on solutions, foams, and pump sprays are highly effective[12], but they can require more frequent administration that other topical insecticides. The rapid 'knock-down' effect can be useful to minimize flea contact and biting behavior in very sensitive animals. Cats are, however, particularly susceptible to permethrin toxicity; these products must be used with care and cats should never be exposed to products designed for use in dogs. Microencapsulated products are safer and have a less rapid knock-down but longer residual activity.

The newer spot-on insecticides fipronil (also available as a pump spray), selamectin, imidacloprid, metaflumizone, and pyriprole are highly effective against fleas, although the killing activity is delayed compared with permethrins[10,13–15]. They are safe products, even in young animals and nursing mothers. They have prolonged residual activity, usually 4–8 weeks but up to 12 weeks for fipronil spray on dogs. Used regularly, these products have also been shown to eliminate environmental infestations[10,13,14,16]. Fipronil and pyriprole, which bind to sebum, and selamectin, which is systemically absorbed, are particularly resistant to bathing and wetting.

Nitempyram is given orally and is an effective adulticide within 15–20 minutes[17]. However, it has poor residual activity and is usually used in association with an IGR.

D-limolene, Tea-tree, Pennyroyal, and other essential oils are repellent and insecticidal, although clinical efficacy remains to be proven[18]. Some essential oils are toxic to cats and should be used with care.

On-animal IGRs

Topical IGRs including methoprene, pyriproxifen, and lufenuron (oral or injectable) can be administered as sole agents, as combination products, or with a separate adulticide[15,16]. They are effective at blocking the life cycle and, therefore, the environmental accumulation of fleas, but the lack of adulticidal activity means that the effect on the overall population takes time. Simultaneous use of an adulticide is therefore recommended at least initially for prompt reduction of the adult population[14,16,19,20].

Other treatments

Although flea control is mandatory, it may not be sufficient to result in complete control of the dermatosis and anti-inflammatory treatment (e.g. antihistamines, glucocorticoids, or essential fatty acids) may be necessary. Short-term treatment can be useful during the initial stages of flea control and to cover any breakdown in the flea management regime.

KEY POINTS

- FBH/FAD is common.
- It may be difficult to convince sceptical owners of the diagnosis in the absence of fleas or feces.
- If you suspect FBH/FAD, evaluate the response to a thorough 6–8-week flea control trial.
- Always use an adulticide on all animals and an environmental adulticide/IGR in the home.

Pediculosis

ETIOLOGY AND PATHOGENESIS

Pediculosis (or louse infestation) (**33**) is more common in Europe than in North America[1]. Infestations are predominantly seen in animals housed together, especially if they are young or debilitated. The most common species that infest dogs is the biting louse (Mallophaga) *Trichodectes canis* (**34**). Other species seen in warmer climates are the sucking lice (Anplura) *Linognathus setosus* (**35**) and *Heterodoxus spineger*. The only species that infests cats is the biting louse *Felicola subrostratus* (**36**).

The entire life cycle is completed on the host within three weeks[1]. Eggs (**37**) are laid on hairs and hatch into nymphs, which undergo several molts to become adults. Transmission occurs by direct contact or by grooming with contaminated brushes or combs. Lice are host specific, but transient contamination of other in-contact hosts, including humans, may be seen.

CLINICAL FEATURES

The clinical appearance is quite variable and can include: asymptomatic carriers; variable scaling with mild pruritus; rough, dry hair coat; alopecia, papules, and crusts with mild to moderate pruritus; and severe inflammation, alopecia, excoriations, and crusting, with extensive pruritus. Occasional cases may mimic miliary dermatitis in cats and flea bite hypersensitivity in dogs. Heavy infestations with sucking lice may result in anemia, especially in young animals.

DIFFERENTIAL DIAGNOSES

- Cheyletiellosis
- Dermatophytosis (cats)
- Sarcoptic mange
- Atopic dermatitis
- Keratinization disorders
- Cutaneous adverse food reactions
- *Neotrombicula* spp. infestation
- Flea bite hypersensitivity (flea allergic dermatitis)

DIAGNOSIS

Diagnosis is based on finding lice or nits on the skin or hair. Lice are wingless, dorsoventrally flattened insects with strong, gripping claws. Biting lice have broad heads, whereas sucking lice have narrow heads. Their eggs ('nits') are large, operculated, and cemented to the hair shaft.

MANAGEMENT

Two treatments 14 days apart using pyrethrin sprays, shampoos, or dips are effective in most cases. Single or multiple treatments with fipronil, selamectin, and imidacloprid are also effective[2-5]. A single ivermectin injection (0.2 mg/kg s/c) has been reported to be effective, but this is not licensed for dogs and cats, and is contraindicated in Collies, Collie crosses, and other herding breeds.

KEY POINT

- Lice are usually easily detected, but they may be missed if not suspected, especially in pruritic animals.

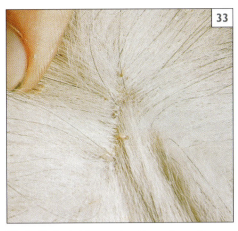

33 Pediculosis. Lice on the skin surface of a heavily infested pup.

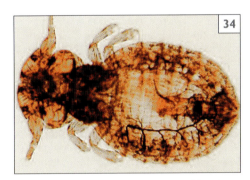

34 *Trichodectes canis.* (Photo courtesy Merial Animal Health)

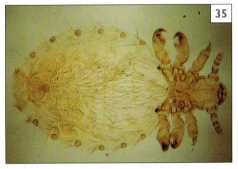

35 *Linognathus setosus.* (Photo courtesy M Geary)

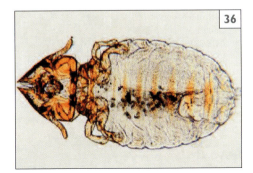

36 *Felicola subrostratus.* (Photo courtesy Merial Animal Health)

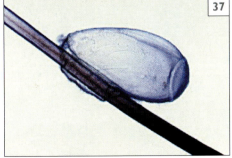

37 Operculated louse egg tightly cemented to the hair shaft. In comparison, *Cheyletiella* eggs are smaller, bound to the hair shaft at the distal egg by silken fibers, and non-operculated. (Photo courtesy Merial Animal Health)

Sarcoptic mange
(scabies, sarcoptic acariosis)

ETIOLOGY AND PATHOGENESIS

Sarcoptic mange is common in dogs but rare in cats. *Sarcoptes scabiei* mites are highly contagious through direct contact, fur, crusts, and fomites, and they will infest a variety of species including humans[1] (**38**), although different varieties are relatively species specific. The mites tunnel through the epidermis, laying eggs that hatch into six-legged larvae, which then molt into eight-legged nymphs and finally into adults that emerge onto the surface. The life cycle takes 14–21 days to complete. Adult females can survive off the host for up to 19 days, but 2–6 days is more usual in normal household conditions.

Initial infection in a naive animal is associated with an asymptomatic period, which is variable but may last 3–6 weeks. Exposure to mites and their allergens induces humoral and cell-mediated hypersensitivity that results in intense pruritus[2]. Animals subsequently infested can exhibit a much shorter lag period.

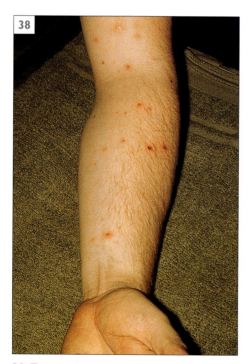

38 Zoonotic lesions of scabies on the forearm of an owner.

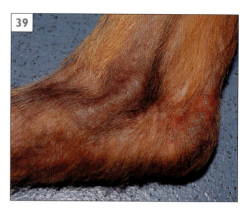

39 Erythema, excoriation, alopecia, and lichenification of the hock in a dog with scabies.

CLINICAL FEATURES

The primary clinical signs are usually acute-onset pruritus and erythematous papules with a grayish-yellow crust. Predilection sites include the pinnal tips and margins, elbows, hocks, ventral chest, and ventral abdomen (**39–42**), but disease can be focal to multifocal and later becomes generalized. Self-trauma results in severe excoriation, lichenification, and patchy alopecia. There may be malaise, weight loss, lymphadenopathy, and crusting in severe long-standing cases. Crusting and scaling are particularly prominent in Norwegian scabies, a variant associated with large numbers of mites, often in immunosuppressed individuals (**43**).

DIFFERENTIAL DIAGNOSES

- Atopic dermatitis
- Cutaneous adverse food reaction
- Bacterial folliculitis
- *Malassezia pachydermatis* dermatitis
- Flea bite hypersensitivity
- Cheyletiellosis
- Otoacariosis
- *Pelodera strongyloides* dermatitis
- Harvest mite (chigger or berry bug) dermatitis

DIAGNOSIS

The history and clinical signs will often allow a tentative diagnosis of scabies. A positive pinnal scratch reflex is highly suggestive of scabies[3]. The diagnosis is confirmed by identifying mites, fecal pellets, or eggs in skin scrapings (**44, 45**). This is poorly sensitive, however, and requires

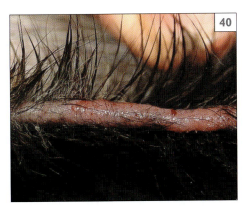

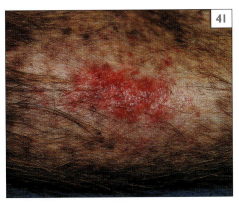

40 Erythema, excoriation, and alopecia of the pinna margin.

41 Erythematous papules, excoriation, and alopecia of the ventral chest.

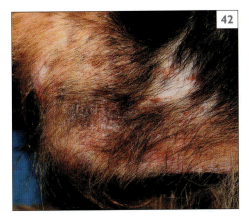

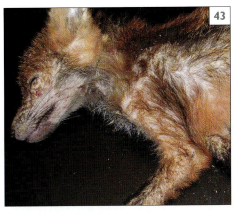

42 Erythematous papules, excoriation, alopecia, and lichenification of the elbow.

43 Severe Norwegian scabies in a Red Fox with generalized scaling, crusting, excoriation, and alopecia. (Photo courtesy M Allington)

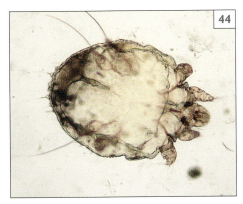

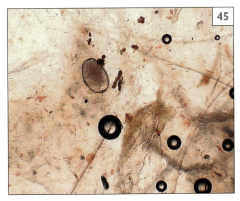

44 Adult female *Sarcoptes scabiei*.

45 *Sarcoptes* eggs and fecal pellets.

examination of multiple skin scrapings, using concentration/flotation techniques, if necessary, from primary lesions at the predilection sites.

Several ELISA tests for *Sarcoptes* specific IgG are available. False-negative results can be seen in early infestations (it takes up to four weeks to develop an adequate titer), and false-positive tests can occur in atopic dogs sensitized to *Dermatophagoides* spp. house dust mites, which share common antigens with *Sarcoptes*[4]. One test subjected to independent scrutiny proved highly sensitive and specific, and did not appear to cross-react with *Dermatophagoides*[2,5]. In one author's (TJN) experience, *Sarcoptes* IgG ELISAs have a very high (99.7%) negative predictive value but a low (29%) positive predictive value because of false-positive results in atopic dogs.

Trial acaricidal therapy is justified in any pruritic dog presented with a history and clinical signs suggestive of scabies, even if skin scrapes and serology are negative.

MANAGEMENT

Miticidal treatment of the affected animal, in-contact dogs, and the environment should be curative[6].

Selamectin and imidacloprid/moxidectin spot-on formulations (given once monthly on 2–3 occasions) are licensed for the treatment of scabies in dogs. At the recommended dose they are safe in Collies, Collie crosses, and other herding breeds sensitive to macrocyclic lactones. There are, however, anecdotal reports of treatment failures and greater efficacy following off-license therapy every two weeks for three applications. Milbemycin oxime (see Canine demodicosis, p. 272) is effective and well tolerated at 2 mg/kg p/o weekly for 3–5 weeks or 1 mg/kg p/o every other day for 2–3 weeks, but is not licensed for canine scabies. Ivermectin (0.2–0.4 mg/kg either weekly p/o or every 14 days s/c for 4–6 weeks) and moxidectin (250 µg/kg s/c every week for 3 weeks or 400 µg/kg p/o twice weekly for 3–6 weeks) are effective, but are not licensed in dogs and should be avoided in avermectin-sensitive breeds.

Topical treatment is more time consuming, requires clipping and/or bathing to remove hair and crusts, and is not necessarily safer. Amitraz dip (see Canine demodicosis, p. 272) is licensed in Europe, Canada, and Australia, and is effective when applied every 7–14 days for 4–6 weeks.

0.25% fipronil solution (see Flea bite hypersensitivity, p. 38) is licensed as an aid to the treatment of canine scabies and can be useful applied at 3–6 ml/kg every 7–21 days for 3–6 weeks in young, pregnant, or nursing dogs, where more potent treatments may be contraindicated. 2.5% lime sulfur (see Dermatophytosis, p. 278) applied weekly for 4–6 weeks is also effective and well tolerated.

KEY POINTS

- Always be alert for scabies.
- Contagious and zoonotic.
- If you suspect scabies, treat it.

51 Six legged, orange-red colored larva of *Neotrombicula autumnalis*, the harvest mite or chigger.

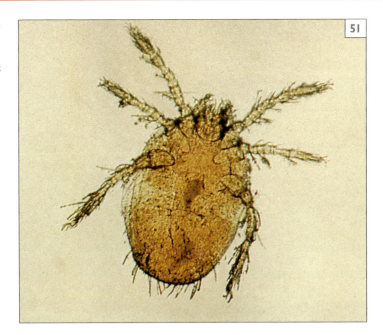

52 Trombiculidiasis. A cluster of trombiculid mites at the medial canthus of a crossbred dog.

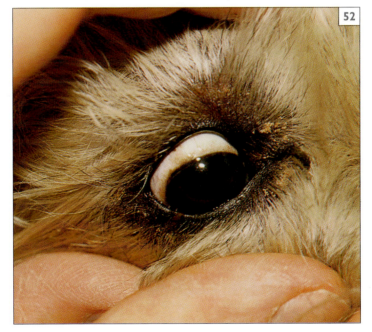

Pelodera strongyloides dermatitis

DEFINITION

Pelodera strongyloides, or rhabditic, dermatitis is an erythematous pruritic dermatitis caused by cutaneous infestation with the larvae of *P. strongyloides*.

ETIOLOGY AND PATHOGENESIS

P. strongyloides is a free-living nematode that has a direct life cycle[1]. It is found in damp soil or moist, decaying organic matter such as straw, leaves, hay, and rice hulls. Larvae may invade skin that comes into contact with the contaminated soil or organic material and initiate cutaneous inflammation.

CLINICAL FEATURES

Lesions associated with this infestation occur in areas of skin that come into contact with the ground or bedding, but their appearance will vary markedly between cases. Focal or diffuse alopecia may be present with or without erythema (**53, 54**). Papules, pustules, and crusts may be present in some cases. In chronic cases the skin may become lichenified and hyperpigmented. Pruritus can vary from minimal to intense.

DIFFERENTIAL DIAGNOSES

- Sarcoptic mange
- Atopic dermatitis
- Cutaneous adverse food reaction
- Contact irritant dermatitis
- Demodicosis
- Ancylostomiasis
- Dirofilariasis
- Dermatophytosis
- Bacterial folliculitis

DIAGNOSIS

Skin scrapings should be performed to demonstrate the small, motile nematode larvae (563–625 μm in length) (**55**)[2]. In some cases the larvae are easy to demonstrate and in others it can be very difficult.

MANAGEMENT

The primary goal of management is to change the animal's environment so as to avoid it coming into contact with soil or bedding harboring the larvae. Old, damp straw, hay, or other organic material should be removed from dog houses, kennels, or yards. After cleaning the inside of dog houses and the surfaces of runs, they can be sprayed with malathion (28 g of 57–59% malathion per 4.5 liters of water) or pyrethroids. New bedding consisting of wood chips, old blankets, or shredded paper can then be placed. Animals should be bathed using a mild shampoo. Systemic antibacterial therapy (see Superficial pyoderma, p. 146) would be appropriate if secondary bacterial infection is present.

Systemic glucocorticoids, such as methylprednisolone (0.4–0.8 mg/kg po q 12 h) or prednisolone and prednisone (0.5–1.0 mg/kg po q 12 h) can be used for 3–10 days, or as necessary, to control severe pruritus. Once the environment is cleaned, the lesions should be self-limiting. Giving affected animals 1–3 weekly parasiticidal dips using medications appropriate for scabies has been previously advocated[1,2]. However, the efficacy of this is not known, as there have been no studies performed to show whether these treatments shorten the course of clinical disease or not.

KEY POINTS

- The pruritus associated with *P. strongyloides* may be refractory to steroid therapy.
- Animal has been in contact with moist decaying organic material containing larvae.
- Is self-limiting when animal is removed from infected environment.

53–55 *Pelodera strongyloides* dermatitis. Extensive alopecia, crusting, lichenification, and hyperpigmentation on the dependent aspects of the body (**53**); alopecia and hyperpigmentation (**54**); a photomicrograph of the nematode *P. strongyloides*, found in skin scrapings (**55**).

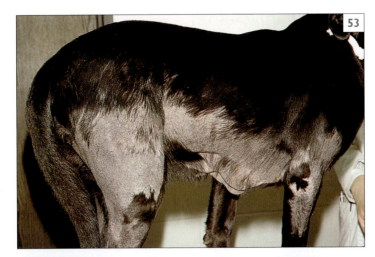

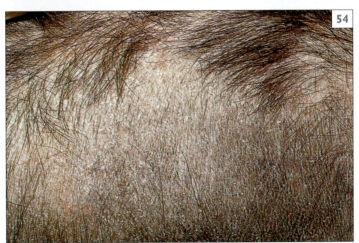

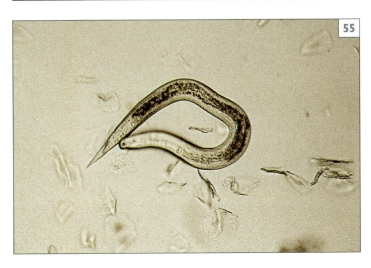

Ancylostomiasis
(hookworm dermatitis)

DEFINITION
Hookworm dermatitis is a condition character-ized by erythematous papular lesions that occur following cutaneous penetration by the larvae of hookworms.

ETIOLOGY AND PATHOGENESIS
The dermatitis develops from the cutaneous penetration of the third-stage larvae of *Uncinaria stenocephala* or *Ancylostoma* spp. located in soil that the animal contacts[1]. Skin lesions are more often associated with *U. stenocephala* infestation than with *Ancylostoma* spp. Larvae enter the skin primarily at areas of desquamation, but occasionally they may enter via hair follicles[2]. In contrast to *Ancylostoma* spp., *U. stenocephala* rarely completes its life cycle by percutaneous penetration[2,3].

CLINICAL FEATURES
The condition is more frequently noted in hookworm-infested dogs housed on dirt runs with poor sanitation. Lesions are primarily located on the feet, but they may be seen on any area of skin that touches the ground. Erythema-tous papules constitute primary lesions, but chronically affected skin often becomes diffusely erythematous and thickened and may exhibit alopecia (**56**). The epithelium of the footpads becomes roughened due to the development of keratinized papillae. Chronically affected foot-pads may eventually become soft and spongy, especially at the pad margins[4]. Nails may grow faster, become ridged, twisted on their long axis, thicker at the base, and, in severe cases, break off. Arthritis of the distal interphalangeal joints may be a sequela[4]. Pruritus is usually mild but can vary in intensity[2,4].

DIFFERENTIAL DIAGNOSES
- Atopic dermatitis
- Demodicosis
- Contact dermatitis
- *Pelodera strongyloides* dermatitis
- Bacterial pododermatitis
- Harvest mite or chigger infestation
- *Malassezia pachydermatis* pododermatitis
- Trauma

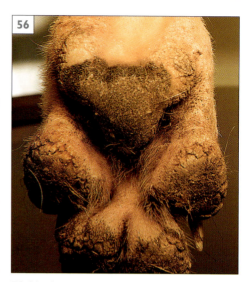

56 Hookworm dermatitis. Note the extensive erythema and scale formation in this chronic case.

DIAGNOSIS
Diagnosis is based on a history of being housed on dirt runs or kennels and poor sanitation, as well as the clinical findings. A positive fecal exam-ination for hookworm eggs provides supporting evidence but does not confirm a diagnosis. Generally, larvae cannot be demonstrated on microscopic examination of skin scrapings.

MANAGEMENT
All affected and associated dogs should be given appropriate anthelmintic treatment and a prophy-lactic program should be started. Frequent removal of feces from the runs and kennels, as well as improved sanitation, should be initiated. If feasible, dirt runs or kennels should be relo-cated so that animals are removed from the para-sitized environment. Sodium borate (0.5 kg/m^2) may be used to destroy larvae on the ground, although owners should be made aware that this treatment will kill vegetation[1].

KEY POINT
- Ancylostomiasis is unusual, although it may occur in certain groups of dogs (e.g. racing Greyhounds).

Intertrigo

DEFINITION
Intertrigo, or skin fold dermatitis, is an inflammatory condition occurring in skin that has intimate contact with adjacent skin.

ETIOLOGY AND PATHOGENESIS
Lip, facial, vulvar, body, and tail fold dermatitides result from inflammation that occurs when skin is closely opposed to skin. There is local abrasion, inflammation, and an accumulation of surface secretions, which result in maceration and secondary infection.

CLINICAL FEATURES
Lip fold dermatitis (**57**) results from the overlapping of redundant skin of the lower lip. The redundant skin forms a crevice, which entraps food particles and saliva, producing an ideal environment for bacterial growth. The resultant surface infection is characterized by a foul odor, which most clients associate erroneously with dental disease. Affected skin is erythematous, at times ulcerated, and occasionally covered by a small amount of exudate.

Facial fold dermatitis (**58, 59**) occurs more frequently in brachycephalic breeds such as Pekingese, English Bulldogs, and Pugs. The interiginous areas between folds of skin over the bridge of the nose and under the eyes become

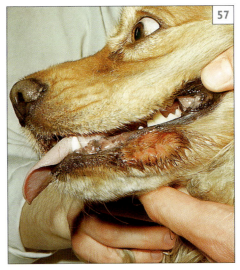

57 Lip fold dermatitis. An extensive patch of erythema and erosion in the lip fold of a Cocker Spaniel.

macerated and inflamed due to epiphora or accumulation of sebaceous or apocrine secretions. A secondary bacterial infection may occur.

Vulvar fold dermatitis is more common in obese animals that have a small vulva deep within a perivulval fold. Accumulation of urine and vaginal secretions causes irritation and maceration

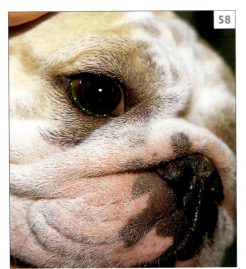
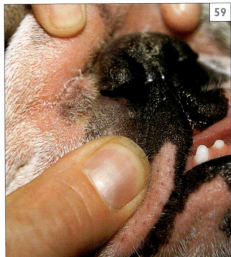

58, 59 Facial folds in an English Bulldog need to be separated to reveal fold pyoderma.

of adjacent skin, resulting in severe inflammation, secondary bacterial infection, and occasional ulceration. Affected animals exhibit increased licking of the vulvar area and this is generally the primary concern of clients.

Tail fold dermatitis (**60**) occurs more often in English Bulldogs, Boston Terriers, and Pugs. The dermatitis results from pressure and friction of their corkscrew tails on the skin of the perineum, as well as maceration, which may occur under skin that folds over the tail.

Body fold dermatitis occurs in those animals that have redundant skin thrown up into folds (e.g. Basset Hounds and Shar Peis). Folds are most frequently found on the limbs and trunk. As in other folds, the accumulation of surface secretions results in inflammation and secondary infection.

DIFFERENTIAL DIAGNOSES
- *Malassezia pachydermatis* infection
- Atopic dermatitis
- Cutaneous adverse food reaction
- Demodicosis
- Mucocutaneous candidiasis
- Epitheliotropic lymphoma

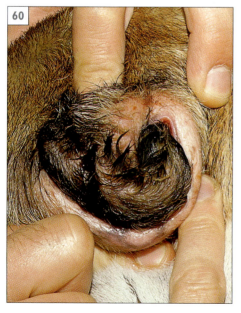

60 Tail fold dermatitis. Erythema and alopecia around the base of the tail in a Bulldog.

DIAGNOSIS
Clinical findings confirm a diagnosis, but impression smears should be taken from affected areas to determine the presence of bacteria or yeast. Skin scrapes should be taken to rule out *Demodex canis*, and impression smears or tape strips should be examined to rule out *M. pachydermatis* and *Candida* spp. Cutaneous lymphoma is rare and only diagnosed by histopathologic examination of biopsy material. *Malassezia* may be present as the only organism in some cases of intertrigo (see *Malassezia* dermatitis, p. 57) and mixed bacterial/*Malassezia* infections can be seen in others.

MANAGEMENT
Soiled hair that is excessive should be clipped and affected areas cleaned with shampoos containing chlorhexidine or ethyl lactate, or with benzoyl peroxide gel. If lesions appear moist, they can be treated 2–3 times a day for five minutes with a drying solution containing aluminum acetate (Burrow's solution). Other antimicrobial washes (see *Malassezia* dermatitis, p. 57 and Superficial pyoderma, p. 146) can be used and in some cases these may be very effective when applied regularly. After cleaning and/or drying, an antibiotic–steroid cream or ointment can be applied. Mupirocin ointment applied twice daily is especially efficacious in treating and controlling the bacterial components of this condition (this drug is not licensed for animals in some European countries and its use in animals may be forbidden). If deep bacterial infection appears to be present, treatment with systemic antibiotics would be indicated.

Owners should be forewarned that medical treatment will only control the condition and that surgical intervention is necessary for a cure. Cheiloplasty and episioplasty are appropriate procedures for lip and vulvar fold dermatitis, respectively. Tail amputation and removal of redundant skin is the preferred approach for tail fold dermatitis. Facial and body folds may also be removed surgically, but they may be considered desirable traits in some show animals and therefore necessitate a careful discussion of the procedure with the clients prior to surgery.

Malassezia dermatitis

ETIOLOGY AND PATHOGENESIS

Like staphylococci (see Superficial pyoderma, p. 146), *Malassezia* spp. yeasts are normal commensals in most dogs and cats. Mucosal reservoirs are an important source of transient contamination and infection, but cutaneous defense mechanisms normally limit colonization and infection. *Malassezia* dermatitis is therefore usually secondary to an underlying condition[1,2]. The vast majority of canine infections are associated with the non-lipid-dependent species *Malassezia pachydermatis*, although *M. furfur* has also been isolated[3]. A wider variety of species including *M. pachydermatis* and the lipid-dependent species *M. sympodialis* and *M. furfur* have been isolated from cats[4,5].

CLINICAL FEATURES

Canine *Malassezia* dermatitis can occur in any breed. Some breeds (e.g. Bassett Hounds and West Highland White Terriers) are predisposed, although this may represent a predisposition to primary causes rather than to *Malassezia per se*. Clinical signs include otitis externa, pruritus, erythema, a rancid, musty or yeasty odor, seborrhea, scaling, alopecia, lichenification, and hyperpigmentation. Clinical signs can be focal or generalized, diffuse or well demarcated. Commonly affected sites include the ears, lips, muzzle, feet, ventral neck, axilla, medial limbs, and perineum (**61, 62**). *Malassezia* can also cause paronychia, with a waxy exudate and discoloration of the nails[2,6].

Pruritus is less common in feline *Malassezia* dermatitis. Clinical signs include: otitis externa; feline acne; seborrheic and scaling facial dermatitis; generalized scaling and erythema; and paronychia with discoloration of the nails (particularly in Devon Rex cats) (**63**). Generalized erythema and scaling have been associated with *Malassezia* dermatitis in cats with thymoma, lymphocytic mural folliculitis, and paraneoplastic alopecia[7].

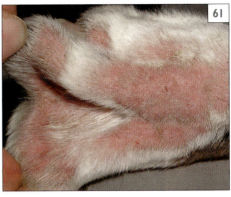

61 *Malassezia* dermatitis affecting the foot of an atopic Boxer with erythema, alopecia, and scaling.

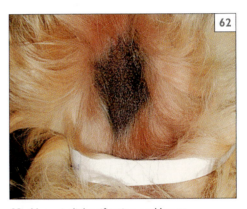

62 Alopecia, lichenification, and hyperpigmentation of the ventral neck caused by *Malassezia* dermatitis in an atopic Golden Retriever.

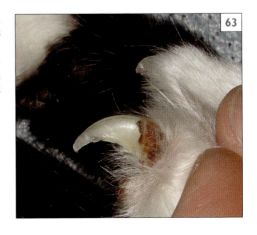

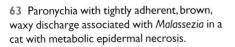

63 Paronychia with tightly adherent, brown, waxy discharge associated with *Malassezia* in a cat with metabolic epidermal necrosis.

64 Numerous oval to peanut-shaped budding *Malassezia* surrounding corneocytes in an impression smear from otitis externa in a dog. Note the variable pink to purple staining. (Diff-Quik, ×400)

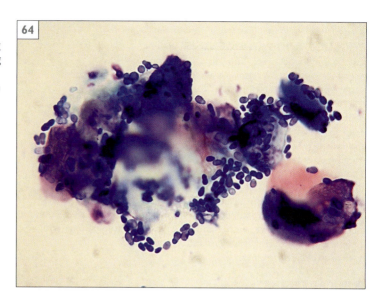

Table 2 Differential diagnoses of *Malessezia* dermatitis	
Diagnosis	**Possible underlying conditions**
Fleas	Body folds
Sarcoptic mange	Sarcoptic mange
Demodicosis	Demodicosis
Dermatophytosis	Atopic dermatitis
Staphylococcal pyoderma	Food allergy
Atopic dermatitis	Endocrinopathies
Food allergy	Keratinization defects
Drug reactions	Superficial necrolytic dermatitis
Contact dermatitis	Zinc responsive dermatosis
Seborrhea oleosa	Feline paraneoplastic alopecia
Seborrheic dermatitis	Feline thymoma
Feline acne/facial dermatitis	FeLV or FIV
Acanthosis nigricans	Feline acne/facial dermatitis
Epitheliotropic lymphoma	Immunosuppressive therapy
	Psychological stress

DIFFERENTIAL DIAGNOSES

A variety of other skin conditions can mimic *Malassezia* dermatitis (*Table 2*), but this is complicated by the fact that many of these can also be a trigger for a secondary *Malassezia* infection[1].

DIAGNOSIS

No agreed criteria have been established, but demonstration of elevated numbers of *Malassezia* with a good clinical and mycological response to antifungal treatment is diagnostic[2]. *Malassezia* are easily visible as small oval to peanut or snowman shapes, often forming rafts on the surface of squames, on cytology of tape-strips, and direct or indirect impression smears. They most frequently stain blue-purple, but can appear red-pink or pale blue (**64**). Some *Malassezia* fail to stain, but their refractile cell wall can be picked out with a closed condenser. There is no standard accepted cut-off value to diagnose *Malassezia* dermatitis, especially as they may not be uniformly distributed across a slide. In practice, only occasional *Malassezia* yeasts are found on healthy skin.

M. pachydermatis will grow on Sabouraud's medium, although the lipid-dependent species require supplemented media such as modified Dixon's agar[8]. However, as *Malassezia* are commensal organisms, isolation, particularly of small numbers, is not necessarily significant[2].

Malassezia can be present in the overlying keratin crust and hair follicles, but are often removed by processing. *Malassezia* can also be incidental findings in skin biopsies from other dermatoses. Histopathology of *Malassezia* dermatitis is characterized by acanthosis, hyperkeratosis, and a superficial inflammatory infiltrate.

Research has shown that a proportion of atopic dogs develop specific IgE titers and intradermal tests to *Malassezia* extracts, suggesting that they may act as allergens[9–11]. *Malassezia* specific serology and intradermal tests are available, although the clinical significance of *Malassezia* hypersensitivity and the efficacy of antiyeast therapy in canine atopic dermatitis are unclear[12].

MANAGEMENT
Topical therapy
Topical therapy is generally the most cost effective and safest treatment (*Table 3*). However, it is also the most labor intensive, and therefore not necessarily the most appropriate in all cases. Localized areas of *Malassezia* dermatitis (e.g. body folds) can be treated with focal application of an antifungal product, but the whole body should be treated in multifocal or generalized cases of *Malassezia* dermatitis[2]. It is particularly important to treat the ears, mucocutaneous junctions, and feet, as these are likely reservoirs of *Malassezia*. Treatment should be continued daily to three times weekly until resolution, then as necessary to maintain the improvement. Treatment with degreasing shampoos or antibacterial products may also be necessary initially. Adverse reactions are uncommon, although most of the antifungal products can be drying and irritating,

and may need to be combined with emollient rinses or shampoos.

Other treatment options include lotions, ointments, and creams containing ketoconazole, clotrimazole, or miconazole, although these are not licensed for use in animals. One per cent terbinafine lotion is effective in human seborrheic dermatitis.

Systemic therapy
Ketoconazole[13] (5–10 mg/kg p/o q24h, not licensed in animals) and itraconazole (5 mg/kg p/o q24h) are highly effective. Clinical improvement should be obvious after 7–14 days, although treatment should be continued for 7–14 days beyond clinical cure. Maintenance doses 2–3 times weekly may be necessary in some cases. Side-effects can include anorexia, vomiting, diarrhea, liver damage, vasculitis, and teratogenicity. Itraconazole is better tolerated than ketoconazole. Systemic terbinafine (30 mg/kg p/o q24h) is also effective and well tolerated, but is not licensed for dogs[14].

Zoonotic infections
Carriage of *M. pachydermatis* in dog owners has been demonstrated[15]. This should not be a concern in healthy individuals, but there are reports of zoonotic infections in immunocompromised neonates and adults[16,17].

KEY POINTS
- The pruritus associated with *Malassezia* may be refractory to steroid therapy.
- Most, although not all, cases are associated with underlying disease.

Table 3 Topical therapy for *Malassezia* dermatitis

Preparation	Advantages	Other considerations
2% miconazole/2% chlorhexidine	Excellent antibacterial and antifungal; residual activity	May be drying and irritating; safe in cats
2–4% chlorhexidine	Good antibacterial and antifungal; residual activity	May be drying and irritating; safe in cats
2% sulfur/2% salicylic acid	Antibacterial, antifungal, keratolytic, keratoplastic, and antipruritic	Well tolerated in long-term use; safe in cats
Piroctone olamine and monosaccharides	Microbial balancing and anti-adherent	Non-drying; safe in cats
1% selenium sulfide	Good antifungal, antiparasitic, and keratolytic agent	Can be drying and irritating; safe in cats
Enilconazole rinse	Good antifungal agent	May be toxic in cats

Epitheliotropic lymphoma
(cutaneous T cell lymphoma, mycosis fungoides)

DEFINITION
Epitheliotropic lymphoma is a rare, cutaneous neoplasm of dogs and cats characterized by epidermotropic T lymphocytic infiltration of the skin.

ETIOLOGY AND PATHOGENESIS
Certain T lymphocytes express membrane receptors, which ensure that they repeatedly migrate through the dermis and epidermis. Epitheliotropic lymphoma results when one, or several, clones of these cells become malignant, although the stimulus for this neoplastic transformation is not known[1,2]. In humans there is speculation that persistent environmental antigens and/or Langerhans cell abnormalities could act as a stimulus for chronic T-cell activation, with proliferation and eventual clonal expansion[3]. Recent studies suggest that atopic dermatitis is a risk factor in dogs[4]. The immunophenotype of canine epitheliotropic T cells is CD8[+], while in man CD4[+] predominates[5]. The neoplastic lymphocytes infiltrate the upper dermis and epidermis, resulting in thickening, hyperkeratosis, plaques, and ulceration.

CLINICAL FEATURES
Epitheliotropic lymphoma is a disease of the older dog and cat and there is no breed or sex predisposition. The most common presentation in both dogs and cats is of a pruritic erythroderma with plaques of silvery-white scale (**65**) that is non-responsive to systemic glucocorticoids[1,6,7]. The condition is pleomorphic and has been divided into four clinical presentations: 1) pruritis and erythema with scaling, loss of pigmentation, and alopecia; 2) mucocutaneous dermatitis with erythema, depigmentation, and ulceration; 3) solitary or multiple plaques or nodules (**66**) that may be covered with scale or crust; 4) oral with ulceration of the gingiva, palate, or tongue[8]. Mixed forms are also seen.

DIFFERENTIAL DIAGNOSES
- Atopic dermatitis
- Cutaneous adverse food reaction
- Sarcoptic mange
- *Malassezia pachydermatis* infection
- Mucocutaneous pyoderma

- Pemphigus vulgaris
- Bullous pemphigoid and other subepidermal blistering dermatoses
- Lupus erythematosus
- Non-neoplastic stomatitis
- Other causes of secondary defects in keratinization should also be considered

DIAGNOSIS
Diagnosis of epitheliotropic lymphoma is made on the basis of histopathologic examination of biopsy samples.

MANAGEMENT
Epitheliotropic lymphoma is often refractory to treatment and the prognosis is poor. Topical mechlorethamine hydrochloride (nitrogen mustard) (10 mg dissolved in 50 ml of water or propylene glycol) applied daily to erythematous scaling lesions may induce temporary resolution. However, this drug should be used with extreme caution as it is carcinogenic and a potent contact sensitizer. The person applying the preparation should wear gloves and there should be no contact between treated areas and human skin. Appropriate informed consent should be obtained if this treatment is to be tried. Safflower oil (3 ml/kg) given orally twice a week or the retinoid isotretinoin (3 mg/kg p/o q24h) may provide temporary remission in some animals[9-11]. In one trial, lomustine (CCNU), used as a sole treatment or in combination with retinoids or other lymphoma protocols, provided complete remission in 17% of the cases and partial response in 61% of the cases, with a mean duration of 88 days[12]. This drug is myelosuppressive (which is accumulative) and hepatotoxic and it can also initiate gastrointestinal signs. A single initial dose of the drug has the potential to result in life- threatening myelosuppression[12]. Because of the potential side-effects it is recommended that lomustine be used under the supervision of an oncologist. Recombinant human interferon alpha has also resulted in remission in a few cases, although it was only for 3–4 months.

KEY POINTS
- The pruritis associated with epitheliotropic lymphoma may be refractory to steroid therapy.
- The initial signs may be so mild that suspicion is not aroused.

65 Pruritic erythroderma with plaques of silvery-white scale in a case of epitheliotropic lymphoma.

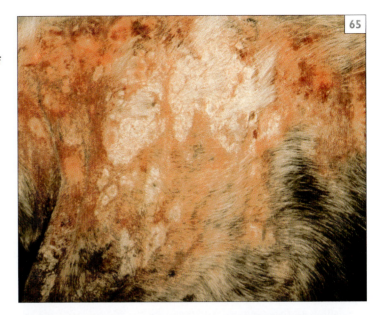

66 Erythematous, ulcerated plaques of mycosis fungoides.

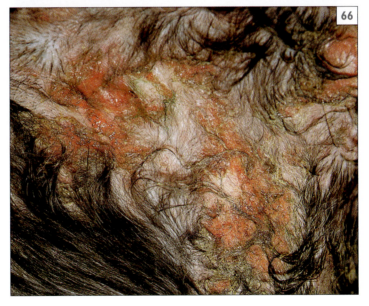

Acral lick dermatitis

DEFINITION

Acral lick dermatitis (ALD; acral lick granuloma, acral pruritic nodule) of the dog is a cutaneous manifestation of an obsessive–compulsive disorder[1,2].

ETIOLOGY AND PATHOGENESIS

Obsessive–compulsive disorders probably represent complex aberrations in neurophysiology, although the fundamental defects are not known[1-3]. In some non-neurological cases it might be that a predisposing cause or initial insult (e.g. hypersensitivity [atopy, food], foreign body, infection, arthritis, osteopathy, puncture wound, or insect bite) induces attention and licking, which then exposes sensory nerves in the lower epidermis, resulting in a continued stimulus to lick. A peripheral, sensory axonopathy has been reported[3] in affected dogs and this may be one explanation for the continued irritation, which initiates the lesions in some dogs. It is important to differentiate true psychogenic ALD, ALD secondary to an organic cause, and ALD-like lesions with other etiologies (see Differential diagnoses)[2,4]. It is, however, recognized that the divisions are far from clear-cut, and that stress and medical triggers can both contribute to the development of ALD in an individual dog. The stereotypical behavior is often further inadvertently reinforced by owner attention[2,5]. All three types of ALD are inevitably secondarily infected, usually with staphylococci, but there can also be gram-negative rods and anaerobes[5]. Chronic folliculitis and furunculosis are important in the pathogenesis, resulting in further inflammation, fibrosis, and self-trauma.

CLINICAL FEATURES

Most cases occur in large breeds. German Shepherd Dogs, Doberman Pinschers, Irish Setters, Labrador and Golden Retrievers, Dalmatians, and Great Danes appear to be predisposed[1,2,6,7]. The lesion typically occurs on the anterior aspect of the forelimb, in the carpal and metacarpal areas. Multiple lesions on more than one limb may be present in some individuals. Alopecia and saliva staining are followed by erosion of the skin, and a firm, thickened, well-circumscribed, often pigmented and, occasionally, ulcerated plaque results (**67**).

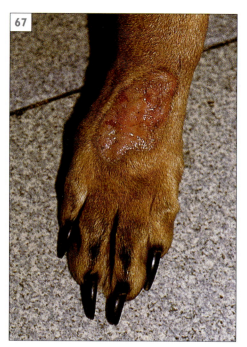

67 Acral lick granuloma. An erythematous, eroded, well-demarcated plaque on the distal aspect of the forelimb of a Doberman Pinscher.

Syringomyelia is a condition in Cavalier King Charles Spaniels associated with abnormal atlanto–axial morphology, altered CSF dynamics, and damage to the spinal cord. This can result in neurogenic pain and pruritus, often manifest as scratching and rubbing of the cranial shoulder and lateral neck.

DIFFERENTIAL DIAGNOSES

- Localized folliculitis and furunculosis or kerion
- Foreign body or pressure point granuloma
- Cutaneous neoplasia
- Demodicosis
- Tick or insect bite reaction
- Deep bacterial, mycobacterial, leishmanial, or fungal infections
- Syringomyelia

Medical triggers for ALD include:
- Hypersensitivities, ectoparasites and other pruritic conditions
- Fractures, implants, osteomyelitis, arthritis, intervertebral disk disease, and other orthopedic lesions
- Traumatic, inflammatory, or degenerative neurologic lesions

DIAGNOSIS

A psychodermatosis is diagnosed by exclusion. A thorough history and clinical examination will help identity underlying conditions and rule out differential diagnoses, although routine hematology and biochemistry, radiography, ultrasonography, CT, and/or MRI will be necessary in some cases. A full neurologic examination and behavioral assessment should be considered in appropriate cases[2]. All acral lick granulomas should be biopsied for histopathology to help eliminate differentials such as neoplasia and infectious granulomas. They exhibit characteristic histopathologic features that can aid diagnosis[5]. Biopsy material should also be sent for bacteriological culture and sensitivity to confirm infection and identify suitable antibiotics[1,5].

MANAGEMENT

Any predisposing causes should be addressed. Dogs exhibiting lesions on multiple limbs are considered to have a poorer prognosis[8], perhaps because they reflect a true psychodermatosis, while solitary lesions reflect alternative etiologies. Antibacterial therapy, preferably based on culture and sensitivity, is essential (see Deep pyoderma, p. 166). The antibiotic should penetrate well into scar tissue and be effective against *Staphylococcus* spp. as well other species identified on cytology or culture. Most cases exhibit a good response within 3–4 weeks, but complete resolution may take 3–4 months, especially if there is furunculosis with multiple free hair shafts and extensive scarring. Topical application of a mixture of a fluorinated glucocorticoid in dimethylsulfoxide used to be recommended[6], but its value is doubtful in many cases[1]. Capsaicin ointment (0.25%) applied once daily is beneficial is some cases. One author (TJN) has successfully used topical 0.1% tacrolimus, topical hydrocortisone aceponate spray, and ciclosporin (cyclosporine) (5 mg/kg) in combination with aggressive bactericidal antibiotic therapy in a few cases. Care should be taken not to exacerbate lesions when combining antibiotic and anti-inflammatory therapy.

Many cases will benefit from control of stress and obsessive–compulsive disorder. No one approach has been shown to be more effective, although it is thought that a combination of behavioral therapy and drug therapy is more beneficial than either alone[2,5]. Clomipramine (1 mg/kg p/o q12h increasing to 1.0–3.5 mg/kg q12h over 3–4 weeks) is licensed to treat behavioral disorders in dogs. Other non-licensed drugs used for behavioral modification include: amitriptyline (1–2 mg/kg p/o q12h increasing to 1–4 mg/kg q12h over 3–4 weeks); a combination of amitryptaline (2 mg/kg q12h) and hydrococodone (0.25 mg/kg p/o q24h); doxepin (1 mg/kg p/o q12h increasing to 1–5 mg/kg q12h over 3–4 weeks); fluoxetine (1 mg/kg p/o q12–24h); sertraline (1 mg/kg p/o q24h); diazepam (0.55–2.2 mg/kg p/o q12–24h); alprazolam (0.05–0.25 mg/kg p/o q12–24h); lorazepam 0.025–0.25 mg/kg p/o q12–24h); oxazepam (0.2–1.0 mg/kg p/o q12–24h); clonazepam (0.05–0.25 mg/kg p/o q12–24h); and naltrexone (2 mg/kg p/o q24h)[2,5,6,7,9]. One small, open study concluded that dextromethorphan (2 g/kg p/o q12h) significantly reduced ALD-associated behavior in dogs with allergic dermatitis[10]. All of these drugs should be used with care – serotonin uptake inhibitors can cause sedation and other central neurologic effects, tachycardia, mydriasis, restlessness, dry mouth, urinary retention, GI tract atony, gastritis, and nausea, and they are contraindicated in hepatic or renal disease. Benzodiazepines can cause sedation and loss of inhibition, memory, and learned behaviors, ataxia, depression, and paradoxical excitement. One randomized, blinded trial found that dog appeasing pheromone (DAP) was as effective as clomipramine in canine separation anxiety[11]. DAP is safe and easy to use, and may therefore be useful in ALD.

Lasers can be used to debride precisely acral lick granulomas. By sealing blood vessels, lymphatics, and nerve endings, laser therapy results in faster healing with less pain and swelling[5,12]. Without concurrent management of the underlying cause, however, most cases will develop new lesions at the original site or another location. Surgical excision is often very difficult, as the site and size of lesions create problems for wound closure and the presence of sutures encourages self-trauma. Devices to prevent the animal from licking a lesion (e.g. Elizabethan collars, neck restraints, or a plastic bucket with a portion of the bottom cut out and then fitted with the animal's head inside and attached to the collar) will often allow healing of lesions, but these should only be used as a short-term solution while further investigations and/or treatments are carried out, as the lesions generally return following removal of the device[2].

Syringomyelia is best diagnosed and managed by a neurologist, as it may involve neurologic tests, radiography, and MRI. Treatment options include surgery, COX-2 inhibitors, glucocorticoids, opioids, and gabapentin[8,13].

KEY POINT
- Resolution of lesions is difficult and may not be possible in some cases.

Schnauzer comedo syndrome

ETIOLOGY AND PATHOGENESIS
This is a follicular keratinization disorder of Miniature Schnauzers characterized by comedo formation along the dorsal midline[1]. The syndrome is probably associated with an inherited developmental defect of the hair follicles leading to abnormal keratinization, comedo formation, follicular plugging and dilation and, in some cases, a secondary bacterial folliculitis.

CLINICAL FEATURES
Lesions develop in young to adult Miniature Schnauzers. They extend laterally from the dorsal midline and are located from the neck to the sacrum. In many cases, lesions are more prominent on the lumbar sacral region (**68**). In early or mild cases the lesions may not be visualized, but small papules can be palpated over the dorsum; these may be crusted and firm or soft and waxy. With progression, there is thinning of the hair and the papular comedones become more obvious (**69**). A secondary bacterial folliculitis may develop and this will often be accompanied by pruritus and pain. Small crusts may develop in association with the infection.

DIFFERENTIAL DIAGNOSES
- Demodicosis
- Bacterial folliculitis
- Dermatophytosis
- Flea bite hypersensitivity
- Contact dermatitis to topical medications

DIAGNOSIS
The history and clinical signs are highly suggestive, and the diagnosis can be confirmed by biopsy and histopathology. Skin scrapes, tape-strip cytology, fungal cultures, and flea control trials can be helpful to rule out the differential diagnoses.

MANAGEMENT
The prognosis is variable, but generally good for most dogs, although on-going treatment will be necessary. Mild cases with few lesions may not require treatment. More severe cases can be managed with keratolytic shampoos used twice weekly to remission and then as necessary. Use milder, less drying products initially and progress to more potent products as required. Most of the

76 Mast cell neoplasia. Solitary, ulcerating nodule on the stifle of a dog.

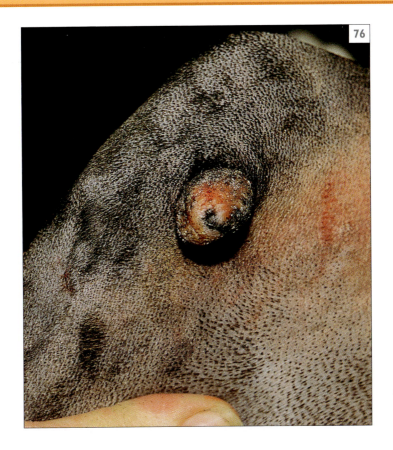

77 Pitting edema (Darier's sign) in a Weimeraner with a mast cell tumor.

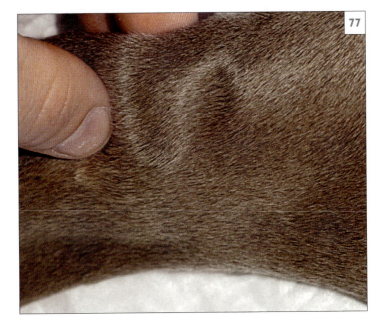

The most common presentation in cats is of a solitary dermal nodule, although multiple lesions may be encountered[3]. They are most commonly seen on the head and neck. Early lesions are usually haired, but later lesions may be erythematous, alopecic, or ulcerated. The majority of mast cell tumors in cats are benign[3,6]. Benign histiocytic mast cell tumors, with multiple, cutaneous papules and nodules, especially on the head, are seen in Siamese kittens and young cats[1]. These usually regress spontaneously.

Urticarial pigmentosa-like lesions, with fluctuating erythema, wheals, papules, and nodules characterized by accumulations of well-differentiated mast cells in the dermis, have been reported in a few dogs and cats. The lesions may resolve spontaneously with or without recurrence, wax and wane, or respond to glucocorticoids[1].

DIFFERENTIAL DIAGNOSES

- Histiocytoma
- Cutaneous or systemic histiocytosis
- Idiopathic sterile pyogranuloma
- Bacterial or fungal granuloma
- Allergic or insect bite reactions
- Foreign body granuloma
- Other cutaneous neoplasms

DIAGNOSTIC TESTS

Mast cells are relatively straightforward to identify by examination of stained needle aspirate samples (**78**). Mast cells typically exfoliate well as individual round cells with moderate to large accumulations of intensely basophilic cytoplasmic granules, although poorly differentiated cells have fewer granules and may be harder to identify. Eosinophils are commonly seen in mast cell tumor aspirates. Cytology is sufficient to confirm mast cell neoplasia, which should prompt the surgeon to take wide (2–3 cm [0.8–1.2 in]) margins, but does not give sufficient information to allow grading of the tumor or the degree of invasiveness, or assess the surgical margins. All excised mast cell tumors should therefore be submitted for histopathology.

Further tests including local lymph node aspiration and/or biopsy, hematology and biochemistry, thoracic radiography, and abdominal ultrasonography with hepatic and splenic aspiration if necessary, and bone marrow aspirates may be required to determine the extent of disease and stage the tumor.

Canine mast cell tumors are graded from I (most benign) to III (most aggressive), although biological behavior, optimum treatment modality, and survival times do not always correlate well with the histopathologic grade. Histopathologic grading in cats does not correlate with prognosis[3,4,7].

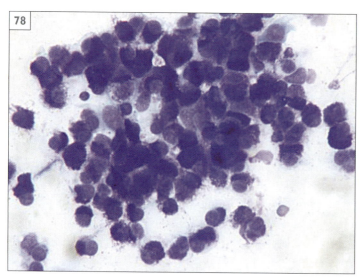

78 Mast cell tumor cytology: numerous round cells with deeply staining blue-purple metachromatic granules that obscure the nucleus. Free granules can be seen in the background.

MANAGEMENT

All canine mast cell tumors should be considered potentially malignant and, for discrete lesions, wide surgical excision is the best treatment. A wide margin of 2–3 cm (0.8–1.2 in) and/or one fascial plane on all surfaces is advised, even for apparently well-demarcated lesions[4,5]. In some areas of the body (the distal limb, for example), this may necessitate sliding or other types of surgical graft. Local hemorrhage and wound breakdown can often complicate surgery. There is little evidence that excision of solitary nodules should be followed up with chemotherapy or radiotherapy, provided that the tumor has been correctly staged and fully excised[8]. If histopathology shows that the tumor has been inadequately resected, further surgery is indicated. Cimetidine (5 mg/kg p/o q6–8h) or ranitidine (2 mg/kg p/o q8–12h) is useful if there is histamine release.

Guidelines for treatment in dogs[1,4,9–11]
Stage 1
One tumor confined to the dermis, with no regional lymph node involvement:
- Wide surgical excision.

Stage 2
One tumor confined to the dermis with regional lymph node involvement:
- Surgical excision of the tumor and affected lymph node, plus radiotherapy or chemotherapy.

Stage 3
Multiple tumors, or large infiltrating tumors, with or without regional lymph node involvement:
- Surgical excision may be palliative, but chemotherapy or radiotherapy will be necessary.

Stage 4
Any tumor with distant metastases:
- Wide excision of primary tumor and affected lymph nodes.
- Chemotherapy.

Radiotherapy
Radiotherapy is an effective option for cutaneous tumors that cannot be adequately excised due to their site and/or infiltration of local tissues[10,12]. Surgery to reduce tumor volume should be considered. Radiotherapy of draining lymph nodes is also an effective adjunct to surgical excision of grade I and II tumors[13]. Tumors on the extremities may respond better than tumors on the trunk[4]. The prognosis for grade III tumors is significantly worse than for grades I or II[1].

Chemotherapy
Prednisolone (40 mg/m^2 p/o q24h for 7 days, then 20 mg/m^2 p/o alternate days) is the mainstay of treatment, although it only achieves short-term remission when used alone[4]. Combination chemotherapy is therefore preferred to improve survival times in prednisolone-responsive tumors. Combination chemotherapy is less effective in prednisolone-resistant tumors, grade III tumors with distant metastases, and with aggressive feline mast cell tumors[3,4,9]. Chemotherapeutic agents used with prednisolone include vinblastine or vincristine and cyclophosphamide:
- Vincristine (0.5 mg/m^2 i/v once weekly): may induce partial remission in some dogs used as a single agent.
- Vinblastine (2 mg/m^2 i/v once every 3 weeks [day 1 of 21-day cycle])[4].
- Cyclophosphamide (250 mg/m^2 p/o divided over 4 days every 3 weeks [days 8, 9, 10, and 11 of 21-day cycle])[4].

Other agents include hydroxyurea and doxirubicin[9]. Intralesional triamcinolone (1 mg/cm tumor diameter) has been suggested as an adjunct treatment at stages 3 and 4. There was interest in the use of intralesional and post-surgical infiltration of the surgical site with deionized water, but this has now been shown to be of no benefit[14].

KEY POINTS
- Potentially a highly malignant neoplasm.
- Very variable clinical appearance and behavior.
- Cytology very useful to identify tumor, but histopathology required for grading.
- Wide excision on all aspects gives the best chance of cure.
- Chemotherapy and radiotherapy recommended for adjunct treatment.
- Use cytology to monitor for recurrence.

Melanocytic neoplasia

DEFINITION
Melanocytic neoplasms are variably malignant tumors that arise from melanocytes within the skin. Melanocytoma refers to all variants of congenital and acquired benign neoplasms arising from melanocytes, while melanoma refers to malignant neoplasms[1]. Lentigo refers to intraepidermal melanocytic hyperplasia of well-differentiated melanocytes[1]. (See Lentigo and lentiginosis profusa, p. 216)

ETIOLOGY AND PATHOGENESIS
In humans, melanocytic neoplasms may be induced by actinic radiation[2]. It has not been determined whether this is so in dogs and cats. The canine tumors are usually benign when they arise on the head and trunk, but malignant when they are intraoral or on the distal limb[3,4]. The reason for this regional pattern of behavior is not known. Feline melanocytic neoplasms are usually malignant, particularly those arising on the eyelid[5].

CLINICAL FEATURES
Melanocytoma
These tumors account for 3–4% of skin tumors in dogs and 0.6–1.3% of skin tumors in cats[6–9]. Incidence is higher in breeds of dogs with heavily pigmented skin. Compound melanocytomas appear as nodules that are <1 cm in diameter and papular, dome-shaped, or plaque-like to pedunculated with a smooth or slightly papillated surface[1]. Dermal melanocytomas appear as 0.5–4.0 cm (0.2–1.6 in) solitary, circumscribed, alopecic, fleshy, dome-shaped masses[1]. The color of melanocytomas can vary from brown to blue-black.

MELANOMA
This tumor accounts for 0.8–20% of all skin tumors and is generally seen in older animals[8,9]. The incidence is higher in breeds of dogs with heavily pigmented skin. In older dogs they are most frequently reported on the lips and eyelids as well as the limbs (**79**) and nail beds[8]. In cats the head, trunk, and tail are the preferred sites[5]. The size can vary, but most melanomas are 1–3 cm (0.4–1.2 in) in size. Most are sessile in shape, but they may be polypoid or plaque-like[1]. They can appear gray, brown, or black in color.

DIFFERENTIAL DIAGNOSES
- Squamous cell carcinoma
- Bacterial and fungal granuloma
- Histiocytosis and sterile pyogranuloma syndrome
- Foreign body granuloma
- Other cutaneous neoplasia

DIAGNOSIS
Aspiration cytology may help to suggest a diagnosis of melanoma, although care must be taken to differentiate them from mast cell tumors[10]. Melanocytes are large round cells that exfoliate well and have abundant brown to black granules. Fewer granules are found in those tumors that are more malignant and less differentiated. However, given the tendency for pedal and digital lesions to behave in a malignant manner, the decision to perform radical excision in cases where significant surgery is indicated should be based on histopathologic criteria and not cytologic criteria. Clinical staging with local lymph node excision, thoracic radiography, and blood panels should follow suspicion of melanoma, given its tendency to metastasize[10].

MANAGEMENT
Truncal melanocytomas are typically benign and excision with a 1 cm (0.4 in) margin is curative in most cases[10]. As tumors arising on the digits are often melanomas, amputation of the digit is preferred to achieve adequate excision with no long-term complications[3,6,7]. The management of melanomas should also involve local excision and, perhaps, local amputation, although owners should be cautioned that most dogs will die of the effects of distant metastasis, typically to the lungs by way of the local lymph nodes[4].

KEY POINTS
- Be prepared to be aggressive in the management of digital masses.
- Treat non-responding digital erythema or ulceration with suspicion.

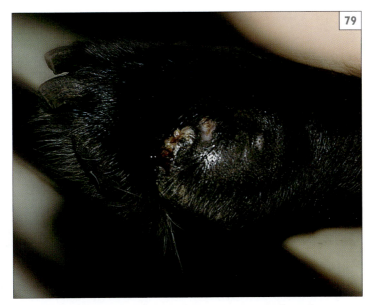

79 Melanoma. Malignant lesion, heavily pigmented, on the foot of a Labrador Retriever.

Basal cell carcinoma
(basal cell epithelioma)

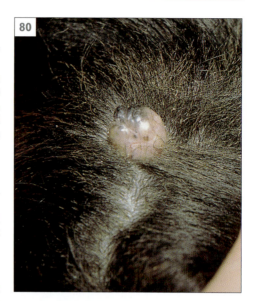

DEFINITION
Basal cell carcinomas are uncommon, benign neoplasms that arise from the basal keratinocytes of the epidermis. Previously these had been included in the broad category of basal cell tumors, which included similar appearing tumors of adnexal structures[1].

ETIOLOGY AND PATHOGENESIS
It is possible that basal cell tumors result from neoplastic change within epidermal stem cells[2]. The stimulus that results in a normally cycling cell changing to a cell with neoplastic potential is not known.

CLINICAL FEATURES
There is no sex predisposition. Most basal cell tumors occur in older dogs and cats, typically on the trunk of dogs and nose, face, and ears of cats[1–4]. The incidence has been reported to be 1.25% of skin tumors in cats and <0.3% in dogs[5,6]. The neoplasms appear as well-circumscribed indurated plaques or umbilicated nodules. Overlying skin may evidence alopecia, crusting, ulceration, and a dark color due to melanin pigmentation (**80**). Tumors tend to be smaller and occasionally multicentric in the cat (**81**). Metastasis has not been reported in the dog and, although metastasis has been reported in the cat, there are too few cases to know the exact incidence[1].

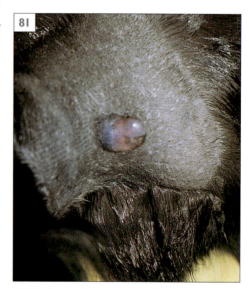

DIFFERENTIAL DIAGNOSES
- Bacterial or fungal granuloma
- Foreign body granuloma
- Follicular cyst
- Other cutaneous neoplasms

DIAGNOSIS
Although the cytologic appearance of basal cell tumors may be characteristic[7], the definitive diagnosis is best made by histopathologic examination of biopsy or excision samples.

80, 81 Basal cell tumor. A small, well-circumscribed, alopecic nodule basal cell tumor on the trunk of a dog (**80**); a cystic, well-circumscribed basal cell tumor on the lateral neck of a domestic shorthair cat (**81**).

MANAGEMENT
Surgical excision is the most effective form of treatment[1].

KEY POINT
- Rare nodular tumor of the skin that is generally benign.

Collagenous nevi

ETIOLOGY AND PATHOGENESIS

A collagenous nevus is a circumscribed developmental defect of the skin, characterized by collagenous hyperplasia. The etiology and pathogenesis are unknown[1].

CLINICAL FEATURES

Collagenous nevi generally appear as firm, well-circumscribed, slowly enlarging nodules of the skin and subcutis, that vary in diameter from 0.5–5 cm (0.2–2 in)[1–3]. Lesions are usually multiple (**82**) and are located more frequently on the head, neck, and proximal extremities. Middle-aged animals are more likely to be affected, but lesions have also been reported in younger animals[2,3]. Slowly enlarging lesions localized to one area of the body have been reported[1].

DIFFERENTIAL DIAGNOSES

- Other cutaneous neoplasms
- Bacterial and fungal granuloma
- Sterile nodular granuloma and pyogranuloma
- Histiocytic lesions

DIAGNOSIS

Cytology is usually non-specific, but may help to eliminate neoplasia. Histopathologic examination of biopsies or excised lesions is diagnostic.

MANAGEMENT

Surgical excision of the nodules is the treatment of choice in most cases. Recurrence occurs rapidly, at an accelerated rate, in those animals with large lesions localized to one area of the body[1–3].

KEY POINT

- Behavior can be unpredictable, but these are essentially benign lesions.

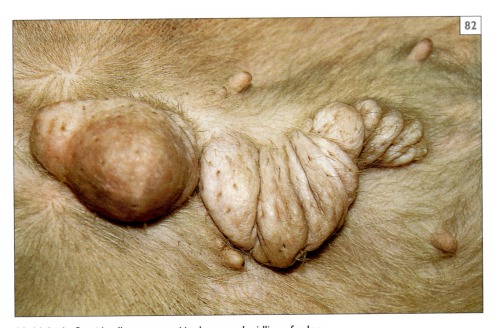

82 Multiple, flaccid collagenous nevi in the ventral midline of a dog.

Canine eosinophilic granuloma

DEFINITION

Canine eosinophilic granuloma is a rare syndrome in which nodules or plaques with a characteristic histopathologic pattern develop in the skin, oral mucosa, or external ear canal.

ETIOLOGY AND PATHOGENESIS

Canine eosinophilic granuloma appears to be a hypersensitivity reaction. The precipitating cause is unknown in many instances, but some cases are suspected of being a hypersensitivity reaction to arthropod bites or insect stings[1-4].

CLINICAL FEATURES

Siberian Huskies and Cavalier King Charles Spaniels are predisposed, but the condition has been reported in other breeds[1-8]. Lesions occur more frequently in the oral cavity, especially on the lateral or ventral surface of the tongue. Oral lesions are friable, bleed easily, and often become ulcerated[3,4,8]. Skin lesions consist of solitary or grouped erythematous papules, nodules, or plaques occurring on the pinna, muzzle, planum nasale, neck, axilla, flank, prepuce, scrotum, or ventral abdomen[1,2,4,6,7].

DIFFERENTIAL DIAGNOSES

- Foreign body granulomas
- Neoplasia
- Bacterial and fungal granulomas
- Sterile nodular granuloma and pyogranuloma
- Histiocytic lesions

DIAGNOSIS

Diagnosis is based on biopsy, cytology, and dermatohistopathology.

MANAGEMENT

Small solitary lesions may regress spontaneously[3,5,7]. Methylprednisolone (0.5–1.0 mg/kg p/o q24h) or prednisone (1–2 mg/kg p/o q12h) may be administered. Lesions generally resolve in 2–4 weeks, after which the dose can be changed to alternate day and then be tapered.

KEY POINT

- Canine eosinophilic granuloma is diagnosed by biopsy and responds well to corticosteroid therapy.

Sterile granuloma and pyogranuloma syndrome

DEFINITION

Sterile granuloma and pyogranuloma syndrome is a disease characterized by skin papules, nodules, or plaques with characteristic histopathologic features.

ETIOLOGY AND PATHOGENESIS

The pathogenesis of sterile granuloma and pyogranuloma syndrome is unknown. However, as no causative agents can be demonstrated and the lesions respond to glucocorticoids and other immunomodulating drugs, an immune-mediated process is suspected[1-3]. In Spain and Italy, where leishmaniasis is endemic, *Leishmania* spp. DNA has been documented by polymerase chain reaction (PCR) and DNA sequencing in 20 of 35 biopsies from dogs that were initially diagnosed as having sterile granuloma and pyogranuloma syndrome[4]. It is therefore important to eliminate *Leishmania* and other infectious agents before concluding that these lesions are sterile.

CLINICAL FEATURES

Lesions consist of firm, non-pruritic (except in cats), non-painful, haired to alopecic papules, nodules, and plaques that occur commonly on the head, particularly the bridge of the nose and the muzzle (**83**). Less frequently, lesions can appear on the pinna, neck, trunk, and extremities (**84**)[1-3]. The syndrome can occur in any breed, but there is a predisposition for the Great Dane, Boxer, Golden Retriever, Collie, and Weimaraner[1-3]. There is no breed predisposition in the cat[5].

DIFFERENTIAL DIAGNOSES

- Neoplasia
- Reactive histiocytosis
- Xanthoma
- Foreign bodies
- Infection: *Leismania* spp., *Nocardia* spp., *Actinomyces* spp., *Blastomyces* spp., *Coccidioides immitis*, *Histoplasma* spp., *Cryptococcus* spp., *Sporothrix* spp., *Basidiobolus* and *Conidiobolus* spp., *Pythium* and *Lagenidium* spp., fast and slow-growing mycobacterial organisms

DIAGNOSIS

Diagnosis is based on dermatohistopathology, with special stains to rule out infectious agents and microbial cultures (tissue) to rule out anaerobic and aerobic bacteria, mycobacteria, and fungi. Serology and PCR may also be appropriate to help rule out infections with some organisms.

MANAGEMENT

The combination of tetracycline and niacinamide (250 mg of each drug p/o q8h in dogs under 10 kg and 500 mg of each p/o q8h in dogs over 10 kg) will cause resolution of lesions in many cases. Doxycycline (10 mg/kg p/o q24h) can be used in lieu of tetracycline. Once the lesions have resolved (6–8 weeks) the interval of dosing can be reduced to twice daily or once daily for maintenance[6,7]. If there is a poor response to tetracycline and niacinamide, or if the lesions are large and extensive, methylprednisolone (0.5–1 mg/kg p/o q12h) or prednisone/prednisolone (1–2 mg/kg p/o q12h) may be administered. Lesions generally resolve in 2–6 weeks. The dose can then be changed to alternate day and, over 8–10 weeks, be tapered to maintenance. Azathioprine (2 mg/kg p/o q24h or q48h) may be used along with glucocorticoids in refractory cases[3]. Azathioprine therapy may also allow for a lower dose of glucocorticoids and, when lesions have resolved, should be dosed on alternate days to minimize side-effects. Azathioprine may result in bone marrow suppression and this should be monitored by performing complete blood counts biweekly for the first eight weeks of therapy and then quarterly. One author (TJN) has had very good results using ciclosporin (cyclosporine) (5 mg/kg p/o q24h to remission, and then tapering the frequency for maintenance).

KEY POINT

• There is generally a good response to therapy, but control rather than cure is the norm.

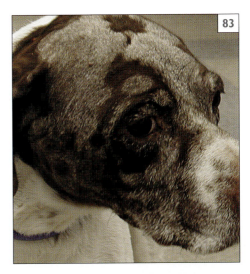

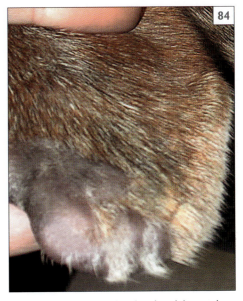

83, 84 Plaques on the head and nodules on the ear of animals with sterile granuloma and pyogranuloma syndrome.

Histiocytic proliferative disorders

ETIOLOGY AND PATHOGENESIS

Most histiocytic diseases in dogs seem to be derived from dendritic cells[1]. Several manifestations have been distinguished on clinical features, morphology, and cell phenotype. They are classed as reactive (cutaneous histiocytosis and systemic histiocytosis) or neoplastic (cutaneous histiocytoma and histiocytic sarcomas). The etiology is unknown, but the phenotype and response to immunosuppressive treatment of the reactive conditions suggest dysregulation of the immune system, possibly a failure of resolution following an inflammatory reaction to pathogens or other triggers. The breed incidence of some conditions suggests there are as yet unknown genetic factors.

CLINICAL FEATURES

Cutaneous histiocytosis

Cutaneous histiocytosis is typically associated with one or more nodules or plaques, especially around the head, neck, perineum and perigenital skin, and extremities (**85, 86**). They can be haired or alopecic and erythematous, but are usually non-painful and non-pruritic. More advanced lesions may undergo central necrosis and scarring. There is no apparent age (range 3–9 years), breed, or sex predisposition[1]. Spontaneous remission may occur, but most cases tend to become slowly progressive.

Systemic histiocytosis

Systemic histiocytosis is most commonly seen in Bernese Mountain Dogs, but also in other breeds including the Golden Retriever, Labrador Retriever, Boxer, and Rottweiler. It usually affects adults (4–7 years), but there is no sex predisposition. Skin lesions are similar to those of cutaneous histiocytosis (see above), but there is also involvement of the conjunctiva, sclera, retrobulbar tissues, nasal cavity, lymph nodes, and internal organs including the liver, spleen, lungs, and bone marrow (**87**).

Cutaneous histiocytoma

Histiocytomas are common tumors, usually seen in dogs less than three years old[2]. They are typically small, non-pruritic, non-painful nodules mostly on the head, ears, neck, and limbs (**88**). They frequently ulcerate, but in the majority of dogs this precedes rapid resolution[2,3].

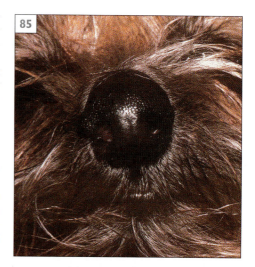

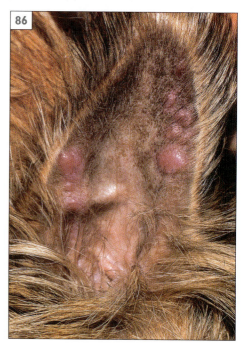

85, 86 Swollen nose (**85**) and erythematous nodules on the pinna (**86**) of a Yorkshire Terrier with cutaneous histiocytosis.

87 Systemic histiocytosis. Poorly defined crusted papules and nodules adjacent to the planum nasale and infiltrating the conjunctiva in a Bernese Mountain Dog.

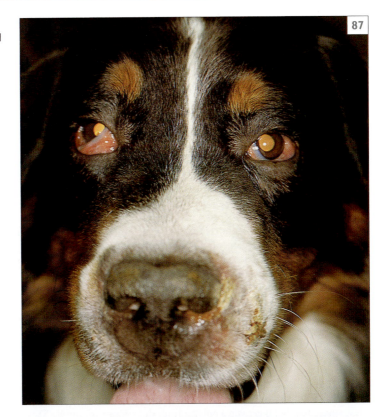

88 Histiocytoma in a young Boxer. The erosion and crusting are typical of nodules that are starting to regress.

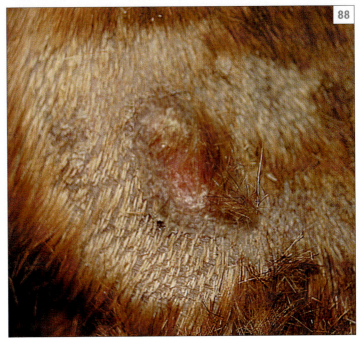

However, ulcerated nodules can become infected or become a focus for self-trauma. Multiple and/or persistent tumors have been recognized, most commonly in Shar Peis. Most cases eventually resolve, although there may be transient lymph node enlargement and infiltration.

Localized histiocytic sarcoma

Localized histiocytic sarcomas are focal, rapid growing, and aggressive tumors. They are usually seen in Bernese Mountain Dogs, Flat Coat Retrievers, Golden Retrievers, Labradors, and Rottweilers, but other breeds can be affected. There is no age or sex predisposition[4]. The lesions tend to affect the skin, subcutis, and deeper tissues on the extremities. Tumors near joints can involve the joint capsule, ligaments, tendons, and muscles. Tumors have also been seen in the liver, spleen, CNS, and lymph nodes. The tumors may undergo focal necrosis and ulceration[4].

Disseminated histiocytic sarcoma (malignant histiocytosis)

This is most widely recognized in Bernese Mountain Dogs[5], but has been seen in other breeds including the Golden Retriever, Labrador Retriever, and Rottweiler. Dogs of any age can be affected and there is no sex predisposition. A large study suggested that there was a polygenic mode of inheritance, with a heritability of 0.298[6]. Disseminated histiocytic sarcoma is an aggressive multisystemic disease that may be a primary multicentric neoplasm or represent rapid and widespread metastasis. In contrast to other histiocytic diseases the skin is rarely affected, but internal organs that are involved can include any combination of the lungs, liver, spleen, kidneys, bone marrow, CNS, muscles, GI system, lymph nodes, and heart. Most dogs present with an acute history of malaise, anorexia, anemia, and weight loss, and other clinical signs depending on the organs affected[4,5,7].

DIFFERENTIAL DIAGNOSES

- Bacterial, mycobacterial or fungal granuloma
- Other cutaneous neoplasia
- Foreign body granuloma
- Idiopathic sterile granuloma and pyogranuloma syndrome

DIAGNOSTIC TESTS

The clinical signs and history of histiocytic disorders are highly suggestive. Cytology and histopathology usually reveal typical histiocytes, with large eccentric, round to oval, indented, vesicular nuclei in cutaneous and systemic histiocytosis. Histiocytomas usually consist of large activated Langerhans cells with large eccentric, round to oval, indented, vesicular nuclei and frequent mitoses and occasional apoptotic cells (**89**)[3]. Histiocytic sarcomas are characterized by variably mixed populations of spindle cells and pleomorphic round cells with a histiocyte-like appearance, multiple, frequently bizarre mitoses, and multinucleate giant cells with marked cytologic atypia[4]. Further investigation may be necessary to demonstrate systemic involvement. Special staining and culture for microorganisms are negative[5].

MANAGEMENT

These can be difficult conditions to manage. In cutaneous histiocytosis, focal lesions can be surgically excised, but others tend to arise elsewhere. There is a variable response to immunosuppressive doses of glucocorticoids with or without azathioprine. Ciclosporin (cyclosporine) and leflunomide have been used with some success more recently[1]. Treatment for systemic histiocytosis is similar, but the prognosis is more guarded as most dogs seem to succumb eventually to systemic involvement.

Most histiocytomas resolve spontaneously. Immunosuppressive drugs could interfere with regression and should be avoided. Surgical excision is usually curative for ulcerated and/or persistent nodules. Persistent malignant histiocytomas with widespread metastases occur in a few dogs and the prognosis for these is very poor.

The prognosis for histiocytic sarcoma is very poor, especially if metastasis to local lymph nodes or internal organs has occurred. Radical surgical excision and/or radiotherapy can be curative for localized tumors[4,5]. Surgical excision and radiotherapy are not appropriate for disseminated histiocytic sarcoma, and there is a poor response to chemotherapy[4].

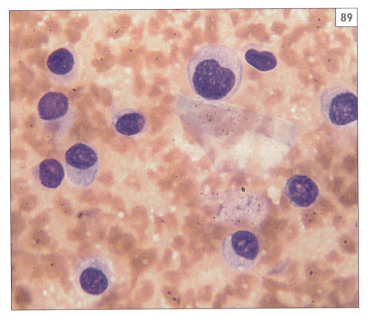

89 Aspirate cytology of a histiocytoma revealing numerous histiocytic cells. (Diff-Quik, ×1000)

HISTIOCYTIC PROLIFERATIVE DISEASES IN CATS

Histiocytic proliferative diseases in cats are much less common and less well characterized than in dogs. Nodular and plaque-like lesions, predominantly of the head and face, with infiltrates of typical histiocytic cells, have been reported. The lesions tend to be persistent, but may respond to immunosuppressive glucocorticoids, vincristine, and interferon. A syndrome similar to disseminated histiocytic sarcoma and multiple histiocytomas has been seen in a few older cats[8].

KEY POINTS

- These are a group of poorly defined conditions.
- Biopsy and histopathologic examination are critical for diagnosis.
- The prognosis is good for cutaneous histiocytosis and histiocytoma.
- The prognosis for systemic histiocytosis and histiocytic sarcoma is poor.

Panniculitis

DEFINITION

Panniculitis is inflammation of the subcutaneous fat.

ETIOLOGY AND PATHOGENESIS

Lipocytes (fat cells) can be damaged by many factors, but the end result of these various etiologies is the release of free lipid into the extracellular space. These lipids undergo hydrolysis into fatty acids, which can incite further inflammation and granulomatous reactions[1,2]. Panniculitis may result from several different etiologies:

- Post-injection panniculitis occurs infrequently in the cat and rarely in the dog. It may be underdiagnosed because clinical signs may not be obvious or may seem inconsequential. This condition has been associated with various vaccines[3] and injection of other medications, including antibiotics. It is postulated that the reaction results from a combination of foreign body and hypersensitivity reactions[3].
- Traumatic panniculitis occurs when blunt trauma, chronic pressure, or decreased blood supply induces focal ischemia[1].
- Infectious panniculitis occurs when bacteria or deep mycotic agents become established in the panniculus.
- Immune-mediated panniculitis can occur with immune-mediated vascular diseases such as systemic lupus erythematosus. It also can occur due to a hypersensitivity to drugs, to infectious agents, or with visceral malignancy[1,2,4]. Erythema nodosum-like panniculitis is a septal panniculitis associated with vascular damage due to systemic hypersensitivity reactions.
- Nutritional panniculitis occurs as feline pansteatitis, which results from a severe, absolute or relative deficiency of vitamin E, often a result of a diet rich in oily fish[5].
- Idiopathic panniculitis encompasses all of the sterile inflammatory diseases of the panniculus that have unknown etiologies. Examples would be idiopathic sterile nodular panniculitis and sterile pedal panniculitis of the German Shepherd Dog[6,7].

CLINICAL FEATURES

Lesions usually occur as solitary nodules[1]. The lesions are variably firm and painful and, in one survey, 35% of nodules were accompanied by fistulous draining tracts[1]. They are most commonly located over the ventrolateral neck, chest, and abdomen[1,2]. There is no age or sex predisposition, but Dachshunds are more frequently affected than other breeds of dogs. Animals with sterile nodular panniculitis are more likely to have multiple lesions (**90, 91**). The larger lesions of these animals, as well as lesions in animals with erythema nodosum-like panniculitis, tend to ulcerate and drain an oily, clear to yellowish-brown liquid[1,2,4].

Sterile pedal panniculitis of the German Shepherd Dog appears as well-demarcated fistulous tracts that have slightly swollen erythematous borders[7,8]. They are most frequently located dorsal to the midline of the tarsal or carpal pad, but lesions have also been associated with other pads. The fistulous tracts drain a small amount of serous to milky, viscid fluid.

Feline pansteatitis is manifested by multiple nodules of varying firmness occurring in the subcutis and abdominal mesenteric fat[5]. Fistulation is rare. Systemic signs such as fever, malaise, and pain may precede or occur in conjunction with the development of nodules.

DIFFERENTIAL DIAGNOSES

- Abscess
- Cutaneous bacterial or fungal granuloma
- Deep bacterial folliculitis and furunculosis
- Cutaneous mycobacterial infection
- Deep mycotic infections
- Cutaneous cysts
- *Cuterebra* spp. infestation
- Cutaneous neoplasia
- Foreign body reactions

DIAGNOSIS

Excision or wedge biopsy, with samples submitted for both histopathologic examination and culture and sensitivity, is the minimal data base for diagnosis.

MANAGEMENT

Panniculitis secondary to systemic disease should resolve when appropriate treatment is instituted. Solitary lesions may be removed surgically. If the panniculitis is due to bacterial or fungal infection, appropriate treatment for the specific agent

90 Panniculitis. Several erythematous nodules on the lateral trunk of a dog.

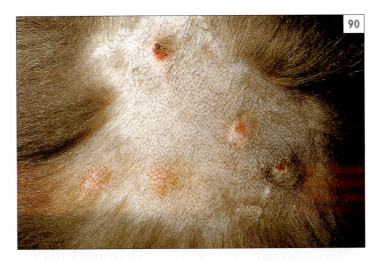

91 Hyperpigmented plaques and sinus formation associated with panniculitis.

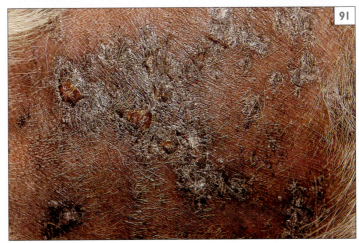

should be instituted based on *in vitro* culture and sensitivity testing. Cats with pansteatitis should be fed a nutritionally balanced diet and, at least until in remission, should be given vitamin E (10 IU/kg) daily. Animals with idiopathic panniculitis respond well to systemic gluco-corticoids[1,2]. Methylprednisolone (0.3–1.0 mg/kg p/o) or prednisolone (2.0 mg/kg p/o) may be given daily until lesions resolve (usually 3–6 weeks), then tapering the dose. There is often long-term or permanent remission. The combination of tetracycline and niacinamide (250 mg of each drug p/o q8h in dogs under 10 kg and 500 mg of each p/o q8h in dogs over 10 kg) may result in resolution of lesions in some animals, or it can be used as maintenance therapy once

the lesions have responded to glucocorticoids. If lesions return, prolonged alternate day steroid therapy may be necessary for control. Daily supplementation with vitamin E (300 IU) may have a steroid-sparing action in some cases[8]. A small number of cases may need a combination of glucocorticoids and cytotoxic agents such as azathioprine for control. (See Pemphigus foliaceus, p. 155, for specific dosing.) Ciclosporin (cyclosporine) (5 mg/kg p/o q24h to remission and then taper frequency) can also be effective.

KEY POINT

- Huge differential. All lesions characterized by sinus and not known to be abscessation should be biopsied.

Cryptococcosis

DEFINITION

Cryptococcosis is a deep mycotic disease resulting from infection with *Cryptococcus neoformans.*

ETIOLOGY AND PATHOGENESIS

Cryptococcus neoformans is a saprophytic, small (1–7 µm), budding yeast with a global distribution. It is characterized by a mucoid, polysaccharide capsule that can vary in size from 1–30 µm. The capsule helps to prevent desiccation and also prevents detection by the immune system of the mammalian host[1]. Although the organism has been isolated from several sources (including soil), it is most frequently associated with pigeon droppings and *Eucalyptus* spp. leaves. Based on circumstantial evidence, the most likely route of infection is through inhalation of airborne organisms[1,2]. They may be deposited in the upper respiratory tract, resulting in nasal granulomas, or proceed to the alveoli and induce pulmonary granulomas. Extension of infection from the respiratory tract occurs by local invasion through the cribriform plates to the CNS or by hematogenous and lymphatic spread[1,3]. Cutaneous infection via traumatic inoculation has also been proposed[4]. Concurrent diseases that are immunosuppressive (e.g. FeLV or FIV infection in cats and ehrlichiosis in dogs) have been associated with cryptococcal infections. However, underlying diseases are uncommon in companion animals with cryptococcosis. *Cryptococcus* will infect humans, but not normally via an animal host, and is therefore not considered a zoonosis.

CLINICAL FEATURES

Cats

Cryptococcosis is the most frequently diagnosed deep mycotic infection in cats. There is no sex predisposition and affected animals range in age from 1–13 years (median five years)[2,3]. Signs of upper respiratory disease occur in 55% of the cases and include a mucopurulent, serous, or hemorrhagic, unilateral or bilateral chronic nasal discharge. Flesh-colored, polyp-like masses in the nostrils or a firm, hard subcutaneous swelling over the bridge of the nose (**92**) will be found in 70% of the cases with a nasal discharge. Skin lesions are present in 40% of the cases and are usually papules or nodules (**93**) that may be either fluctuant or firm and range from 1–10 mm (0.04–0.4 in) in diameter. Larger lesions often ulcerate, leaving a raw surface with a serous exudate[2,4]. Neurologic signs occur in 25% of the cases and may include depression, amaurotic blindness, ataxia, circling, paresis, paralysis, and seizures[1,3]. Ocular involvement may also be present. Regional lymphadenopathy, low-grade fever, malaise, anorexia, or weight loss may occasionally occur[1].

Dogs

Cryptococcosis is less frequently diagnosed in the dog than in the cat. Clinical signs related to ocular and CNS lesions are the most common abnormalities[3]. Skin lesions consisting of papules, nodules, ulcers, abscesses, and draining tracts occur in 25% of the cases and often involve the nose, tongue, gums, lips, hard palate, or nail beds[3].

DIFFERENTIAL DIAGNOSES

- Deep pyoderma and bacterial abcessation
- Other deep mycotic infections
- Cutaneous neoplasia
- Histiocytic lesions and sterile nodular granuloma and pyogranuloma (in dogs)

DIAGNOSIS

Cytologic examination of nasal or skin exudate or CSF and tissue aspirates generally reveals pleomorphic (round to elliptical, 2–20 µm diameter) organisms that are characterized by a capsule of variable thickness, which forms a clear or refractile halo (**94**). The latex cryptococcal antigen test (LCAT) is a serologic method for detecting capsular polysaccharide antigen in serum, urine, and CSF. Titers parallel the severity of infection and may be used to monitor response to therapy[1]. Histopathologic examination of excision or biopsy samples is diagnostic.

MANAGEMENT

Fluconazole (50 mg/cat p/o q12h for 2–4 months) is the recommended therapy[5]. Therapy should be continued for 1–2 months beyond clinical resolution of lesions or until the LCAT titers are negative. Itraconazole (10 mg/kg p/o q12h) and ketoconazole (10 mg/kg p/o q24h) have also been reported to be effective[4–6].

KEY POINT

- *Always* obtain a histopathologic report on nodules biopsied or excised from cats. Many cutaneous nodules in the cat are malignant but some will be cryptococcosis and will be treatable.

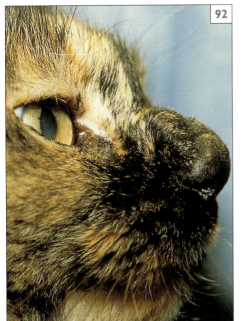
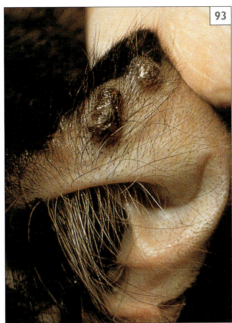
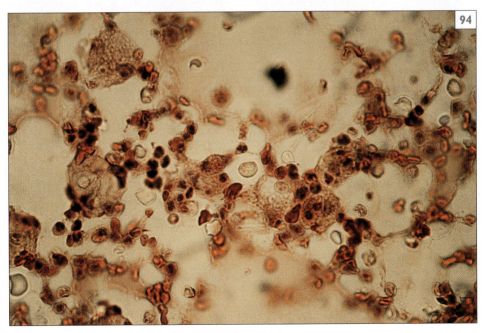

92–94 Cryptococcosis. A nodular lesion on the face of a domestic shorthair cat with cryptococcosis (**92**); papules and nodules on the pinna of a domestic shorthair cat with cryptococcosis (**93**); a photomicrograph of *Cryptococcus* spp. demonstrating the refractile, clearly defined capsule around the yeast (**94**).

Phaeohyphomycosis

DEFINITION

Phaeohyphomycoses are infections caused by dematiaceus (darkly pigmented) fungi[1].

ETIOLOGY AND PATHOGENESIS

Phaeohyphomycoses are ubiquitous saprophytes. Examples of dematiaceus fungi reported to cause dermatologic disease in animals (usually cats) include *Alternaria* spp.[2], *Bipolaris* spp., *Cladosporium* spp., *Curvularia* spp.[3], *Drechslera* spp.[4], *Exophiala* spp., *Moniliella* spp., *Ochroconis* spp., *Phialemonium* spp., *Phialophora* spp., *Pseudomicrodochium* spp., *Scolecobasidium* spp., *Staphylotrichum* spp., *Stemphyllium* spp., *Fonsecaea* spp., and *Cladophyalophora* spp.[3]. Subcutaneous infection results from traumatic implantation and local infection. Granulomatous inflammation ensues and nodules or ulcerative or fistulous lesions may develop[2,4].

CLINICAL FEATURES

Animals present with painless cutaneous papules or subcutaneous nodules, which may develop discharging tracts. Lesions typically are located on the feet or limbs (**95**), although the head and trunk may be affected. There may be local lymphadenopathy, but animals are not usually pyrexic. The lesions are refractory to systemic antibacterial therapy. Dissemination from the site of inoculation is rare, but has occurred in both dogs and cats[3]. This can be associated with immunosuppression following chemotherapy or systemic disease.

DIFFERENTIAL DIAGNOSES

- Abscess following a bite wound
- Staphylococcal furunculosis
- Cutaneous neoplasia
- Sterile nodule pyogranuloma
- Arthropod-bite granuloma
- Blastomycosis and other deep fungal infections
- Nocardiosis and other deep bacterial or mycobacterial infections

DIAGNOSIS

Microscopic examination of 10% potassium hydroxide preparations from exudate or affected tissue will reveal darkly pigmented, septate hyphae (**96**), some of which display occasional bulbous distensions[5]. Brown, black, green, or blue fungal elements are also visible on Diff-Quik-stained cytology smears prepared from fine needle aspirates or draining sinus tracts. Fungal culture on appropriate media will allow a definitive diagnosis, although this may require the expertise of a specialized mycology laboratory. Histopathologic examination of affected tissue will reveal a pyogranulomatous response and may allow identification of hyphae, but definitive diagnosis is not possible. Multinucleate giant cells are common on both cytology and histopathology.

MANAGEMENT

Surgical excision of affected tissue is curative[5]. In areas where excision may be difficult (e.g. the nasal region), systemic antifungal agents such as ketoconazole, flucytosine (50 mg/kg p/o q6h), or amphotericin B may be prescribed, although their use has met with variable success[2,6]. *Drechslera spicifera* infection in a cat has been treated successfully by one of the authors (PJM) using itraconazole (10 mg/kg p/o q24h) for eight weeks. Fluconazole (5 mg/kg p/o q12h) for six months was reported to be successful in treating *Cladophyalophora bantiana* infection in a cat[7]. One author (TJN) has successfully used terbinafine (30 mg/kg p/o q24h) in a dog with an infection refactory to itraconazole.

KEY POINT

- A rare infection.

95, 96 Phaeohyphomycosis. A crusted nodule on the distal limb of a domestic shorthair cat (**95**); a photomicrograph demonstrating the dark-staining branching hyphae (**96**).

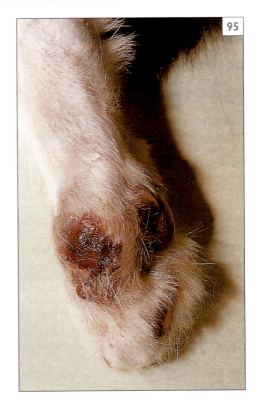

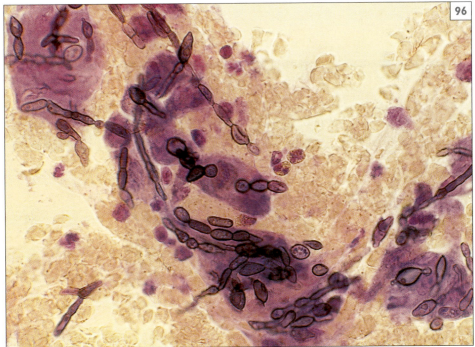

Cuterebra spp. infestation

DEFINITION
A nodular lesion of the skin due to the presence of *Cuterebra* spp. larvae.

ETIOLOGY AND PATHOGENESIS
Adult *Cuterebra* spp. flies are large, resemble a bumble bee, and neither feed nor bite. Females lay their eggs along rabbit runs and near rodent burrows. If a host brushes up against these eggs, they hatch instantaneously and the first-stage larvae crawl into the host's fur[1,2]. From here they enter the host through natural body openings. Migration occurs to the skin, where the third stage becomes clinically noticeable in the subcutaneous tissue[1,2]. Larvae may also undergo aberrant migrations in the brain, pharynx, nostrils, and eyelids[2–4].

CLINICAL FEATURES
Lesions are generally noted in late summer or autumn as 1–2 cm (0.4–0.8 in) nodules located over the head, neck, and trunk (**97**). A fistula develops from which the larva eventually escapes.

DIFFERENTIAL DIAGNOSES
- Dracunculiasis
- Cutaneous neoplasia
- Bacterial or fungal granuloma
- Deep mycotic infections
- Panniculitis
- Foreign body granuloma
- Infected wound

DIAGNOSIS
Opening a fistula reveals the 2.5–4.5 cm (1.0–1.8 in) dark brown to black, heavily-spined larva.

MANAGEMENT
Removal of the larva through the enlarged fistula. If not removed intact, parts of the larva left in the cavity may result in allergic or irritant reactions[1].

KEY POINT
- A rare dermatosis.

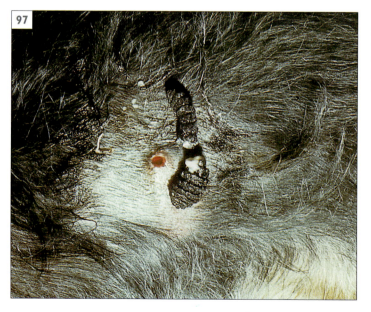

97 Cuterebriasis. A fistulated nodule in the groin of a puppy, with the extracted larva adjacent to the lesion.

Dracunculiasis

DEFINITION

Dracunculiasis is a nodular dermatosis produced by the development of *Dracunculus* spp. adults in the subcutaneous tissue.

ETIOLOGY AND PATHOGENESIS

Dracunculus medinensis (guinea worm) has been reported in humans, dogs, cats, horses, cattle, and other animals in Africa and Asia[1,2]. *Dracunculus insignis* is a parasite of dogs, raccoons, mink, fox, otter, and skunks in North America[2]. The intermediate hosts are small crustacean copepods that inhabit bodies of fresh water worldwide[2]. The copepods ingest first-stage larvae that have been released into water. In the copepods the larvae molt twice over a 12–14 day interval to become the infective third-stage larvae. Animals become infected when drinking water that contains these copepods. Third-stage larvae are released in the process of gastric digestion and migrate to the subcutaneous tissue, where adults develop in 8–12 months.

CLINICAL FEATURES

Animals are presented with single or multiple nodules that either develop draining fistulae or ulcerate (**98**). Urticaria, pruritus, pain, inflammation and, occasionally, pyrexia may be noted[1]. Lesions are generally located on the limbs, head, or abdomen.

DIFFERENTIAL DIAGNOSES

- *Cuterebra* spp. infestation
- Infected wound
- Foreign body
- Cutaneous neoplasia
- Deep mycotic infection
- Panniculitis

DIAGNOSIS

Impression smears of discharge from the fistulae or ulcers may reveal the rhabdiform first-stage larvae, which are between 500 and 760 µm in length. Enlarging and exploring the fistulae may allow demonstration of the adult worms (**98**).

MANAGEMENT

The treatment of choice is surgical excision and removal of the adult worm.

KEY POINT

- May be relatively common in some regions, but is generally rare.

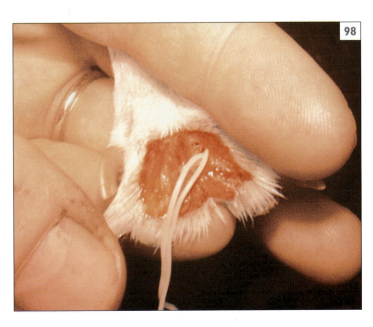

98 Dracunculiasis. A lesion in the interdigital region of a dog, with the adult worm clearly visible.

Calcinosis circumscripta

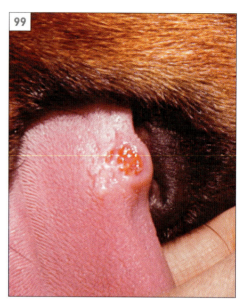

99

DEFINITION
Calcinosis circumscripta is seen as tumor-like nodules resulting from dystrophic calcification.

ETIOLOGY AND PATHOGENESIS
Lesions appear at sites of repetitive or previous trauma such as pressure points, footpads, or sites of injury[1-3]. The specific mechanism of calcium salt deposition is not understood. Hypercalcemia is not present in most dogs.

CLINICAL FEATURES
Lesions occur more frequently in young, rapidly growing dogs, with German Shepherd Dogs, Boston Terriers, and Boxers being predisposed[2]. Firm, well-circumscribed, generally single, nodules ranging from 0.5–7 cm occur in the subcutaneous tissue at sites of pressure points, footpads, chronic injury, or the tongue (**99**)[1-3]. Ulceration may occur in larger lesions or with repeated trauma. Lesions are non-painful, except for those occurring in the footpads. White gritty or pasty material may extrude from the lesions[2].

99 Ulcerated nodule of the tongue of a dog with calcinosis circumscripta.

DIFFERENTIAL DIAGNOSES
- Metastatic calcification occurring secondary to chronic renal failure. This is more likely to be seen in older dogs and several footpads would be affected
- Calcinosis cutis associated with hyperadrenocorticism or systemic steroid therapy. However, this tends to occur as plaque-like lesions on the trunk
- Neoplasia
- Granulomas due to parasites or foreign bodies

DIAGNOSIS
- Cytology
- Biopsy
- Radiology, if necessary, to demonstrate deposits of calcium if the nodules are deep within the metacarpal or metatarsal pads
- Further investigation including hematology, serum biochemistry, and ionized calcium may be necessary in individual cases, but most affected animals are otherwise normal

MANAGEMENT
Surgical excision.

KEY POINT
- Surgical excision is curative.

Ulcerative dermatoses

General approach

- Avoid empirical use of steroids without establishing a diagnosis
- Most ulcers involve infections, neoplasia, or immune-mediated conditions
- Biopsy and histopathology are key to diagnosis
- Always make a definitive diagnosis – the treatment and prognosis depend on it

Common conditions

- Feline eosinophilic granuloma complex
- Feline idiopathic ulcerative dermatitis
- German Shepherd Dog pyoderma
- Cutaneous lupus erythematosus (discoid lupus erythematosus)
- Calcinosis cutis
- Decubital ulcers (pressure sores)
- Squamous cell carcinoma

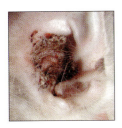 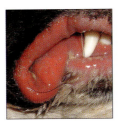 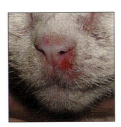 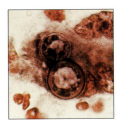

German Shepherd Dog pyoderma

DEFINITION

German Shepherd Dog (GSD) pyoderma is an idiopathic, chronic, recurrent ulcerative and exudative disease predominantly seen in GSDs and GSD crosses[1,2]. Whether it is a true primary pyoderma or primarily an immune-mediated disease is controversial.

ETIOLOGY AND PATHOGENESIS

GSD pyoderma is a distinct condition separate from the pyodermas occurring secondary to flea allergic dermatitis (FAD), atopic dermatitis, adverse reaction to food, demodicosis, or hypothyroidism[1–4]. Nevertheless, FAD, atopic dermatitis, cutaneous adverse food reactions, hypothyroidism, and ehrlichiosis have been recognized as triggers for the condition[3–5].

Staphylococcus intermedius is the most commonly isolated organism, but affected animals are not hypersensitive to staphylococcal antigens[6]. Although immunologic abnormalities have been suggested as predisposing factors, chemotaxis and killing capacities of neutrophilic leukocytes and complement and immunoglobulin levels, with the possible exception of low IgA, are normal, and no specific immunoglobulin or complement deposits have been found in affected skin[7–10]. Decreased levels of T cells, a CD4:CD8 imbalance, and a decrease in the numbers of CD21+ B cells have been demonstrated in the skin of affected dogs compared with healthy dogs. This suggests that the immunologic imbalance may be associated with defective T helper cells[7,9–11]. The histopathology of affected skin is dominated by mononuclear cell infiltration and it is also hypothesized that a defect in the skin barrier and/or innate immune system allows bacteria to penetrate the stratum corneum, be exposed to the adaptive immune system, and initiate a massive cell-mediated inflammatory reaction.

CLINICAL FEATURES

GSD pyoderma occurs most commonly in middle-aged animals, but may be seen at any age[3]. There appears to be no sex predisposition. Lesions generally start over the lateral thighs and dorsal lumbosacral areas, but any area of the body may be affected. Typical lesions include erythematous to violaceous papules, pustules, epidermal collarettes, furuncles, erosions, ulcers, crusts, and sinuses (**100–102**), which drain a hemopurulent material[3,4]. Varying degrees of alopecia and hyperpigmentation may be noted and the peripheral lymph nodes are generally enlarged. Lesions may be pruritic and/or painful. Affected dogs may also have anal furunculosis (see Anal furunculosis, p. 174) and/or pedal panniculitis (see Panniculitis, p. 88), suggesting that these may be clinical manifestations of a similar etiology.

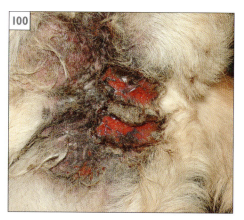

100 German Shepherd Dog pyoderma with ulceration, purulent discharge, and crusting in the groin.

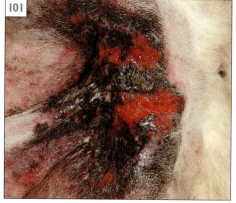

101 Same dog as in **100**; the hair has been clipped to show the extent of the lesions. Note the ill-defined margin, hyperpigmentation, and scarring.

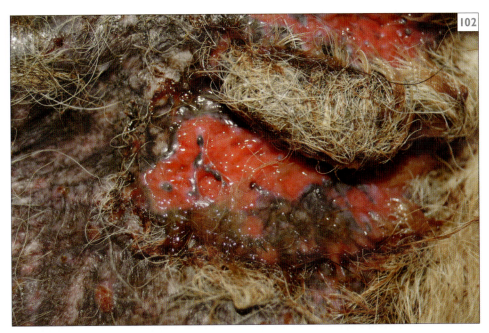

102 Close-up of the dog in **100** showing the typical 'melting' necrosis and underrunning of affected skin.

DIFFERENTIAL DIAGNOSES

- Demodicosis
- Deep pyoderma secondary to other diseases
- Cutaneous infections secondary to systemic mycosis
- Cutaneous infections of subcutaneous or opportunistic fungi or oomycetes
- Opportunistic mycobacterial, filamentous or gram-negative bacterial infection
- Neoplasia
- Drug eruption (Stevens–Johnson syndrome or toxic epidermal necrolysis)

DIAGNOSIS

The history and clinical findings are highly suggestive but not pathognomonic. Skin scrapes, cytology, biopsy and histopathology, bacterial and fungal culture, and antimicrobial sensitivity should be performed to confirm the diagnosis and eliminate the differentials[3]. Flea control trials, food trials, and allergy testing may be indicated in dogs with other clinical signs supportive of FBH/FAD (see Flea bite hypersensitivity, p. 38), cutaneous adverse food reactions (see Cutaneous adverse food reaction, p. 31) or atopic dermatitis (see Canine atopic dermatitis, p. 20). It is important to identify and control possible trigger factors and underlying diseases[4].

MANAGEMENT

Therapy has traditionally revolved around intensive antibiotic therapy[3,4,12]. This usually requires ongoing treatment to maintain remission and could involve:

- Bactericidal antibiotics, preferably on the basis of antibacterial culture and sensitivity. Therapy should continue for two weeks past clinical cure: this may mean 6–12 weeks treatment or longer.
- Antibacterial shampoos and washes to reduce the bacterial load, remove crusts, enhance drainage of purulent material, and ameliorate pain and pruritus.
- Relapsing cases can be treated with staphage lysate (SPL; Delmont Laboratories) or autogenous vaccines (speak to the bacteriology laboratory about this as individual requirements and protocols may differ).

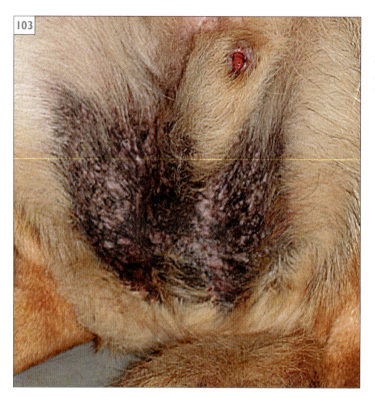

103 Same dog as in **100**; complete resolution following treatment with ciclosporin, but note the extensive scarring.

- Some cases may require pulse antibiotic therapy. This should involve a bactericidal antibiotic that is not prone to induce rapid resistance (e.g. potentiated amoxicillin, cefalexin, or fluoroquinolones). Pulse therapy regimes include:
  - One week on full dose: X weeks off.
  - X days/week on full dose: Y days/week off.
  - 'Weekend' therapy (i.e. full dose for 2–3 days each week) is effective and popular due to its simplicity and high compliance[13,14].
- There is little rationale for chronic low or sub-therapeutic dosing and this is not recommended.
- Dietary management may be necessary with chronic administration of broad-spectrum antibiotics, but most dogs tolerate treatment well.

(See Superficial pyoderma, p. 146 for further discussion of antibacterial treatment options.)

Many cases, however, fail to respond adequately to antibacterial treatment. One author (TJN) routinely uses ciclosporin (cyclosporine) (5–7.5 mg/kg q24h to remission and then as often as necessary to maintain remission) (**103**). The use of this drug suggests that some cases have an immune-mediated etiology, although the response to glucocorticoids and other immuno-suppressive agents is variable.

KEY POINTS
- Poorly understood.
- Many cases require long-term antibacterial therapy.
- Consider ciclosporin in cases with a poor response to antibacterial therapy.

Feline idiopathic ulcerative dermatosis

DEFINITION
Feline idiopathic ulcerative dermatosis is a rare disease of cats resulting in non-healing ulcers of the dorsal neck or back between the scapulae.

ETIOLOGY AND PATHOGENESIS
The etiology and pathogenesis are unknown[1,2]. Some cases appear to follow application of topical, spot-on flea control products or injection of vaccines and depot products, although no firm link can be established in most cases.

CLINICAL FEATURES
The lesion is a 2–5 cm (0.8–2 in) well-demarcated single ulcer located on the caudal dorsal neck or area between the scapulae (**104**). There is a firm elevated border with peripheral swelling and erythema. Cats often self-traumatize the lesion[1,2]. If self-trauma is minimal, a thick crust will form over the lesion.

DIFFERENTIAL DIAGNOSES
- Trauma
- Burn
- Injection reaction
- Foreign body reaction
- Localized hypersensitivity reaction (flea, adverse reaction to food, atopy)
- Eosinophilic granuloma
- Neoplasia

DIAGNOSIS
The clinical features of this condition are highly suggestive. Other differentials can be ruled out and dermatohistopathology might provide supporting evidence.

MANAGEMENT
The lesions are often refractory to medical treatment, are too large for surgical removal, or return after removal. The following are anecdotal reports relating to attempted treatments:
- Ciclosporin (cyclosporine)[3] (microemulsified): 5 mg/kg p/o q24h.
- Applying silver sulfadiazine to the lesion twice daily and either bandaging or fashioning a shirt for the cat to wear so the area is not traumatized by scratching.
- Pentoxifylline: 10 mg/kg p/o q12h.
- Dexamethasone: 0.3 mg/kg p/o q24h.
- Methylprednisolone acetate: 4 mg/kg s/c every 2–3 weeks until healed and then every 2–3 months for control.
- Clomipramine: 1.25–2.5 mg/kg p/o q24h.
- Laser surgery to ablate affected tissue.

KEY POINT
- Be aware that this is a condition that is often refractory to treatment.

104 Crusted ulcer on the dorsal neck of a cat with feline idiopathic ulcerative dermatitis.

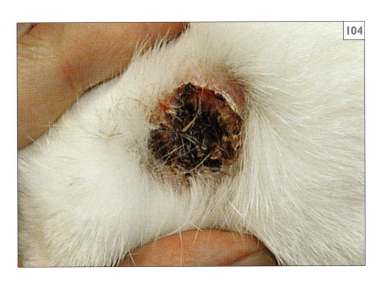

Feline eosinophilic granuloma complex

ETIOLOGY AND PATHOGENESIS

The eosinophilic granuloma complex (EGC) comprises three major forms: eosinophilic or collagenolytic granuloma, eosinophilic or indolent ulcer, and eosinophilic plaque[1,2]. These have distinct clinical and histologic features. EGC is not necessarily a specific diagnosis, however, and the lesions may represent different reaction patterns to the same underlying causes. Some cats suffer single episodes, others exhibit recurrent lesions, and a few present with refractory lesions. Combinations of different lesions can be seen in an individual cat.

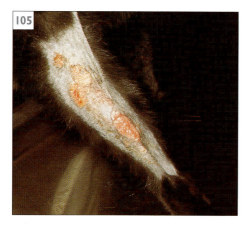

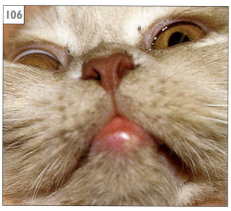

105, 106 Collagenolytic (eosinophilic) granulomas. The linear form (**105**) and the localized form on the mandible of a cat (**106**).

The etiology of these dermatoses is unknown. Local, uncontrolled recruitment of eosinophils results in the release of potent inflammatory mediators, which initiate ongoing inflammation[1,3]. A variety of underlying conditions (see below) have been associated with EGC lesions, but many cases remain idiopathic[2,3]. EGC lesions have also been reported in specific pathogen-free cats in which atopic dermatitis and cutaneous adverse food reactions were ruled out and no underlying cause could be established[4]. Norwegian Forest cats may be predisposed[5].

CLINICAL FEATURES

Eosinophilic or collagenolytic granulomas

These are the only true granulomas within this complex. There are no breed, age, or sex predispositions, although the linear form is more common in cats less than two years of age[1,5]. Recent studies have shown that collagen is normal, indicating that these are true eosinophilic lesions and that the term collagenolytic should be dropped[3]. They are often associated with a circulating eosinophilia. Lesions are associated with allergic or parasitic diseases, they may have a genetic basis in certain colonies, but they are often idiopathic. Pruritus is variable.

Lesions may be single or grouped, nodular, linear or papular and present anywhere on the body. Linear lesions commonly affect the medial forelimbs and caudal thighs, which may represent grooming pathways. There is a distinct form associated with the chin and lower lip ('pouting' or 'button lip') that may wax and wane. The dorsum of the nose, the pinnae, and the footpads are also common sites. The lesions are usually erythematous and alopecic, raised and nodular to elongated, and cord-like. There may also be erosion, ulceration, and necrosis, with pale, gritty foci evident (**105, 106**).

Mosquito bite hypersensitivity

This is a distinct, seasonal pruritic dermatitis associated with mosquito bites[6,7]. Clinical signs include papular, erosive to ulcerating and crusting dermatitis of the nose, muzzle, pinnae, preauricular region, flexor carpi, and the junction of the footpad and haired skin (**107**). Chronic lesions may be depigmented. Affected footpads can be ulcerated, swollen, and hypopigmented. There may be a peripheral eosinophilia and marked peripheral lymphadenopathy.

Eosinophilic plaques

These are well-circumscribed, ulcerated, moist lesions typically found on the ventral abdomen, medial thighs, or caudal trunk[1,2] (**108**). There may also be pedal (**109**) and, rarely, otic lesions (**110**). There is no breed or sex incidence, although young cats may be predisposed. Adjacent lesions may coalesce, presenting as very large, plaque-like areas. Eosinophilic plaques are usually associated with pruritus, although this may not be evident from the history.

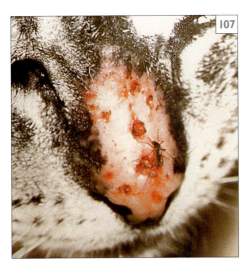

107 Feline mosquito bite hypersensitivity. (Photo courtesy K Mason)

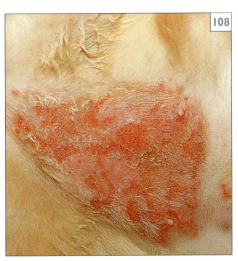

108 Eosinophilic plaque on the ventral abdomen of a cat.

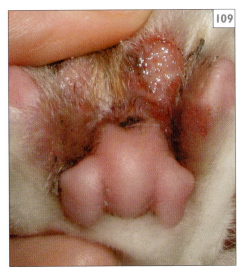

109 Eosinophilic plaque affecting the interdigital skin.

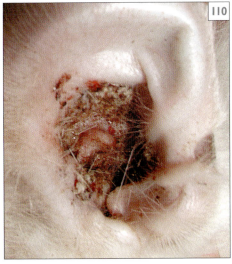

110 Eosinophilic plaques, erosions, and crusts in the vertical ear canal.

Eosinophilic or indolent ulcers

These are well-demarcated unilateral or bilateral ulcers, occurring at the philtrum of the upper lip or adjacent to the upper canine tooth[1,2,5] (**111**). The periphery is raised and surrounds a pinkish to yellow ulcerated center. Large lesions can be very destructive and deforming, but the lesions do not seem to be pruritic or overly painful. Unlike other EGC lesions, eosinophils may not be the predominant finding on cytology or histopathology, and peripheral eosinophilia is rare.

DIFFERENTIAL DIAGNOSES

The differential diagnosis can be quite varied depending on the clinical presentation[2], although many EGC lesions have a very characteristic appearance. Possible differentials include:

- Trauma
- Actinic dermatitis
- Cutaneous neoplasia, especially squamous cell carcinoma
- Dermatophytosis
- Rodent or cat bites
- Feline cowpox infection
- Calicivirus or herpesvirus infection
- Mycobacterial infection
- Deep fungal infection
- Immune-mediated diseases (drug reactions, pemphigus foliaceus, cutaneous lupus)

It is also important to eliminate any potential underlying causes before assuming that the lesions are idiopathic. Underlying causes include[2]:

- Cutaneous adverse food reaction
- Atopic dermatitis
- Flea bite hypersensitivity/flea allergic dermatitis
- Other ectoparasites
- Chronic self-trauma
- FeLV (uncommon and the relationship is now questioned)
- Bacterial infection (usually secondary, although some cases of indolent ulcers may respond to broad-spectrum antibiotics)

DIAGNOSIS

The clinical signs are very characteristic, but cytology, biopsy, and histopathology are diagnostic if necessary. Clinical history and examination will narrow the differentials. Skin scrapes, flea control trials and/or trial antiparasitic therapy (see Flea allergic dermatitis, p. 38), cytology for bacterial infection (see Superficial pyoderma, p. 146), hair plucks, Wood's lamp examination and fungal cultures (see Dermatophytosis, p. 278), and food trials (see Cutaneous adverse food reaction, p. 31) should be performed. Allergen-specific intradermal or serologic tests can be performed to identify allergens for avoidance and

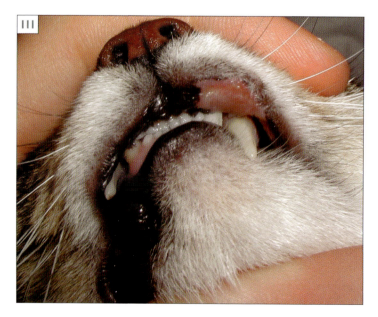

111

111 Indolent ulcer.

immunotherapy (see Canine atopic dermatitis, p. 20), although the value of these in cats is disputed.

MANAGEMENT

The prognosis and long-term treatment depend on the underlying trigger. However, many cases are idiopathic and require symptomatic treatment. Symptomatic treatment may also be necessary to control acute flares in animals on long-term therapy. Certain lesions, particularly indolent ulcers, may be refractory to treatment. Some lesions, especially linear granulomas in young cats, may spontaneously resolve[1,5]. Essential fatty acids and antihistamines (see Canine atopic dermatitis, p. 20) have been reported to be useful, especially if an allergic trigger is suspected, although more potent treatment may be needed initially to get the lesions in remission.

Most cases will respond to systemic prednisolone (2 mg/kg q24h) or methylprednisolone (0.8× prednisolone dose). Once in remission this can be tapered to a maintenance dose given every other day. Some cats may respond better to dexamethasone (0.15× prednisolone dose) or triamcinolone (0.25–0.8× the prednisolone dose), especially in the initial stages of treatment, although neither drug is licensed for cats[1]. Treatment can either be switched to prednisolone or methylprednisolone for maintenance, or be tapered to a maintenance dose given every three days. Depot injections of methylprednisolone (given every 2–4 weeks until remission, then every 6–8 weeks for maintenance) are best reserved for cats that cannot be treated orally. Intralesional triamcinolone can be useful for solitary, well-defined lesions[1].

Surgical excision, cryosurgery, laser surgery, and irradiation have been recommended for single, well-defined lesions refractory to medical therapy[1]. This is often successful, particularly for indolent ulcers, although recurrence or the development of new lesions is common.

Immune modulation with recombinant feline interferon omega (5 million IU s/c 3 times weekly for 3 weeks) or recombinant human interferon alpha (30–60 IU/cat p/o q24h for 30 days) has been successful in a small number of cats, although the lesions recurred following cessation of therapy.

Ciclosporin (cyclosporine) (5–7.5 mg/kg q24h to remission, then taper frequency) has been successful and well tolerated in a range of eosinophilic skin diseases in cats[8]. Adverse effects are similar to those seen in dogs (see Canine atopic dermatitis, p. 20). A small number of cats have developed fatal toxoplasmosis following therapy[9]. There appears to be a small risk of naive cats acquiring infection, but recrudescence in seropositive cats is unlikely. At present the authors recommend pretreatment serology, discuss the risks with the owners, and advise feeding processed foods and treats. Keeping treated cats indoors is not always feasible. Ciclosporin is not at present licensed for use in cats.

Other drug options[1,2] that can be used in recalcitrant cases, with or without glucocorticoids, include: chlorambucil (0.1–0.2 mg/kg q24h tapered to every other day); aurothioglucose (gold salt therapy/chrysotherapy; 1 mg/kg weekly i/m until remission and then monthly) (**Note:** Give 1 mg test dose i/m initially and monitor for bone marrow suppression and skin eruptions); and progestagens, such as megestrol acetate, which have very potent glucocorticoid activity. (**Note:** Long-term use is associated with polyuria, polydipsia, mammary gland hyperplasia and neoplasia, diabetes mellitus, and iatrogenic hyperadrenocorticism, including ventral abdominal alopecia, which could confuse the clinical presentation. Some of these effects may be irreversible.)

Hydrocortisone aceponate has been effective and well tolerated in a small number of cats with eosinophilic plaques.

KEY POINTS

- Clinically well recognized, but poorly understood.
- It is important to control underlying triggers.
- Many cases require symptomatic treatment.

Drug eruptions

ETIOLOGY AND PATHOGENESIS

Drug eruptions are rare conditions in which pleomorphic cutaneous lesions, with or without systemic signs, occur as a result of exposure to a chemical compound. They may reflect immunologic or non-immunologic reactions[1]. The animal may become sensitized to, or react to, medications, preservatives, or even dyes within drug formulations or foods. Reactions may occur to systemic or topical medications. Most drug eruptions result in extensive lesions and are unpredictable in nature. Rarely, a repeatable, localized reaction may be noted (fixed drug eruption) (**112**)[1].

CLINICAL FEATURES

There is no breed, age, or sex predisposition to cutaneous drug eruption, although Dobermanns are predisposed to sulfonamide-induced reactions[2,3]. Certain drugs, particularly penicillins and sulfonamides[4,5], appear to be commonly implicated (which may simply reflect volume of use), but it should be remembered that any drug can induce a drug eruption[1,5]. Clinical signs include urticaria and angioedema (**113**), contact dermatitis, erythematous macules (**114**), papules or crusted vesicles, exfoliative dermatitis, vasculitis and vasculopathy (**115**), pemphigus or pemphigoid and Stevens–Johnson syndrome (**116**), or toxic epidermal necrolysis[1–9] (**117**).

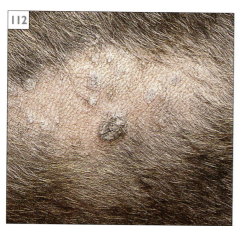

112 Fixed drug eruption on the lateral flank of an Airedale Terrier.

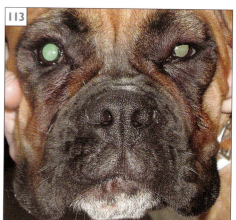

113 Urticaria and angioedema in a Boxer following methadone administration.

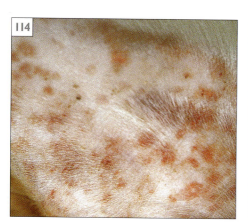

114 Erythematous macules and patches following Imodium (loperamide) treatment.

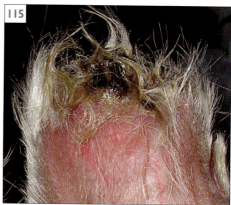

115 Ear tip necrosis in a West Highland White Terrier following treatment with fenbendazole.

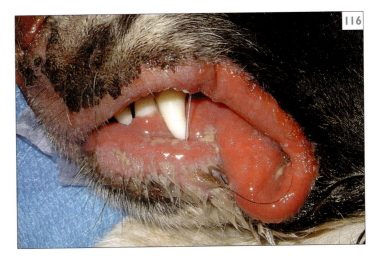

116 Severe ulceration of the muzzle and nose in a Springer Spaniel with Stevens–Johnson syndrome following trimethoprim-sulfonamide treatment.

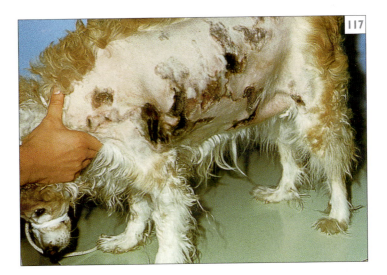

117 Toxic epidermal necrolysis secondary to drug eruption.

Pruritus is usually absent, but is occasionally marked. Systemic abnormalities can include anemia, thrombocytopenia, bone marrow suppression, hepatopathy, pancreatitis, nephrotic syndrome, keratoconjunctivitis sicca, arthropathy, uveitis, and neurologic signs[1,4,5,9,10].

DIFFERENTIAL DIAGNOSES
- Superficial to deep bacterial infections
- Irritant or contact dermatitis
- Pemphigus group, systemic lupus erythematosus, and other immune-mediated dermatoses
- Cutaneous neoplasia

DIAGNOSIS
Drug eruption may be tentatively diagnosed on the basis of known exposure to the drug, compatible clinical signs, the presence of compatible histologic features on examination of biopsy samples, and resolution of the signs after withdrawal of the suspected drug[1]. Definitive diagnosis, however, is only possible with provocative exposure, which is inadvisable, since it may precipitate severe systemic or generalized signs.

MANAGEMENT

Removal of the offending agent and appropriate supportive therapy are sufficient in cases exhibiting only moderate signs of reaction. All drugs should be stopped: if treatment is essential (e.g. antibiotics), a drug pharmacologically distinct from the suspect agent should be selected. One author (TJN) frequently sees cases that fail to respond to withdrawal of medication. This may be because of persistent antigenic stimulus or because once initiated the immune-mediated reaction becomes self-perpetuating. The goals of therapy are therefore to stop the ongoing condition, if present, and manage residual skin lesions (see the appropriate chapters for treatment of defined immune-mediated syndromes). Intravenous human immunoglobulin (ivHIG; 0.5–1.5 g/kg i/v over 6–12 hours) can be useful in arresting Stevens–Johnson syndrome and toxic epidermal necrolysis[8] (see Toxic epidermal necrolysis, p. 194). This is well tolerated, although there is a risk of sensitization and anaphylaxis with multiple exposure.

Some cases, such as those with extensive open skin lesions or toxic epidermal necrolysis, will require aggressive fluid therapy and anti-shock regimes. Areas with necrotic skin should be treated with topical silver sulfadiazine ointment, activated silver, and other appropriate dressings to prevent infection and encourage wound healing. The value of systemic glucocorticoids is disputed[11], since most of the damage is irreversible and ongoing at the point of diagnosis. Clinicians should also bear in mind that drug reactions can occur to steroid and other anti-inflammatory medications, and that individuals with an ongoing drug reaction may be primed for further reactions.

The prognosis is variable. It is generally good with mild cutaneous lesions and worsens with more severe lesions and systemic involvement. The patient's records should indicate drug sensitivity and clearly identify drugs that should be avoided.

KEY POINTS

- Drug eruption is probably under-recognized.
- Do not re-challenge to confirm your diagnosis.

Cutaneous lupus erythematosus
(discoid lupus erythematosus)

DEFINITION

Cutaneous lupus erythematosus is a dermatosis in which localized, photoaggravated skin lesions occur.

ETIOLOGY AND PATHOGENESIS

The etiology of cutaneous lupus erythematosus is unclear. It has been proposed that in genetically predisposed, susceptible individuals, actinic radiation induces an inflammatory cascade that damages dermal and epidermal components, provoking a localized, chronic, immune-mediated reaction[1]. The inflammation results in erythema, scale, crusting, and depigmentation[2].

CLINICAL FEATURES

There is no age predilection, but females and some breeds of dogs (e.g. Shetland Sheepdogs, Rough Collies, German Shepherd Dogs, and Siberian Huskies) are predisposed[3,4]. Cutaneous lupus erythematosus is very rare in cats[5]. The most common sites for lesions are the nose and planum nasale[2,3] (**118, 119**). The lips, periorbital regions, pinnae, nails, and scrotum are also affected in some cases[2,3]. Interestingly, the pinnae are more commonly affected in cats[5]. Rarely, the sheath and digits exhibit lesions[3]. Lesions are usually alopecic and erythematous and display varying degrees of depigmentation. In active lesions there may be a fine scale and even small, adherent crusts. In long-standing lesions scarring can occur and severe lesions may become ulcerated. Mucocutaneous lesions are very rare in cutaneous lupus erythematosus.

DIFFERENTIAL DIAGNOSES

- Actinic dermatitis
- Dermatophytosis
- Nasal pyoderma
- Demodicosis
- Pemphigus complex
- Drug eruption
- Systemic lupus erythematosus
- Uveodermatologic syndrome
- Mucocutaneous pyoderma
- Proliferative nasal arteritis/vasculitis
- Parasympathetic nasal dermatitis
- Idiopathic nasal depigmentation
- Proliferative arteritis of the nasal philtrum

DIAGNOSIS

Clinical history and examination will demonstrate that the lesions are localized and that there are no systemic signs[3]. The cardinal observation in narrowing the huge differential diagnosis is whether the lesion affects the planum nasale or not. It is very unusual for dermatoses other than immune-mediated diseases to affect the planum nasale: they may affect adjacent haired skin, but they do not cross the border. Histopathologic examination of biopsy samples is usually diagnostic[3,4] and immunofluorescence is rarely necessary. Antinuclear antibody tests are nearly always negative[3,4].

MANAGEMENT

The combination of tetracycline and niacinamide (250 mg of each drug p/o q8h in dogs under 10 kg and 500 mg of each p/o q8h in dogs over 10 kg) (doxycycline 10 mg/kg p/o q24h may be used instead of tetracycline) will control a majority of cases[6]. Topical 0.1% tacrolimus ointment applied twice daily may be used as an adjunct treatment. Cases that are less severe may respond to tacrolimus ointment as the sole therapy[7]. Systemic prednisolone will induce remission, and low-dose alternate day prednisolone will keep most animals in remission[3,4]. Topical sun-blocking creams and sun avoidance will help to keep the dose as low as possible. Some cases may be kept in remission with topical hydrocortisone cream or more powerful topical glucocorticoids, or with a sun blocker alone. Megadoses of vitamin E (400–800 IU daily) have been reported as useful in a proportion of cases, although there is a 1–2 month lag phase[3]. Ciclosporin (cyclosporine) (5.0–7.5 mg/kg p/o q24h to remission and then tapering for maintenance) can also be effective in cases with more severe or widespread lesions.

KEY POINTS

- The most common immune-mediated dermatosis.
- Try to avoid inducing Cushingoid changes for what is usually a localized problem.

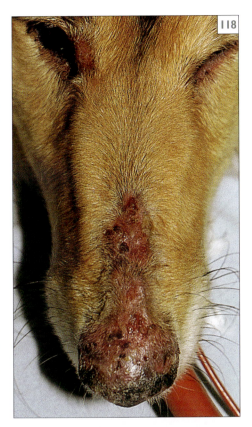

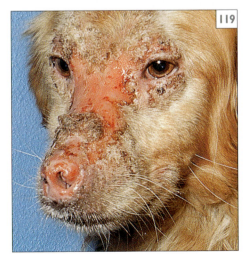

118, 119 Cutaneous lupus erythematosus. Lesions on the rostral face (**118**); more extensive lesions on the face (**119**).

Systemic lupus erythematosus

ETIOLOGY AND PATHOGENESIS

Systemic lupus erythematosus (SLE) is a rare, multisystemic immune-mediated disease that is part of the lupus group of conditions. Many of the immunologic mechanisms have been elucidated, but the initiating causes remain obscure. Genetic factors, systemic disease, neoplasia, viruses, hormones, drugs, and environmental conditions (e.g. exposure to sunlight) have all been implicated[1-5]. The primary immunologic events may be associated with defective suppressor T cell function[6], leading to a polyclonal gammopathy and the unrestrained production of autoantibodies, and T cell activation with a decreased CD4+:CD8+ ratio[2].

These responses may be cell or tissue specific, directed against erythrocytes, platelets, and leukocytes, or they may be directed against ubiquitous nuclear antigens[1]. Antinuclear antibodies (ANA) can combine with free DNA to form immune complexes. These may be deposited in glomeruli, causing a membranous glomerulonephritis; in arteriolar walls, resulting in local fibrinoid necrosis and fibrosis; or in synovia, provoking arthritis. Both cell/tissue specific and non-specific autoantibodies may be found either separately or in combination, leading to the diverse clinical presentation of SLE[1].

CLINICAL FEATURES

Canine SLE occurs in middle-aged animals. Rough Collies, Shetland Sheepdogs, Beagles, Afghan Hounds, German Shepherd Dogs, Old English Sheepdogs, Poodles, and Irish Setters may be predisposed[1,7]. There is no general sex predisposition, although entire females and male German Shepherd Dogs may be at more risk[7]. Clinical signs may appear suddenly or gradually, and will often wax and wane, making diagnosis difficult[1]. Lameness, due to polyarthritis and/or polymyositis, is the most common clinical sign, seen in 75–91% of cases[1,7,8]. Other systemic signs include pyrexia of unknown origin, glomerulonephritis and proteinuria, hemolytic anemia, thrombocytopenia, neutropenia, myocarditis, thyroiditis, splenomegaly, lymphadenopathy, and CNS disorders[1,3,7]. Skin changes occur in 50–60% of cases[1,7]. They may be localized or generalized and involve the face, ears, limbs, body, mucocutaneous junctions, and mucosae. Lesions are varied and unpredictable and include alopecia, erythema, ulceration, crusting, scarring, leukoderma, cellulitis, panniculitis, and furunculosis[1,3,7] (**120–123**). SLE has also been associated with generalized bacterial infection[3].

SLE is rare in cats and generally presents as an autoimmune hemolytic anemia. Other clinical signs include pyrexia, skin lesions (alopecia, erythema, scaling, crusting, and scarring, especially of the face, pinnae, and paws), thrombocytopenia, and renal failure[9,10].

DIFFERENTIAL DIAGNOSES (for the skin lesions)

- Dermatophytosis
- Demodicosis
- Cutaneous (discoid) lupus erythmatosus (including exfoliative and vesicular CLE)
- Epitheliotropic lymphoma
- Necrolytic migratory erythema
- Leishmaniasis
- Erythema multiforme
- Dermatomyositis
- Stevens–Johnson syndrome and toxic epidermal necrolysis
- Drug eruption
- Vasculitis
- Infectious or sterile (immune-mediated) panniculitis
- Pemphigus vulgaris
- Pemphigus foliaceus
- Bullous pemphigoid
- Epidermolysis bullosa

Note: Several of these conditions may be considered trigger factors and/or clinical manifestations of SLE, which complicates the diagnosis[2,4].

DIAGNOSIS

Diagnosis of SLE is challenging because of the unpredictable clinical signs and lack of a specific test[8]. Diagnosis is based on history and clinical findings suggestive of a multisystemic immune-mediated disorder plus supporting laboratory findings[2]. Routine hematology, biochemistry, and urinalysis can reveal anemia (non-regenerative or hemolytic), thrombocytopenia, leukopenia or leukocytosis, gammaglobulinemia, hypoalbuminemia, and proteinuria[2]. Coombs, platelet factor-3, and anti-platelet antibody tests are variably positive.

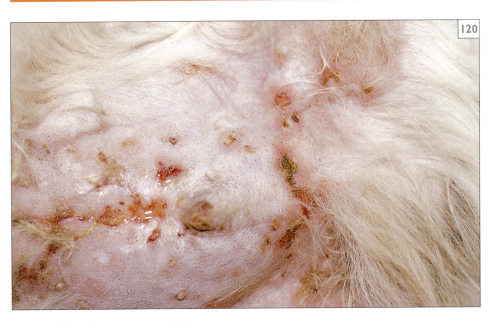

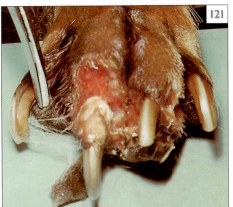

120, 121 Systemic lupus erythematosus. Ulcers and fistulas on the ventral abdomen (**120**) and paronychia (**121**) in a dog.

122, 123 Cutaneous (**122**) and oral (**123**) ulceration in a dog with systemic lupus erythematosus.

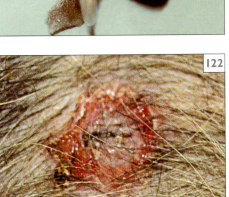

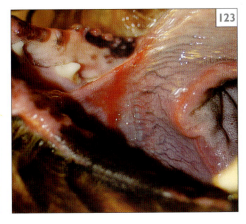

ANA test

This is an indirect immunofluorescent test that measures the titer of serum antibodies specific for nuclear antigens such as ANA, PCNA, anti-histone, and anti-double and anti-single stranded DNA antibodies[2,3,7,8,11–13]. ANA is the most specific and sensitive test for SLE. However, some normal dogs and cats, dogs undergoing treatment with certain drugs (griseofulvin, penicillin, sulfonamides, tetracyclines, phenytoin, procainamide) and dogs with other immune-mediated, infectious and neoplastic diseases may also have detectable ANA[2,9,10]. Strictly, a diagnosis of SLE needs a positive ANA test, but it may be negative in animals that have received glucocorticoids.

Biopsy and histopathology

This is often non-specific, but typical findings include interface dermatitis with basal cell vacuolation and necrosis of basal cells with the formation of colloid or Civatte bodies. Lesions may also involve the hair follicle outer root sheaths. Lichenoid inflammation of the dermis without basal cell involvement, vasculitis, atrophic changes, and necrosis may also be present[2]. Direct immunofluorescence can reveal immunoglobulin (IgA and/or IgM) or complement (C3) at the basement membrane zone in 50–90% of cases, although these may be found in other skin diseases[2]. Cytologic analysis of synovial fluid from animals with lameness may show increased numbers of non-degenerated neutrophils and occasional mononuclear cells[2].

LE cell test

LE cells are polymorphonuclear neutrophils with phagocytosed nuclei from dead and dying cells. The presence of LE cells is not a reliable feature of SLE because there is a high incidence of both false-positive and false-negative results[2].

Major and minor signs

In view of the difficulty in establishing a reliable diagnosis, a rating of the diagnostic signs has been suggested (see *Table 4*)[2,7,9,10]. Definite SLE requires either two major signs or one major and two minor signs in addition to serologic evidence of SLE. Probable SLE requires one major or two minor signs together with serologic evidence. Other authors regard four clinical signs as necessary for diagnosis.

Table 4
Rating of the diagnostic signs

Major signs	Minor signs
Non-erosive polyarthritis	Pyrexia of unknown origin
Dermatologic lesions	CNS signs such as seizures
Coombs positive anemia	Pleuritis (non-infective)
Significant thrombocytopenia	Pericarditis (non-infective)
Glomerulonephritis (proteinuria)	Altered CD4+:CD8+ ratio
Polymyositis	Polymyositis
Marked neutropenia	
ANA positive	

MANAGEMENT

Systemic corticosteroids such as prednisone, prednisolone, or methylprednisolone (2.0–4.0 mg/kg p/o q12–24h) are the initial therapy of choice. If significant improvement does not occur within ten days, concurrent administration of azathioprine (1.0–2.0 mg/kg p/o q24–48h) can be instituted. Azathioprine must not be used in cats; chlorambucil (0.2 mg/kg p/o q24h, then q48h) can be used instead. Other drugs that could be considered include cyclophosphamide (50 mg/m² body surface area q48h or 4 consecutive days/week), chrysotherapy (aurothioglucose, 1.0 mg/kg i/m weekly), niacinamide/tetracycline (dogs <10 kg, 250 mg of each q8h; dogs >10 kg, 500 mg of each q8h), and levamisole[2,7,9,10]. Gene therapy using recombinant canine CTLA-4 and IgA domains to down-regulate lymphocyte activation was successful in one study[14].

Once clinical control has been achieved, the drug dosage schedules should be decreased to the lowest schedule that keeps the disease in remission. The prognosis for SLE is guarded, as 40% of cases die within one year due to either the disease or drug complications[2]. The prognosis is better if an inciting condition can be identified and corrected.

KEY POINT

• A disease that is very hard to diagnose definitively, particularly if the animal was previously exposed to steroid therapy.

Vesicular cutaneous lupus erythematosus of the Shetland Sheepdog and Collie

DEFINITION
This is an autoimmune syndrome of the Shetland Sheepdog and Collie resulting in ulcers of the groin and axilla that have undulating serpiginous borders.

ETIOLOGY AND PATHOGENESIS
This condition was previously known as ulcerative dermatosis of the Shetland Sheepdog and Collie[1]. However, it has been determined that affected animals have circulating antibodies to extractable nuclear antigens in 82% of the cases and direct immunofluorescence revealed deposition of immunoglobulins bound to the dermal–epidermal junction in 50% of the cases[2]. In addition, there is a T lymphocyte-rich interface dermatitis. These findings correlate with the vesicular variant of subacute cutaneous lupus erythematosus in humans[2].

124 Serpiginous ulcers on the abdomen of a Collie with vesicular cutaneous lupus erythematosus.

CLINICAL FEATURES
The syndrome affects adult Shetland Sheepdogs and Rough Collie breeds or crosses thereof[1,2,3]. Lesions usually first appear in the summer months[3]. Vesicles and bullae are the primary lesions, but they are transient and may only be noted in histologic sections of early lesions. Ulcers are formed over the groin, axilla, and ventral abdomen. In some cases they may involve the mucocutaneous junctions and concave aspects of the pinnae[1,3]. The ulcers are coalescing and may be annular, but they are more often polycyclic or serpiginous (**124**)[1,3].

DIFFERENTIAL DIAGNOSES
- Bullous pemphigoid
- Epidermolysis bullosa acquisita
- Pemphigus vulgaris
- Systemic lupus erythematosus
- Erythema multiforme–toxic epidermal necrolysis syndrome
- Drug reaction

DIAGNOSIS
Diagnosis is based on history, clinical findings, and compatible histologic findings. Routine antinuclear antibody (ANA) testing is negative. However, in research situations, special techniques can be used to demonstrate circulating antibodies to extractable nuclear antigens in a majority of cases[2].

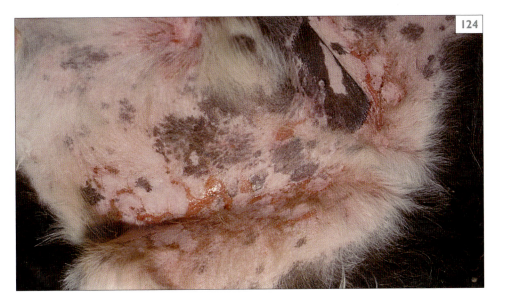

124

MANAGEMENT

The first step in the treatment is to resolve the clinical signs; the second step is the maintenance of clinical remission. Suppression of clinical signs is achieved with immunosuppressive doses of methylprednisolone or prednisolone (1.1–2.2 mg/kg p/o q12h)[4]. Azathioprine (1 mg/kg p/o q48h) is generally used in conjunction to allow for a lower maintenance dose of corticosteroids[4]. Once clinical signs have resolved, the methylprednisolone or prednisolone dose is tapered, at three-week intervals, to daily and, if remission is maintained, to every other day dosing. Further reduction of the alternate day steroid dose can then be attempted to find the least amount that prevents recurrence of lesions. Azathioprine may result in bone marrow suppression and this should be monitored by performing complete blood counts bi-weekly for the first eight weeks of therapy and then quarterly. (See Pemphigus foliaceus, page 155, and other immune-mediated diseases for further details on therapeutic options.)

If secondary bacterial infection occurs, treatment should be instituted with appropriate systemic antibacterial agents.

Sun avoidance has been advocated, although the exact role of sunlight in the pathogenesis of this condition is unknown[5].

There are anecdotal reports of and one case report of ciclosporin (cyclosporine) (5 mg/kg p/o q24h) being an effective therapeutic option[5,6].

KEY POINT

- Be aware that this is a condition that is not cured and some cases can be difficult to control.

Pemphigus vulgaris

ETIOLOGY AND PATHOGENESIS

Pemphigus vulgaris (PV) is a rare, vesicular and ulcerative condition of the skin and mucosae. IgG autoantiboides are thought to bind to plakins and desmoglein 3 (dsg3), components of the desmosome cell junctions in the basal epidermis[1,2]. Disruption of desmosomes leads to loss of cohesion between the keratinocytes and acantholysis[1]. Primary lesions are vesicles, which rapidly rupture and ulcerate.

CLINICAL FEATURES

There is no breed, age, or sex predisposition[1,3]. Most cases present with mucocutaneous and oral ulceration and exhibit systemic signs such as pyrexia, depression, and anorexia. Cutaneous lesions comprise erosions and ulceration (**125, 126**), particularly in the axilla and groin, and the nail bed and nasal planum[3–5]. Lesions in cats are concentrated in the oral cavity and the head, and systemic signs are less common. Nikolsky's sign may be present.

DIFFERENTIAL DIAGNOSES

- Bullous pemphigoid (BP)
- Epidermolysis bullosa (EB)
- Drug eruption
- Stevens–Johnson syndrome and toxic epidermal necrolysis
- Systemic lupus erythematosus (SLE)
- Cutaneous neoplasia
- Mucocutaneous candidiasis

DIAGNOSIS

The clinical signs are highly suggestive of an immune-mediated disease. The history can reveal possible drug exposure and/or evidence of a multisystemic disease (e.g. SLE). Impression smear cytology of fresh lesions of PV may demonstrate acanthocytes, which are not present in BP or EB. Cytology may, however, only reveal non-specific inflammation and secondary infection. Biopsy and histopathology are usually diagnostic[1,3,5], although immunohistochemistry may be needed in some cases. Unlike BP and EB, clefts occur above the basement membrane, leaving isolated adherent basal cells ('cling-ons' or 'tombstones' – i.e. suprabasilar acantholysis)[1,3].

MANAGEMENT

PV has a guarded prognosis[3]. The aim of treatment is to induce remission as quickly as possible. High-dose prednisolone (2–4 mg/kg p/o q12–24h; double this in cats) is the cornerstone of most therapeutic protocols. Dexamethasone (0.15× the prednisolone dose) or triamcinolone (0.8× the prednisolone dose) can be effective in animals that do not respond to prednisolone or methylprednisolone, particularly cats. Severe cases can be given glucocorticoid pulse therapy (11 mg/kg i/v in saline over 1–3 hours for 1–3 days). There is, however, a high incidence of severe side-effects at these doses, and gut protectants (e.g. sucralfate, H1 antagonists, and omeprazole) should be considered.

If a clinical improvement is not evident within 7–14 days, other immunosuppressive agents should also be used. Many dermatologists advocate cytotoxic agents in conjunction with prednisolone from the outset. Azathioprine (1–2 mg/kg q24h to every other day; do not use in cats) is most commonly used, although full clinical effects may take 2–6 weeks to become apparent. Other options include chlorambucil (0.1–0.2 mg/kg q24h), cyclophosphamide (50 mg/m² body surface area q48h or 4 consecutive days/week), chrysotherapy (aurothioglucose 1.0 mg/kg i/m weekly), dapsone (1 mg/kg q8–12h), sulfasalazine (22–44 mg/kg q8h), and niacinamide/tetracycline (dogs <10 kg, 250 mg of each p/o q8h; dogs >10 kg, 500 mg of each p/o q8h)[3,5]. Mycophenolate mofetil (22–39 mg/kg p/o divided q8h) has been used in conjunction with glucocorticoids to successfully manage pemphigus vulgaris in humans[6] and 50% of a small number of dogs with pemphigus foliaceus. (See Pemphigus foliaceus, p. 155, for general principles of cytotoxic therapy and adverse effects.)

Antimicrobial treatment during the initial phases of immunosuppression improves the prognosis in canine pemphigus foliaceus, although outcomes for pemphigus vulgaris have not been reported[7].

Once remission is attained, the drug doses are slowly tapered to the minimum required to maintain remission. Prednisolone and methylprednisolone are more suitable for long-term maintenance than triamcinolone and dexamethasone, which have a longer duration of activity and are more likely to induce iatrogenic hyperadrenocorticism even given every 48–72 hours.

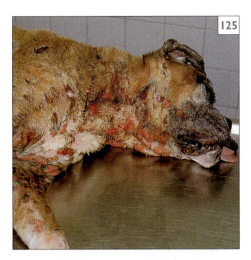

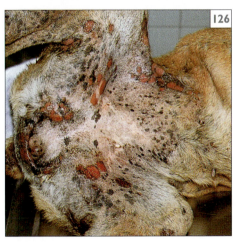

125, 126 Pemphigus vulgaris. Erosions, ulcers, and crusts on the ventral aspects of the neck (**125**) and the abdomen (**126**) in a Boxer.

Euthanasia may be necessary if acceptable remission cannot be achieved and/or there are unacceptable adverse effects from treatment.

KEY POINTS

- A potentially devastating disease that requires aggressive treatment.
- Generally has a poor prognosis.

Bullous pemphigoid

DEFINITION
Bullous pemphigoid is a rare, vesicobullous and ulcerative condition affecting the skin and oral mucosa. It is the most well known and best characterized of the subepidermal blistering diseases, although many cases may have been erroneously diagnosed as bullous pemphigoid before such conditions as epidermolysis bullosa acquista and vesicular cutaneous lupus erythematosus were recognized in animals[1,2].

ETIOLOGY AND PATHOGENESIS
The etiology is unknown, although genetic susceptibility to environmental triggers and adverse drug reactions may both be factors. The condition is characterized by autoantibodies directed against 180 kDa type XVII collagen (BP180, BPAG2) and/or the 230kD plakin epidermal isoform BPAGle (BP230) in the hemidesmosomes and, possibly, the basement membrane zone of the skin and the mucosa[2,4,5]. Mucous membrane or cicatricial pemphigoid is a variant that especially targets collagen XVII in the basement membrane of mucous membranes and mucocutaneous junctions[1]. This results in disruption of dermoepidermal cohesion, separation, and subepidermal vesicle formation. The vesicles quickly rupture and most animals present with ulcers and crusting[4]. The condition has been reported in both dogs and cats[5].

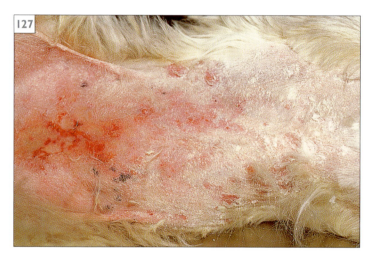

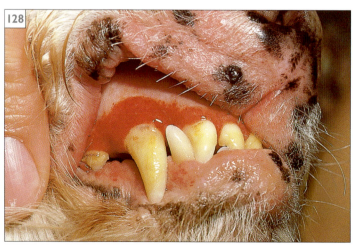

127, 128 Bullous pemphigoid. Ulcerations and erosions on the ventral abdomen (127) and within the oral cavity (128).

CLINICAL FEATURES

Collie breeds appear to be predisposed, although case series are small owing to the rarity of the condition. Most cases present with rapid or acute onset of ulcers and erosions (**127**), which may be confluent and very extensive[4,5]. Predilection sites for lesions include mucocutaneous junctions, axillae, and groin[1,5]. Most cases have ulcerations within the oral cavity (**128**). Pyrexia, septicemia, bacteremia, dehydration, and shock may occur in acute cases with widespread ulceration. Affected animals are usually anorexic and depressed. Occasional cases may have a more chronic course, where crusting is more prominent than ulceration.

DIFFERENTIAL DIAGNOSES

- Pemphigus vulgaris
- Epidermolysis bullosa acquista
- Systemic lupus erythematosus
- Vesicular cutaneous lupus erythematosus
- Drug eruption (Stevens–Johnson syndrome and toxic epidermal necrolysis)
- Cutaneous neoplasia

DIAGNOSIS

The clinical signs are very suggestive of a subepidermal, ulcerating immune-mediated disease. The history may be consistent with a drug eruption, and the presence of polysystemic disease can suggest systemic lupus erythematosus. Clinical examination will confirm the absence of Nikolsky's sign and impression smear cytology will fail to demonstrate acantholysis. Definitive diagnosis usually rests on histopathologic examination of biopsy samples[4,5]. Routine histopathology, however, can only identify a subepidermal disease, and immunologic techniques are necessary to differentiate them[1,5].

MANAGEMENT

The aim of treatment is to induce remission as quickly as possible. High doses of prednisolone (2.0–4.0 mg/kg p/o q12–24h) are key to most therapeutic protocols[4]. The high incidence of severe side-effects at these doses means that if the clinical signs do not improve within 7–14 days, other adjunctive agents should be used in an attempt to reduce the dose of prednisolone. Typically, azathioprine (1.0–2.0 mg/kg p/o q24h to every other day; do not use in cats) is used, although full clinical effects may take 2–6 weeks to become apparent. Other options include chlorambucil (0.1–0.2 mg/kg q24h), cyclophosphamide (50 mg/m^2 body surface area q48h or 4 consecutive days/week), chrysotherapy (aurothioglucose 1.0 mg/kg i/m weekly), dapsone (1 mg/kg q8–12h), sulfasalazine (22–44 mg/kg q8h) and niacinamide/tetracycline (dogs <10 kg: 250 mg of each q8h; dogs >10 kg: 500 mg of each q8h) (doxycycline 10 mg/kg p/o q24h may be used instead of tetracycline)[6-8]. Mycophenolate mofetil (22–39 mg/kg divided q8h) has been used in conjunction with glucocorticoids to manage pemphigus vulgaris successfully in humans[9] and reduce lesions by 50% in a small number of dogs with pemphigus foliaceus, and it may be worth considering in recalcitrant cases. (See Pemphigus foliaceus, p. 155, for general principles of cytotoxic therapy and adverse effects.)

Once remission is attained, the drug doses are slowly tapered to the minimum required to maintain remission. Affected skin will often heal with scarring. The prognosis for bullous pemphigoid is guarded, and in some cases the dosage of medication necessary to maintain remission is still sufficient to produce unacceptable side-effects. Euthanasia may therefore be necessary.

KEY POINTS

- A rare but potentially devastating disease.
- Needs aggressive management, but a very guarded prognosis is appropriate.

Epidermolysis bullosa acquisita

DEFINITION

Epidermolysis bullosa acquisita (acquired epidermolysis bullosa) is an autoimmune blistering disease.

ETIOLOGY AND PATHOGENESIS

In epidermolysis bullosa acquisita, circulating IgG and IgA target the globular aminoterminal NC1 domain of collagen VII in anchoring fibrils that bind to the basement membrane zone[1]. This results in dermoepidermal cleavage. The condition was thought to be rare, but further immunologic studies have shown it to represent up to 25% of subepidermal blistering diseases[2]. Previously, many of these cases may have been misdiagnosed as bullous pemphigoid.

CLINICAL FEATURES

Lesions consist of erythematous macules and urticarial plaques from which transient vesicles develop and rapidly rupture, resulting in ulcers. Lesions develop in the oral cavity, mucocutaneous junctions, and intertriginous or frictional areas such as the face, axillae, and abdomen[2,3]. In rare instances, lesions can develop on the nasal planum and footpads (**129**), and sloughing of the nails may occur[3]. Affected dogs can become febrile and lethargic. Great Danes appear to be predisposed and the disease often develops in animals under 15 months of age[2].

DIFFERENTIAL DIAGNOSES

- Bullous pemphigoid
- Vesicular cutaneous lupus erythematosus of Collies and Shetland Sheepdogs
- Pemphigus vulgaris
- Erythema multiforme
- Bullous drug eruptions
- Hereditary epidermolysis bullosa

DIAGNOSIS

Dermatohistopathology can be suggestive, but is not specific. Definitive diagnosis can be made with direct immunofluorescence studies and antigen immunomapping with collagen IV-specific monoclonal antibodies to demonstrate the specific area of cleavage[1].

MANAGEMENT

Treatment protocols have not been established, but treatment as prescribed for immune-mediated skin conditions may be helpful (see Pemphigus foliaceus, p. 155). Skin trauma should be avoided. Appropriate systemic antibiotics should be given for for secondary bacterial infection if present. Mild cases can be compatible with life, but the prognosis for severe cases is poor.

KEY POINT

- This is an ulcerative skin disease that can be difficult to distinguish from other autoimmune skin diseases that result in ulceration.

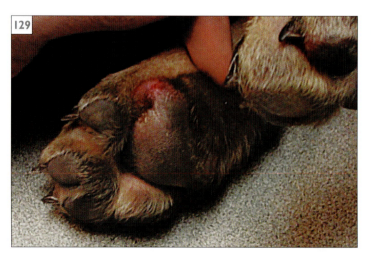

129 Ulceration of the footpad in a dog with epidermolysis bullosa acquisita.

Plasma cell pododermatitis of cats

DEFINITION
Plasma cell pododermatitis is a rare disorder of cats associated with plasma cell infiltration into one or more footpads[1].

ETIOLOGY AND PATHOGENESIS
The cause of the disease is not known, although the presence of elevated serum globulin concentrations, lymphocytosis, plasma cell involvement, and dermoepidermal immune complex deposition suggests an immune-mediated disorder[2,3]. The gradual accumulation of plasma cells and granulation tissue results in soft, poorly defined swelling of the affected pad. Ulceration and secondary infection of the protruding tissue usually follow.

CLINICAL FEATURES
There is no breed, age, or sex predisposition. Usually only a single pad is affected, typically the central metacarpal or metatarsal pad[1]. Occasionally, a digital pad or several pads may be affected[1,2]. Initially, there is a soft, painless swelling of the affected pad (**130**), accompanied by hyperkeratotic, interlacing striae. A pale blue or violet discoloration may be apparent. If the pad ulcerates, a mound of hemorrhagic granulation tissue protrudes. There may be local lymphadenopathy, but discomfort and pain are rare. Secondary infection may ensue in some cases[1] and, rarely, hemorrhage may be significant[2]. Affected cats are generally reported to be negative for feline leukemia virus (FeLV) and feline immunodeficiency virus (FIV). However, in one report, 50% of the cats were FIV positive[4]. Some cats may also develop swelling over the bridge of the nose.

DIFFERENTIAL DIAGNOSES
The clinical presentation is almost unique. Other causes to consider include:
- Bacterial or fungal granuloma
- Collagenolytic granuloma
- Squamous cell carcinoma
- Feline herpesvirus or calicivirus respiratory infection

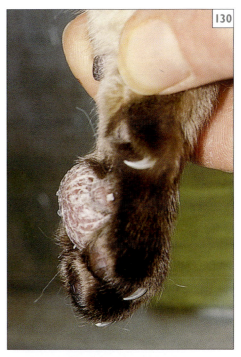

130 Plasma cell pododermatitis. Globose central pad immediately prior to ulceration.

DIAGNOSIS
Stained impression smears may reveal plasma cells. Histopathologic examination of biopsy material is diagnostic.

MANAGEMENT
Doxycycline (5 mg/kg p/o q8h for 4–8 weeks) will cause resolution in a majority of cases[5]. A number of other therapeutic regimes have been reported such as systemic antibacterial agents, glucocorticoids, surgical excision, bandaging, chlorambucil, and chrysotherapy[1–3]. However, they are not as consistently effective as doxycycline.

KEY POINT
- Almost pathognomonic appearance.

Idiopathic ear margin vasculitis (proliferative thrombovascular necrosis of the pinna)

DEFINITION

Idiopathic ear margin vasculitis is a rare disease characterized by ulcerative lesions localized to the margins of the pinna.

ETIOLOGY AND PATHOGENESIS

The pathogenesis of this disease is unknown. However, it is probably an immune-mediated vasculitis caused by immune-complex disease (type III hypersensitivity)[1,2].

CLINICAL FEATURES

Dachshunds are predisposed to this condition, but other breeds may also be affected. Too few cases have been documented to determine if there is an age or sex predisposition. Affected animals first develop alopecia along the margins of the pinna. Then, skin in focal areas (0.2–2.0 cm/0.08–0.8 in) along the very edge of the pinna becomes darkened, slightly thickened, and undergoes necrosis resulting in ulcers (**131**). Typically, both ears are involved and each will have from one to eight lesions. Occasionally, 0.2–0.5 cm (0.08–0.2 in) ulcers will be noted on the inner aspects of the pinna. Lesions do not appear to be painful or pruritic and no other skin lesions or systemic signs are present. The ulcers will slowly enlarge if left untreated.

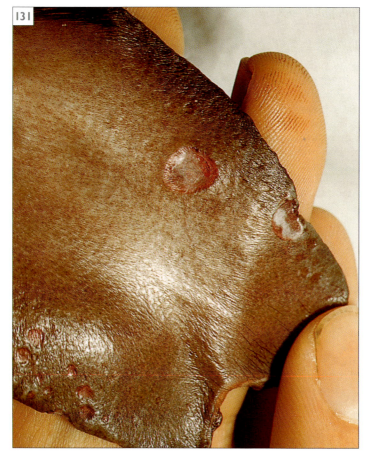

131 Idiopathic ear margin vasculitis. Focal, well-demarcated 'punched-out' lesions on the pinna.

DIFFERENTIAL DIAGNOSES
- Frostbite
- Septic vasculitis
- Immune-mediated vasculitis secondary to other diseases
- Proliferative thrombovascular necrosis[2]
- Disseminated intravascular coagulation
- Cold agglutinin disease
- Cryoglobulinemia
- Ischemic necrosis associated with toxins
- Drug eruption

DIAGNOSIS
Diagnosis is based on history, clinical findings, and histopathologic examination of biopsy samples. Several biopsies may be necessary to demonstrate the classic leukocytoclastic pattern of vasculitis.

MANAGEMENT
The following drugs have been advocated for the treatment of ear margin vasculitis:
- Sulfasalazine (10–20 mg/kg p/o q8h). Once controlled the dose can be reduced to q12h or q24h. (**Note:** Side-effects of this drug include keratoconjunctivitis sicca and hepatotoxicity, therefore animals should be monitored using the Schirmer tear test and liver enzymes tests.) One author (PJM) prefers this treatment option.
- Tetracycline and niacinamide (250 mg of each drug p/o q8h in dogs under 10 kg and 500 mg of each drug p/o q8h in dogs over 10 kg) (doxycycline 10 mg/kg p/o q24h may be used instead of tetracycline). Niacinamide may occasionally cause nausea.
- Pentoxifylline (10–40 mg/kg p/o q8–12h). May occasionally cause nausea. One author (TJN) prefers this drug with or without prednisone.
- Prednisone, prednisolone, or methylprednisolone (1.0–4.0 mg/kg p/o q12h) may also result in resolution of lesions.
- Dapsone (1.0 mg/kg p/o q8h) stops the progression of lesions so that re-epithelialization occurs. Once the lesions have been controlled, the frequency of dosage can be reduced to the least amount necessary to maintain remission. Blood dyscrasias, thrombocytopenia, and hepatotoxicity may occur with dapsone therapy; however, some affected animals will only respond to dapsone[3]. Therefore, hemograms and chemistry profiles should be performed every two weeks during the first six weeks of therapy and monthly thereafter. Toxic changes are generally reversible if the dapsone administration is discontinued.
- Other cytotoxic agents may be considered in recalcitrant cases (see Pemphigus foliaceus, p. 155).

Tissues do not fill back in after undergoing necrosis, therefore the ear margins will still have punched-out areas present even with successful treatment. In most cases the condition is controlled rather than cured. Surgery may be necessary to remove necrotic tissue and one author (PJM) has observed cases resolve, without further treatment, when the ears were cropped.

KEY POINT
- A rare dermatosis, which may be difficult to manage effectively.

Proliferative arteritis of the nasal philtrum

DEFINITION

Proliferative arteritis of the nasal philtrum is a disease that results in ulcers of the nasal philtrum. It may be associated with extensive hemorrhage.

ETIOLOGY AND PATHOGENESIS

The etiology of the arteritis is not known. It is speculated that inflammation of the arterial walls leads to progressive thickening, resulting in partial occlusion, local tissue ischemia, necrosis, and ulceration[1].

CLINICAL FEATURES

Four of five dogs in the original report were Saint Bernards and one was a Giant Schnauzer[1]. It has also been reported in a Newfoundland[2]. Linear ulcers varying from 3–5 cm (1.2–2 in) in length and 2–5 mm (0.8–2 in) in width are found spanning the nasal philtrum (**132**). Arterial bleeding from the ulcers is often noted and may be so severe that it requires surgical repair.

DIFFERENTIAL DIAGNOSES

- The lesions are distinctive, but early lesions may have some features of discoid lupus erythematosus or parasympathetic nasal dermatitis limited to the nasal philtrum
- Trauma

DIAGNOSIS

Diagnosis is based on history and clinical findings.

MANAGEMENT

One author (PJM) has successfully treated these cases with a combination of tetracycline and niacinamide (500 mg each p/o q8h for animals over 15 kg) (doxycycline 10 mg/kg p/o q24h can be used instead of tetracycline) and tacrolimus ointment (0.1%) applied twice daily. Prednisone (1.1 mg/kg p/o q12h) has also been used with or without topical application of flucinolone in dimethyl sulfoxide[2]. Cases unresponsive to the preceding treatments may respond to topical tacrolimus along with cytotoxic drugs such as azathioprine and prednisone/prednisolone. (For specific doses see Pemphigus foliaceus, p. 155.) Surgical intervention may be necessary if there is severe hemorrhage, and removal of the lesion may be curative in some cases.

KEY POINT

- Arterial bleeding from the ulcer can be severe.

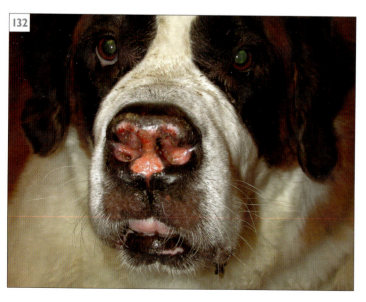

132 Ulceration of the nose in a Saint Bernard with proliferative arteritis of the nasal philtrum.

Vasculopathy of Greyhounds

DEFINITION

Vasculopathy of Greyhounds (cutaneous and renal glomerular vasculopathy, Alabama rot, Greenetrack disease) is a condition characterized by ulcerative skin lesions and renal disease.

ETIOLOGY AND PATHOGENESIS

The pathogenesis is postulated to be due to a Shiga-like toxin produced by *Escherichia coli*[1]. This may be similar to the acute renal failure associated with *E. coli* 0157 infections in humans.

CLINICAL FEATURES

Vasculopathy of Greyhounds is observed predominantly in young adult racing Greyhounds that are often fed a raw meat diet. However, it has also been reported in a Great Dane[2]. The majority of lesions occur on the hindlimbs, but they can occasionally be seen on the forelimbs, trunk, and inguinal region[1]. Edema of the skin is the initial finding, which is followed by erythema[1]. The erythematous skin darkens and becomes black as it becomes necrotic. Sloughing of the skin results in deep ulcers that range from 1–5 cm (0.4–2.0 in) in diameter[1]. Renal involvement can vary in severity, as well as concomitant clinical signs of lethargy, malaise, fever, polydypsia, polyuria, vomiting, and diarrhea[1].

DIFFERENTIAL DIAGNOSES

- Breed, history, clinical signs, and renal disease make the diagnosis obvious
- Drug reactions
- Erythema multiforme
- Immune-mediated vasculitis and other immune-mediated ulcerating diseases
- Venomous snake or spider bite

DIAGNOSIS

Diagnosis is based on history and clinical findings. A serum biochemistry profile can be taken to evaluate renal function and a hemogram to evaluate for thrombocytopenia and anemia. Biopsy can also be performed.

MANAGEMENT

The exudates or crusts should be soaked off with warm water or a solution containing chlorhexidine or other effective antimicrobial. Silver sulfadiazine cream is applied every 12 hours until healed. Appropriate systemic antibacterial therapy is given for control of secondary infection. Supportive fluid therapy should be given. A poor prognosis is warranted for those animals with renal involvement[1].

KEY POINT

- Ulcerative skin disease of Greyhounds that often has concomitant renal disease.

Feline cowpox infection

ETIOLOGY AND PATHOGENESIS

Feline cowpox infection is due to infection with an Orthopox virus indistinguishable from cowpox. It is believed that the virus exists within a reservoir population of small, wild mammals[1]. Cats are infected, presumably by bite wounds, and there is local multiplication at the site of inoculation. Viremia then occurs, with multiple, generalized papulocrustous lesions appearing over the subsequent 7–10 days. These lesions gradually resolve and the cats usually make a complete recovery[2]. A fatal variant with a fulminating generalized infection and vasculitis has been recently described[3].

CLINICAL FEATURES

There is no breed, age, or sex predisposition, but hunting cats are most likely to be affected[1]. Most cases are seen in the late summer and autumn period. The primary lesion, a papulovesicle, is usually on the head or forelimb and may become secondarily infected. Multiple (usually >10) secondary lesions follow, most occurring on the head and trunk[1,2]. These secondary lesions begin as small, firm papules, which enlarge to become flattened, crusted, alopecic areas between 0.5 and 2.0 cm (0.2 and 0.8 in) in diameter (**133**). Occasionally, secondary lesions are erythematous and exudative[1,2]. In most cases the lesions heal within four weeks. The primary lesions may be mildly irritating, but pruritus is not a major feature of this condition.

Systemic complications are rare unless cats are treated with systemic glucocorticoids or other immunosuppressive agents[4] and/or are systemically immunosuppressed (e.g. FIV)[5], although fulminant and fatal cases have been described in the UK[3]. Systemic involvement can include pulmonary lesions (**134**), widespread vasculitis, and secondary bacterial infection (**135**)[6].

DIFFERENTIAL DIAGNOSES

- Cat bite abscess
- Flea bite hypersensitivity
- Dermatophytosis
- Superficial pyoderma
- Mycobacterial infection (feline leprosy)
- Miliary dermatitis
- Eosinophilic granuloma
- Systemic fungal infection

DIAGNOSIS

The history, clinical signs, and local knowledge are suggestive and the diagnosis can be confirmed by biopsy and histopathology, serology, electron microscopy, and virus isolation[4,7,8].

MANAGEMENT

Therapy is supportive and may include fluids, nutritional support, and antibiotics[1,4,5]. Cowpox is zoonotic and barrier precautions should be instituted[9].

KEY POINTS

- Do not give steroids to these cats.
- Potentially zoonotic.

133 Soft, eroding and crusting secondary lesion ('pox') in a cat with cowpox infection.

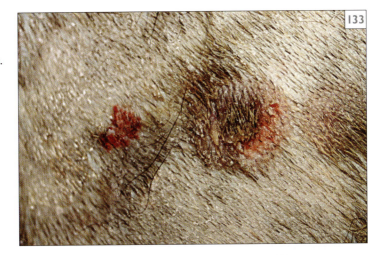

134 Pulmonary lesions in the cat in **133**.

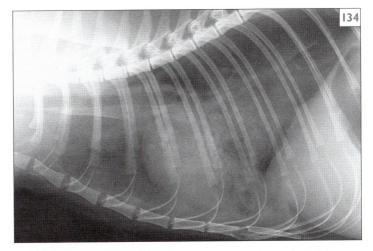

135 Severe secondary infection, cellulitis, and edema in a cat with a highly virulent, fulminant form of cowpox.

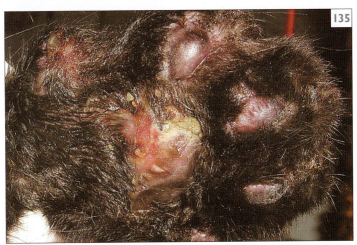

Feline cutaneous herpesvirus and calicivirus infections

ETIOLOGY AND PATHOGENESIS

Feline herpesvirus (feline viral rhinotracheitis virus/FHV) and feline calicivirus (FCV) usually cause upper respiratory tract infection, keratitis, and oral ulceration[1,2]. On rare occasions, cats with active or recent infection develop cutaneous lesions from which virus particles may be isolated[1]. Whether the virus is inoculated during grooming, acts as a secondary invader after ulceration occurs, or arrives by hematogenous or neurogenic spread is not known. However, the virus does multiply within the local epidermis and is not merely a contaminant[3,4]. Immunosuppression associated with poor body condition, stress, FIV or FeLV, and steroids or other immunosuppressive treatments may predispose cats to more generalized viral infections with cutaneous involvement[1]. Highly virulent, systemic strains associated with edema, cutaneous ulceration, and high mortality have recently been described[2,4].

CLINICAL FEATURES

Cats infected with either feline herpesvirus or calicivirus may exhibit concurrent oral ulceration and/or upper respiratory tract infection[1,2,5]. Lesions usually occur on the distal limbs (**136**) or head (**137**, **138**) (particularly the periocular skin), although they may be more generalized. The most common cutaneous lesions are poorly defined moist ulcers, although more discrete crusted lesions are occasionally seen[4–6]. Lesions may appear to be mildly pruritic, especially in the early stages. There may also be local lymphadenopathy.

DIFFERENTIAL DIAGNOSES

- Irritant contact dermatitis
- Cat bite abscessation
- Feline poxvirus infection
- Eosinophilic granuloma syndrome

DIAGNOSIS

The presence of oral or upper respiratory tract viral infection with cutaneous ulceration, particularly if there has been treatment with glucocorticoids and/or any form of stress, is highly suggestive. Affected animals should be checked for FeLV and FIV infection. Histopathologic examination of affected tissue can identify cytopathic changes typical of viral infections[4,5]. Viral isolation from affected tissue, particularly if it is disinfected before sampling, may help confirm active viral infection rather than simple contamination[1,2,4]. Immunohistochemistry, *in-situ* hybridization, and PCR can be used to detect FHV-1 antigen and DNA in affected skin[3,5,6].

MANAGEMENT

Affected cats should not be given systemic glucocorticoids. Systemic broad-spectrum antibacterial drugs should be administered to prevent secondary infection. Cats should be fed a high-quality diet and kept as free from stress as possible. Topical administration of 5-iodo-2'-deoxyuridine solution may be helpful in cases of feline herpesvirus infection. Lysine (500 mg q24h), which can prevent herpesvirus replication, is very safe and easily administered, but it does not destroy the virus or clear infection[7]. Interferon omega (1.5 million IU divided into perilesional and s/c injections given once to twice weekly) successfully resolved facial FHV-1 dermatitis in one cat[8]. Other unproven treatment options include topical idoxuridine or acyclovir and sublingual recombinant human interferon alpha (30 IU)[7]. The dose and efficacy of systemic acyclovir are limited by nephrotoxicity. New antiviral drugs may prove to be more efficacious and better tolerated[7]. Affected cats may become persistent virus carriers[1]. Immunosuppression or stress can trigger recurrent infections.

KEY POINT

- Do not give steroids to cats with skin ulcers.

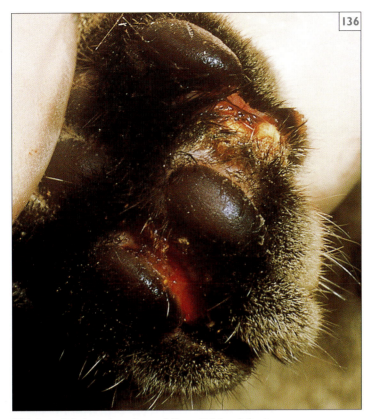

136 Interdigital erosions due to feline calicivirus infection.

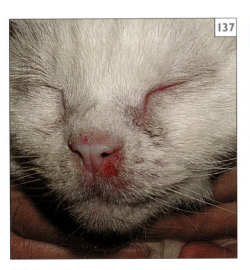

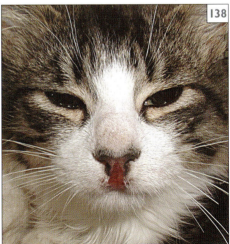

137 Facial ulceration and photophobia due to feline herpesvirus.

138 Ulceration of the nasal philtrum due to feline calicivirus.

Mucocutaneous pyoderma

DEFINITION

Mucocutaneous pyoderma is a syndrome resulting from bacterial infection of the mucocutaneous junctions.

ETIOLOGY AND PATHOGENESIS

The pathogenesis of mucocutaneous pyoderma has not been determined. However, response to systemic and topical antibacterial therapy would indicate the role of bacterial infection in the etiology.

CLINICAL FEATURES

Lesions are most frequently noted on the lips and perioral skin, but they can also be located in the perianal area, planum nasale, eyelids, vulva, and prepuce (**139, 140**). They are characterized by erythema, swelling, and crusts, which are bilaterally symmetrical (they may be unilateral in the nares)[1]. Fissuring, erosions, ulceration, and crusts may occur in severe cases. Depigmentation often occurs and may be prominent[2]. Lesions may be painful and self-trauma can occur. Age or sex predilections have not been noted, but German Shepherd Dogs and GSD crosses may be predisposed[1].

DIFFERENTIAL DIAGNOSES

- Lipfold pyoderma (however, lesions of lipfold pyoderma are generally located in the triangular fold on either side of the lower lip)
- Cutaneous (discoid) lupus erythematosus and other immune-mediated diseases
- Atopic dermatitis (if lesions are confined to the lips)
- Zinc responsive dermatosis
- Localized demodicosis (with demodicosis, lesions usually involve the haired skin)
- *Malassezia* dermatitis
- Epitheliotropic lymphoma
- Metabolic epidermal necrosis

DIAGNOSIS

Diagnosis is based on history, clinical findings, ruling out other differentials, and response to antibiotic therapy.

MANAGEMENT

- Soak off exudates or crusts with warm water or a solution containing chlorhexidine.
- Apply topical antibiotics (e.g. mupirocin, polymyxin B, fusidic acid) every 12 hours until healed, then three days per week or as needed for control.
- If lesions are severe or do not respond to the mupirocin ointment, give systemic antibacterial therapy as described for superficial pyoderma (see Superficial pyoderma, p. 146). Treatment may need to be continued on two or three consecutive days per week for control.

KEY POINT

- Be aware that this is a condition that is generally controlled but not cured.

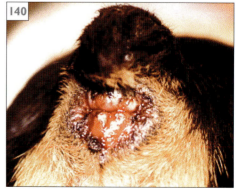

139 Excoriation at commissure of the lips of a dog with mucocutaneous pyoderma.

140 Ulceration of the anus of a dog with mucocutaneous pyoderma.

Nocardiosis

DEFINITION
Nocardiosis is a pyogranulomatous infection due to *Nocardia* spp. organisms.

ETIOLOGY AND PATHOGENESIS
Nocardia spp. are saprophytic aerobic bacteria that enter the body through soil contamination of wounds, inhalation, or ingestion[1,2]. Plant awns may also serve as a means of introducing the organism into tissues. Immunosuppression may predispose animals to infection. Species isolated from lesions of dogs and cats include *N. asteroides*, *N. brasiliensis*, and *N. caviae*[1]. All have a worldwide distribution except *N. brasiliensis*, which is confined to Mexico, Central America, and South America[1]. *Nocardia asteroides* is the species most often associated with lesions in dogs and cats.

CLINICAL FEATURES
Cutaneous infection typically occurs after a wound is contaminated with soil. Draining fistulous tracts, ulcers, abscesses, and subcutaneous nodules are the most common clinical findings (**141, 142**). Additional signs of fever, weakness, lethargy, pyothorax, and dyspnea may develop. Discharge from tracts, ulcers, and abscesses can vary from serosanguineous to sanguinopurulent, and is often described as 'tomato sauce colored'. *Nocardia* spp. may also produce oral lesions.

DIFFERENTIAL DIAGNOSES
- Deep pyoderma
- Pyoderma secondary to other diseases
- Cutaneous infections of systemic fungi
- Cutaneous infections of opportunistic fungi or algae
- Opportunistic mycobacterial infection
- Penetrating foreign bodies
- Panniculitis

DIAGNOSIS
A tentative diagnosis can be made by finding gram-positive, partially acid-fast, branching, filamentous rods on either impression smears or histopathologic examination of biopsy material. Definitive diagnosis is made by culture, which may be difficult[1]. Laboratories to which the samples are submitted should be notified that *Nocardia* spp. have been included in the differential diagnosis, since specialized culture is required.

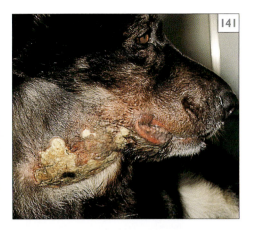

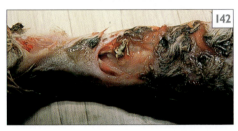

141, 142 Nocardiosis. Lesions on the ventral face and neck of a dog (**141**) and on the forelimb of a cat (**142**).

MANAGEMENT
Drainage should be established for all lesions. The *in vitro* susceptibility of *Nocardia* spp. does not necessarily predict *in vivo* efficacy[1]. Sulfadiazine (80 mg/kg p/o q8h) is effective for the majority of cases. Alternatives include minocycline (5–25 mg/kg p/o q12h), erythromycin (10 mg/kg p/o q8h), clindamycin (11 mg/kg p/o q12h), and ampicillin (20–40 mg/kg p/o q6h). Amikacin (8–12 mg/kg i/m or s/c q8h) is also highly effective[1]. Treatment will generally take at least six weeks and should be continued one month beyond clinical cure. Owners should be warned that some cases will not respond and that relapses may occur.

KEY POINT
- Cats with non-responsive abscessation should be checked for FeLV infection and samples should be submitted for culture and sensitivity testing (both aerobic and anaerobic).

Blastomycosis

DEFINITION

Blastomycosis occurs as a consequence of infection by *Blastomyces dermatidis*.

ETIOLOGY AND PATHOGENESIS

Cutaneous lesions usually occur as a consequence of hematologic spread after inhalation of spores[1,2]. Therefore, in addition to cutaneous lesions, most cases have internal granulomas, especially in the lungs. However, primary cutaneous infection may occur after inoculation of wounds[1,2]. Large, adult, entire male hunting and sporting dogs are predisposed to blastomycosis[3], presumably because of the risk of traumatic inoculation. The organism is presumed to be a soil saprophyte, more likely to be found in moist, acidic, or sandy soil containing decaying wood, animal feces, or other organic enrichment[4]. The disease has a geographic distribution within river valleys of Southern Canada and the Midwestern United States. Humans may be infected from the same sources as animals, but they are not commonly infected following exposure to animal tissues and the disease is not therefore considered a true zoonosis.

CLINICAL FEATURES

Most clinical signs are slow to develop, with little signs of pain, except perhaps lameness. The clinical signs will vary according to the degree of systemic involvement and the organs affected. However, pulmonary signs are seen in 65–85% of cases. Wide dissemination to lymph nodes, skin, oral and nasal mucosae, gastrointestinal tract, bones, and central nervous system may be seen in a small number of animals[1,2], and these animals might be expected to show weight loss, anorexia, and lethargy in addition to signs referable to specific organ involvement. The cutaneous signs include subcutaneous nodules and masses, draining tracts, and recurrent abscessation (**143**)[1,2].

DIFFERENTIAL DIAGNOSES

- Penetrating foreign body
- Demodicosis
- Panniculitis
- Feline leprosy and atypical mycobacterial infection
- Other subcutaneous mycoses
- Cuterebriasis or dracunculiaisis
- Cutaneous neoplasia
- Histiocytic lesions
- Sterile nodular granuloma and pyogranuloma

DIAGNOSIS

Diagnosis is usually made by cytologic examination of exudates and aspirates, which reveal 5–20 µm refractile double-walled, broad-based budding yeast (**144**), by histopathologic examination of excised tissues, and by serologic methods[1,2], although diagnosis by serologic means alone is not recommended. However, submission of urine for *Blastomyces* antigen detection by enzyme immunoassay has a sensitivity of 95.5%[5]. Thoracic radiographs will often show a generalized interstitial to nodular infiltrate[4].

MANAGEMENT

Systemic mycoses require systemic medication and treatment may be necessary for several months. Amphotericin B (see Leishmaniasis, p. 198), alone or in combination with 5-fluorocytosine or ketoconazole, has been recommended[1,2,6]. Amphotericin B is nephrotoxic and 5-fluorocytosine is a bone marrow depressant; therefore, clinicians considering the use of these agents should read the detailed references. Currently, the treatment of choice is itraconazole (10 mg/kg p/o q24h). The treatment should be continued 30 days beyond clinical and radiologic resolution of the lesions.

KEY POINT

- If you diagnose this disease, be sure to ensure that there are no systemic lesions; do not treat it as just a skin disease.

143, 144
Blastomycosis. A discharging sinus and nodular lesion in the groin of a Labrador Retriever due to blastomycosis (143); a photomicrograph demonstrating the refractile, spheroid shape of *Blastomyces* spp. (144).

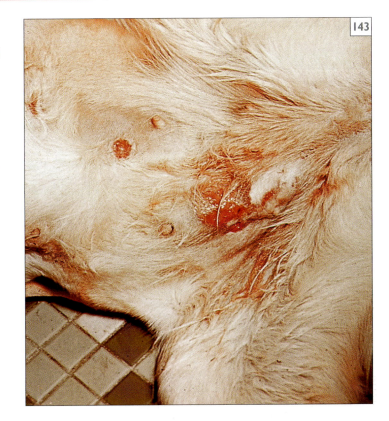

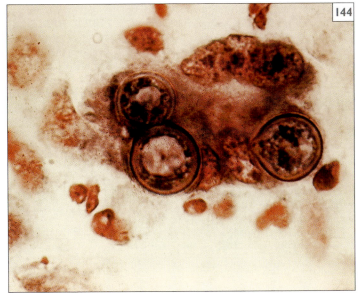

Sporotrichosis

DEFINITION

Sporotrichosis is a subacute or chronic pyogranulomatous infectious disease of dogs and cats caused by the dimorphic fungus *Sporothrix schenckii*.

ETIOLOGY AND PATHOGENESIS

The organism is found worldwide and grows as a saprophytic mycelial fungus in moist organic debris[1]. Infection occurs via inoculation of the fungus into the skin by thorns or plant material, or by contamination of open wounds or broken skin with exudates from infected animals[1]. In a host the organism establishes infection in the yeast form. The number of organisms found in draining fluids is much greater in cats than in other species, which increases the risk of transmission to other animals or humans[2]. Motile organisms have been found to penetrate intact human skin[3].

CLINICAL FEATURES

Typical lesions appear as papular or nodular swellings 3–5 weeks after inoculation[1]. Lesions become alopecic, crusted, and ulcerated, draining a reddish-brown serosanguineous fluid[2]. They are more common on the dorsal aspects of the head and trunk, but the extremities may also be involved (**145, 146**). Regional lymphadenopathy is common and affected lymph nodes may fistulate. Occasionally, lesions may extend along the lymphatics or become disseminated to bone, eyes, GI tract, CNS, and other visceral organs[1].

DIFFERENTIAL DIAGNOSES

- Cutaneous infections of systemic fungi
- Subcutaneous mycoses or algal infections
- Demodicosis
- Deep pyoderma
- Opportunistic mycobacterial infection
- Penetrating foreign bodies
- Panniculitis
- Histiocytic or sterile pyogranuloma or granuloma syndrome lesions

DIAGNOSIS

Impression smears or biopsies may reveal the round, oval, or cigar-shaped yeast, which may be extracellular or within macrophages or inflammatory cells. Organisms are often present in small numbers and may be difficult to demonstrate with routine stains. Preferred stains for demonstration of the organism are PAS or GMS. Fluorescent antibody techniques are helpful for demonstration of the organisms. Diagnosis can also be made by culture or by inoculation of laboratory animals.

MANAGEMENT

Potassium or sodium iodide is the treatment of choice. In the dog, sodium iodide solution (44 mg/kg of a 20% solution p/o q8h) is given for 7–8 weeks or one month beyond clinical cure[1]. The dose in cats is decreased (22 mg/kg q8h or q12h) due to the marked sensitivity of the feline species to iodine preparations[1]. Signs of iodide toxicity include fever, ptyalism, ocular and nasal discharges, anorexia, hyperexcitability, dry hair coat with excess scaling of the skin, vomiting or diarrhea, depression, twitching, hypothermia, and cardiovascular failure. Itraconazole (10 mg/kg p/o q24h) has been used successfully in dogs[4] and in cats, and its use may be preferable from the outset.

PUBLIC HEALTH SIGNIFICANCE

As there are documented cases of humans acquiring sporotrichosis by contact with ulcerated wounds or fluids from lesions, extreme care should be taken in handling infected animals, exudates, or contaminated materials. There is a greater risk associated with cats.

KEY POINT

- Zoonotic potential.

145, 146
Sporotrichosis.
Generalized cutaneous
lesions in a dog (**145**);
nodular form on the
face of a cat (**146**).

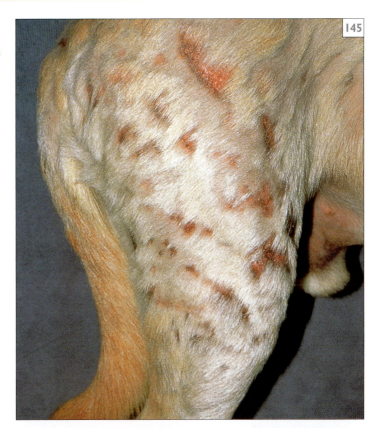

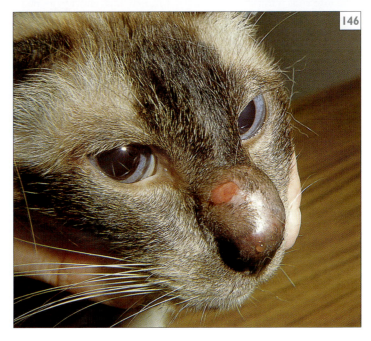

Calcinosis cutis

DEFINITION

Calcinosis cutis results from dystrophic mineralization of the dermal and adnexal elastin and collagen fibers, and is virtually pathognomonic for hyperadrenocorticism (see Hyperadrenocorticism, p. 237)[1].

ETIOLOGY AND PATHOGENESIS

Calcinosis cutis has not been reported in cats. The mechanism that results in the deposition of soluble calcium and phosphate ions onto the collagen and elastin matrix is not known, but probably involves steroid-induced abnormalities in parathyroid hormone metabolism. A chronic, granulomatous, inflammatory response is commonly induced by the mineralization[1]. Calcinosis cutis is more commonly associated with iatrogenic hyperadrenocorticism rather than the naturally occurring disease[2]. The reason for this is not known. Calcinosis cutis occurs in a variable proportion of cases (1.7–40%[3,4]), presumably reflecting the various proportions of iatrogenic to naturally occurring disease in case series. In rare instances calcinosis cutis can be idiopathic or secondary to inflammatory diseases.

CLINICAL FEATURES

Calcinosis cutis is usually found on the dorsum or in the axillae or groins[4]. Dogs typically present with erosive, crusted, ulcerated, and gritty-feeling patches of erythema and erythematous or crusted papules (**147, 148**). It may also present as yellow-pink hard plaque-like lesions. Close examination may reveal an accumulation of pale mineral within intact lesions. The affected areas are often secondarily infected, particularly if mineral is being slowly eliminated through the skin, and these cases are usually extremely pruritic, failing to respond to both systemic antibacterial and glucocorticoid therapy.

DIFFERENTIAL DIAGNOSES

- Pyotraumatic dermatosis
- Superficial or deep pyoderma
- Other causes of dystrophic or metastatic calcification
- Irritant dermatitis
- Cutaneous neoplasia

DIAGNOSIS

The degree of pruritus is often the first indication that these lesions are not simply pyoderma. Many, but not all, dogs will have other signs suggestive of internal disease (e.g. polyuria/polydipsia, muscle wasting, and exercise intolerance), which will raise suspicion of hyperadrenocorticism. Close examination and palpation of the lesions will often allow an appreciation of mineralization. This is even more apparent when skin scrapes and biopsy samples are taken. Histopathologic examination of biopsy samples may be necessary to provide a definitive diagnosis. Once calcinosis cutis is identified, a search for the underlying cause should be made.

MANAGEMENT

Identify and attend to the underlying cause of the mineralization. If the cause is iatrogenic, animals should be weaned from glucocorticoid therapy. Complete resolution is to be anticipated provided the underlying problem is treatable. There are anecdotal reports that application of dimethyl sulfoxide (DMSO) to lesions twice daily will hasten resolution. If DMSO is applied to extensive lesions, blood calcium levels should be monitored, as mobilization of calcium from the skin lesions may cause hypercalcemia. One author (TJN) has noted several cases of calcinosis cutis that either worsened or first appeared following discontinuation of glucocorticoid therapy or effective medical or surgical management of spontaneous hyperadrenocorticism. Lesions in these cases eventually resolved.

KEY POINT

- The pruritus associated with this dermatosis may be refractory to steroid therapy.

147 Calcinosis cutis causing ulceration, crusting, and papules in the groin and medial thighs of a dog with iatrogenic hyper-adrenocorticism.

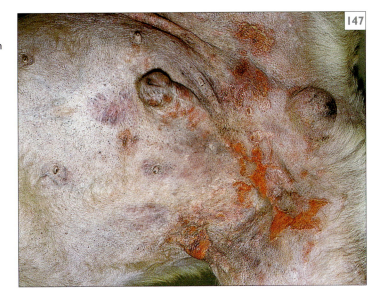

148 White papules and plaques of calcinosis cutis.

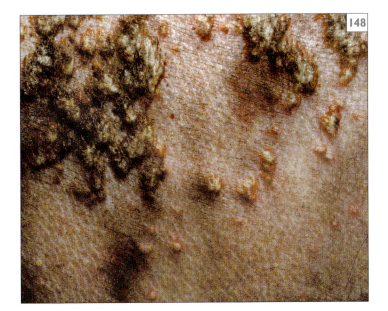

Squamous cell carcinoma

ETIOLOGY AND PATHOGENESIS

Squamous cell carcinoma (SCC) is a common, malignant neoplasm of dogs and cats arising from epidermal squames. Long-term exposure to actinic radiation is a major risk factor, particularly in lightly pigmented skin[1-4]. UVB radiation is oncogenic and locally immunosuppressive, inhibiting local immune surveillance[2]. Undoubtedly, there are other factors involved in the etiology of cases not directly attributable to actinic radiation[3]. SCC has been associated with chronic inflammatory disease and other epithelial tumors[1,5]. Multicentric SCC in situ (Bowen's-like disease) has been associated with chronic immunosuppression with prednisolone and ciclosporin (cyclosporine) in a dog[6] and in cats with FIV[7]. SCCs arise in the epidermis, are locally invasive, but have a low metastatic potential[3,4].

CLINICAL FEATURES

SCCs tend to occur in older animals. Dalmatians, Bull Terriers, Boxers, and white-haired cats are predisposed[3]. Early signs of actinic damage in exposed sites include erythema, lichenification, scaling, and cutaneous horns. In dogs, SCCs tend to occur on the trunk and limbs (**149, 150**) rather than on the head, whereas in cats the head, especially the pinnae (**151**), is a predisposed site[3,4]. Clinically, there appear to be two presentations: a proliferative, vegetative form that is often ulcerated (**152**) and, less commonly, an erosive ulcerating form[3,4]. Pedal SCCs have a more aggressive nature and metastasize early[8]. Black Standard Poodles are predisposed to digital SCCs at the junction of the skin and nail[8]. More than one toe on several feet may be involved. Digital SCC is easily mistaken for paronychia in the early stages[8] (see Disorders of the nails, p. 268).

DIFFERENTIAL DIAGNOSES

- Traumatic injury
- Localized pyoderma
- Dermatophytosis
- Demodicosis
- Subcutaneous mycobacterial, filamentous bacterial, and fungal infections
- Other cutaneous neoplasms

DIAGNOSIS

The clinical signs are highly suggestive, particularly if actinic changes are present. Impression smears, however, can be misleading because of non-specific surface inflammation and bacterial contamination. Neoplastic keratinocytes can nevertheless be seen on representative smears from scraped samples or after removing scales and cutaneous horns[9]. Biopsy and histopathology are diagnostic and will help determine the grade and invasiveness of the tumor.

MANAGEMENT

SCCs should be staged for local invasion and distant metastasis before treatment[4,8]. Surgical excision with wide margins is usually curative[3,4,10,11]. Digital SCCs may be managed with digital or limb amputation, but they tend to metastasize to the local lymph node and the lungs relatively early[8]. Adequate surgical resection and reconstruction and facial lesions can be difficult, particularly in cats[3,11]. Photodynamic therapy using topical EI aminolevulinic acid cream with exposure to red light of 635nm[12], or aluminum phthalocyanine tetrasulfonate with irradiation power densities of 100 mW/cm^2 and energy densities of 100 J/cm^2 [13], appears to be effective in cats. Radiotherapy with megavoltage irradiation[10], hypofractionated radiation[14], or strontium 90[15] is effective in appropriate cases without spread to local lymph nodes. Laser therapy and cryosurgery are best reserved for early, shallow lesions, as it is difficult adequately to ablate all neoplastic cells in later lesions[8].

KEY POINTS

- Non-responsive ulceration should be biopsied.
- Most SCCs are locally invasive but not metastatic; however, they should be staged before treatment.

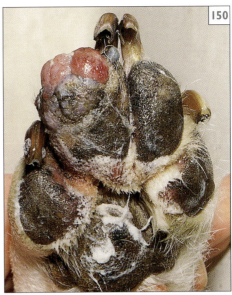

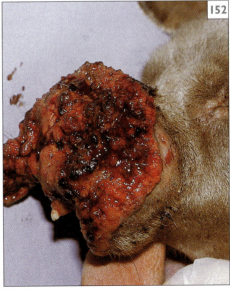

149 Squamous cell carcinoma on the precrural fold of a dog.

150 Ulcerated nodule of squamous cell carcinoma on the toe of a dog.

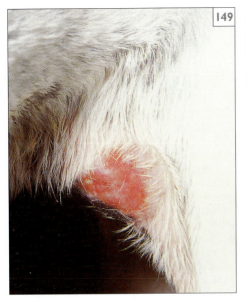

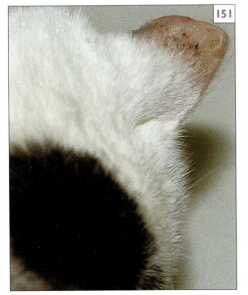

151 Squamous cell carcinoma on the pinna of a cat.

152 Squamous cell carcinoma on the face of a Weimaraner. Note the very proliferative nature of this neoplasm.

Metabolic epidermal necrosis

DEFINITION

Metabolic epidermal necrosis is an uncommon skin disorder variously known as diabetic dermatopathy, hepatocutaneous syndrome, necrolytic migratory erythema, and superficial necrolytic dermatitis.

ETIOLOGY AND PATHOGENESIS

Metabolic epidermal necrosis is associated with metabolic diseases such as a hepatopathy, diabetes mellitus, and glucagon-secreting pancreatic tumors (glucagonoma)[1–4]. It is uncommon in dogs[1] and very rare in cats[5]. The syndrome in humans is generally associated with hyperglucagonemia resulting from a glucagon-secreting pancreatic islet cell tumor[1,4]. Although cases of metabolic epidermal necrosis due to glucagon-producing pancreatic tumors have been reported in dogs[2,6], the majority of cases do not have a pancreatic neoplasm. Abnormalities of the liver characterized by moderate to severe vacuolation of hepatocytes, parenchymal collapse, and nodular regeneration are present in the majority of cases[4,7]. However, most animals with liver disease do not have metabolic epidermal necrosis, which suggests that the pathogenesis involves a specific underlying metabolic dysfunction rather than primary liver disease. In one report, 44% of cases were associated with phenobarbital administration[7]. Increased plasma glucagon may play a role, even though levels are generally normal in dogs in which they have been evaluated[4,6]. Explanations for this include poor sensitivity or specificity of the assay, poor correlation of plasma glucagon levels with increased pancreatic secretion, or a non-immunoreactive enteric form of glucagon. Hyperglycemia and diabetes mellitus are noted in many dogs, but these tend to occur after hepatic and cutaneous disease and are not therefore thought to be involved in the pathogenesis[4]. Most affected dogs have markedly decreased plasma amino acid levels, which may lead to epidermal protein depletion and necrolysis[4,7,8]. Other potential factors involve decreased levels or altered metabolism of zinc and essential fatty acids[4].

CLINICAL FEATURES

Metabolic epidermal necrosis is a disease of older dogs, and cutaneous changes generally precede systemic illness. No sex predisposition has been noted[1,4,7], although the condition may be more frequent in West Highland White Terriers and Shetland Sheepdogs[8]. Some dogs may have a history of weight loss. Hyperkeratosis, scaling, crusting, and cracking of the digital pads are the most consistent clinical findings (**153, 154**)[1,4,6,7] and may result in lameness.

The scales are typically large, thick, and tightly adherent. Erythema, scaling, erosion, ulceration, and crusting (**155**) occur on the muzzle, mucocutaneous junctions, ears, pressure points (elbows, hocks, hips, and stifles), genitalia, abdomen, and axillae[1,4,6,7,9]. Ulcerations of the oral cavity are seen in some cases. Dullness, inappetence, and polyuria/polydipsia may occur in the later stages, with overt hepatic failure and/or diabetes mellitus. Rarely, animals may present in a ketoacidotic crisis. Secondary pyoderma and *Malassezia* dermatitis are common[1].

DIFFERENTIAL DIAGNOSES

- Pemphigus foliaceus
- Cutaneous or systemic lupus erythematosus
- Zinc responsive dermatosis
- Superficial bacterial or fungal infections
- Epitheliotropic lymphoma
- Primary keratinization defect
- Demodicosis

DIAGNOSIS

The history and clinical signs are highly suggestive. Histopathology of skin biopsies reveals a typical 'red, white, and blue' pattern consisting of parakeratosis and parakeratotic crusts, acanthosis with prominent intracellular edema in the mid-epidermis, and a lichenoid mononuclear cell infiltrate[1,6,7,9]. Several biopsies may be necessary, as these findings are variable and inconsistent in any one sample. Hematology and biochemistry usually reveal elevated glucose, AP, and ALT, with abnormal bile acid stimulation tests[1], but most cases do not have overt liver failure[7]. These parameters may, however, be normal. Plasma amino acids may be low[6–8], and plasma glucagon

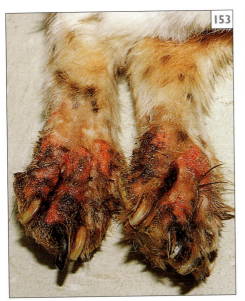

153 Metabolic epidermal necrosis. Erythema, erosions, crust, and alopecia on the distal limbs of a Springer Spaniel.

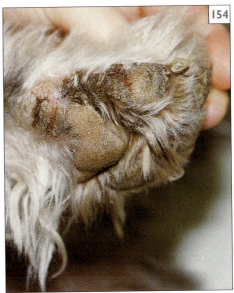

154 Metabolic epidermal necrosis. Pedal lesions characterized by severe crusting of the footpads.

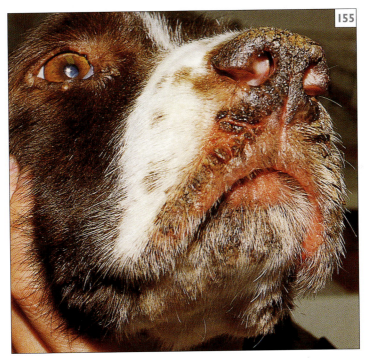

155 Metabolic epidermal necrosis. Erythema, erosions, crust, and alopecia on the face of a Springer Spaniel. (Photo courtesy S Torres)

may be elevated if a glucagonoma is present[2,6]. Radiography is non-specific, but affected livers have a typically mixed hyper- and hypoechoeic, 'honeycomb'-like appearance on ultrasonography[7,9]. Further investigation including ultrasound-guided biopsy may be necessary to confirm liver pathology consistent with hepatocutaneous syndrome (parenchymal necrosis and nodular regeneration). Hepatic cirrhosis may be present in some cases[9]. Other tests may be required to detect a glucagonoma or diabetes mellitus.

MANAGEMENT

Metabolic epidermal necrosis due to causes other than glucagonoma is associated with serious internal disease and the prognosis is poor, with most dogs dying or being euthanased within five months of the development of cutaneous lesions[1,7]. Despite this, aggressive therapy can result in prolonged survival times for a year or more in some dogs[9].

The evidence for aberrant protein, zinc, and/or essential fatty acid (EFA) metabolism suggests that nutritional support should be beneficial. Critical care or liver specific prescription diets with high-quality proteins[9] can be fed as the main diet if the dog will accept a change of food. High-quality protein supplements include 3–6 egg yolks, powdered casein, or proprietary amino acid combinations[9]. Zinc (see Zinc responsive dermatosis, p. 204) and EFA supplements can also be given[9]. Intravenous amino acids have been very successful in some dogs. Most protocols use 8–10% solutions given at 25 ml/kg over 6–8 hours using a jugular catheter. (One author [TJN] routinely uses cephalic or saphenous catheters.) Dogs should be monitored for signs of hepatic encephalopathy and plasma ammonia should be monitored every 2–4 hours if possible. Other therapies for hepatic disease that may be of benefit include S-adenosylmethionine and ursodeoxycholic acid, although the evidence is largely anecdotal. Colchicine may aid dogs with hepatic cirrhosis[9].

If a glucagonoma is diagnosed, surgical removal is the treatment of choice, although the surgery can be difficult and is associated with significant postoperative mortality[2,6]. The somatostatin analog octreotide, which inhibits glucagon release, may temporarily ameliorate clinical signs if surgery is not appropriate or if metastases are present.

Hair should be clipped from moist lesions to avoid matting and crusting. Gentle bathing with anti-scaling and/or antimicrobial shampoos will facilitate resolution of secondary infections and open lesions. Keratolytic and emollient products may help reduce scaling and fissuring. Systemic antimicrobials may be necessary in some cases, but care should be taken to avoid drugs that require hepatic metabolism and excretion.

KEY POINTS
- History and clinical signs are usually enough to suggest the diagnosis, but histopathologic examination of a biopsy sample is mandatory.
- The prognosis is guarded to poor, but prolonged survival times can be achieved with aggressive therapy.

Decubital ulcers
(pressure sores)

DEFINITION
Decubital ulcers (pressure sores) occur mainly over bony prominences because of continual localized pressure to the skin.

ETIOLOGY AND PATHOGENESIS
Animals that are recumbent due to neurologic deficits or musculoskeletal problems are predisposed to decubital ulcers. Compression of the skin and subcutaneous tissue collapses blood vessels, resulting in ischemia, necrosis, and subsequent ulceration. Laceration, friction, burns from heating pads, irritation from urine or fecal material, malnutrition secondary to inadequate diet, anemia, or hypoproteinemia may also be contributing factors[1]. Cutaneous atrophy due to spontaneous or iatrogenic hyperadrenocorticism, including topical drugs, may also predispose to ulcers.

CLINICAL FEATURES
The initial clinical finding is hyperemia. Tissue necrosis and ulceration follow if the pressure is not relieved. Lesions most frequently occur in skin overlying the scapular acromion, lateral epicondyle of the humerus, tuber ischii, tuber coxae, trochanter major of the femur, lateral condyle of the tibia (**156**), and the lateral sides of the fifth digits of the forelimbs and hindlimbs. Secondary bacterial infection can lead to undermining of the skin beyond the ulcer edges. Osteomyelitis can develop in bone underlying the ulcer.

DIFFERENTIAL DIAGNOSES
- Cutaneous neoplasia
- Pyoderma
- Deep mycotic or mycobacterial infection

DIAGNOSIS
Diagnosis is based on clinical findings and histopathologic examination of biopsy samples. Appropriate testing may be necessary if an underlying disease is suspected.

MANAGEMENT
Ideally, decubital ulcers should be prevented by turning the recumbent animal frequently (every two hours) and providing soft bedding such as a water mattress. Providing adequate nutrition and keeping the skin clean, via twice daily bathing or whirlpool baths, is also important, particularly in the long-term hospitalized patient. Particular attention should be paid to protecting the skin from contact with urine by using a cage rack and applying petrolatum to areas of skin that urine is likely to contact[2]. Once ulcers have developed, they may be managed by either non-surgical or surgical means. Non-surgical management consists of wound lavage and topical antibacterial therapy such as silver sulfadiazine[2]. Doughnut bandages can be placed over the ulcer to avoid direct pressure on the wound. Surgical treatment is accomplished by debridement of necrotic and infected tissue and wound closure to heal by primary intention[1]. The preventive measures previously mentioned must be strictly adhered to following surgery.

KEY POINT
- Be aware that decubital ulcers can occur in hospitalized patients.

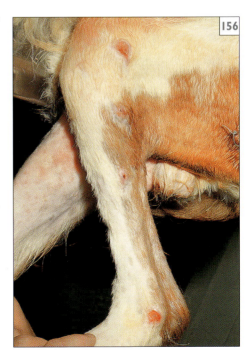

156 Decubital ulcers overlying bony prominences on the lateral stifle and hock of a dog.

Ehlers–Danlos syndrome
(cutaneous asthenia, dermatosparaxis)

DEFINITION
Ehlers–Danlos syndrome comprises an inherited group of congenital connective tissue dysplasias characterized by loose, hyperextensible, abnormally fragile skin that is easily torn by minor trauma.

ETIOLOGY AND PATHOGENESIS
Several forms of this syndrome, with different clinical, genetic, and biochemical changes, have been recognized in dogs, cats, man, cattle, and sheep[1]. All of these forms have a common basis in that they are accompanied by connective tissue weakness due to abnormalities in biosynthesis or post-translational modifications of collagen[1]. The main form of Ehlers–Danlos syndrome in the dog is a dominantly inherited collagen packing defect characterized by focal or diffuse areas of severely disorganized fibers with many abnormally large fibrils[1]. The tensile strength of affected skin is 4% of that of non-affected skin[1]. Two forms of the syndrome have been reported in the cat: a dominant form similar to the collagen packing defect of dogs, and a recessive form characterized by a deficiency of N-procollagen peptidase enzyme, which results in collagen that is in the form of twisted ribbons instead of cylindrical fibrils and fibers[2,3].

CLINICAL FEATURES
Ehlers–Danlos syndrome has been documented in the Beagle, Boxer, English Setter, English Springer Spaniel, Greyhound, Irish Setter, Keeshond, Saint Bernard, German Shepherd Dog, Manchester Terrier, Welsh Corgi, Red Kelpi, Soft-coated Wheaten Terrier, Toy Poodle, Garafiano Shepherd Dog, Fila Brasiliero, mixed breed dogs, and Himalayan and domestic long- and shorthair cats[4]. One author (TJN) has also seen this syndrome in a Staffordshire Bull Terrier and a Neapolitan Mastiff. Fragility, hyperextensibility, and sagging or loose skin since birth are the most characteristic clinical findings (**157**). Animals may be presented with multiple scars or tears in the skin (**158**). Joint laxity may be an additional finding in some animals and can result in osteoarthritis.

DIFFERENTIAL DIAGNOSES
The syndrome is distinctive for dogs. Cats may develop fragile skin due to naturally occurring or iatrogenic hyperglucocorticoidism, diabetes mellitus, with excessive use of megestrol acetate, and with feline acquired skin fragility syndrome[5].

DIAGNOSIS
Diagnosis is based on history, clinical findings, biopsy for light or electron microscopy, cell culture, and biochemical study of collagen.

MANAGEMENT
Any tears of the skin that are present should be sutured and the animal's lifestyle adjusted so as to minimize trauma to the skin. Affected animals should not be used for breeding.

KEY POINT
• Rare congenital disease characterized by fragility and hyperextensibility of the skin.

157 Hyper-extensibility of the skin in a cat with cutaneous asthenia.

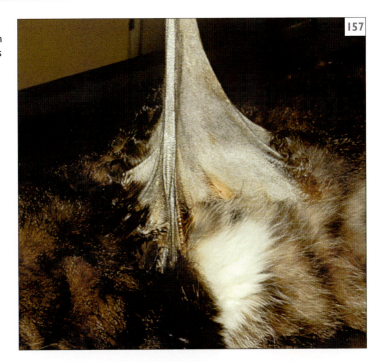

158 Crusts and ulcers resulting from minor trauma in the fragile skin of a cat with cutaneous asthenia.

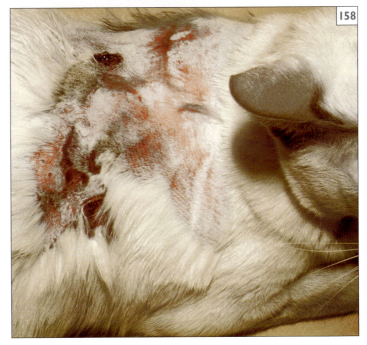

Papular and pustular dermatoses

General approach

- These conditions are common, but intact pustules are uncommon in dogs and cats
- Superficial pyoderma is common and frequently misdiagnosed
- Multiple pustules and crusts in sites unusual for pyoderma suggest pemphigus foliaceus
- Pustules may also be seen in demodicosis, dermatophytosis, deep pyoderma, calcinosis cutis, drug eruptions, and rare sterile pustular immune-mediated conditions

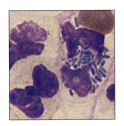
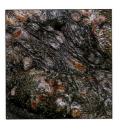
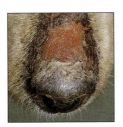
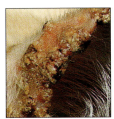

Superficial pyoderma

ETIOLOGY AND PATHOGENESIS

Superficial pyoderma describes cutaneous bacterial infection that is confined to the stratum corneum of the interfollicular skin and hair follicles. Normal canine and feline skin is colonized by a variety of resident bacterial and fungal organisms. These are not normally pathogenic and they may help prevent colonization by pathogenic species through niche competition. Potential pathogens such as coagulase-positive staphylococci frequently colonize mucocutaneous junctions from where they are seeded to the skin by licking and grooming. Mucosal reservoirs are, therefore, an important source of transient contamination and potential infection[1]. Infection with gram-negative species can result from oro-fecal or environmental contamination[2].

Most skin infections develop when a combination of virulence factors and alterations to the cutaneous microenvironment allow the microorganisms to overwhelm the physical, chemical, and immunologic skin defenses (*Table 5*). Primary or idiopathic recurrent superficial pyoderma is rare and most recurrent pyodermas are secondary to underlying cutaneous or systemic disorders such as ectoparasites, hypersensitivities, endocrinopathies, and keratinization defects[3]. The phenomenon of quorum sensing, however, enables staphylococci to turn on virulence factors (including coagulase, superantigens, protein A, and hemolysins) once a certain population density is reached. This results in epidermal damage, inflammation, and changes to the microenvironment that permit further bacterial colonization and proliferation[4,5]. Staphylococci and *Malassezia* may also produce mutually beneficial growth factors.

The vast majority of canine pyodermas are associated with coagulase-positive staphylococci. The most common species is *Staphylococcus intermedius*, although *S. aureus*, *S. hyicus*, and *S. schleiferi* have also been isolated, particularly in North America[6–8]. It is possible that these species have been underestimated, as some laboratories do not speciate coagulase-positive staphylococci isolated from dogs. Superficial pyoderma is much less common in cats, and is associated with a wider range of organisms including *S. intermedius*, *S. felis*, *S. aureus*, *Pasteurella multocida*, and anaerobes (although the latter are more common in abscesses)[9].

Methicillin-resistant species including *S. intermedius*, *S. aureus*, and *S. schleiferi* have been recently isolated from dogs and cats[10–12]. The latter two species were more likely to be associated with deeper, opportunistic infections compared with *S. intermedius*[13].

Table 5 Primary causes of skin infections	
Underlying condition	**Etiology**
Allergic, pruritic, and inflammatory dermatoses	Self-trauma degrades cutaneous barrier; increased skin humidity and temperature; seeding of staphylococci and *Malassezia* by licking; increased staphylococcal adherence to atopic keratinocytes; immunosuppressive treatment
Keratinization defects and seborrhea	Disordered desquamation and degraded cutaneous barrier; altered sebum; follicular hyperkeratosis and obstruction
Endocrinopathies and metabolic diseases	Immunosuppression; keratinization defects
Immunosuppression	Congenital or acquired immunodeficiency; anti-inflammatory or immunosuppressive treatment
Anatomy	Body folds, thick coats, etc. that increase temperature and moisture
Iatrogenic	Overbathing removes sebum and macerates the skin; poor nutrition affects skin, hair, sebum, and immunity; dirty environment

159 Bullous impetigo in a dog with hyper-adrenocorticism.

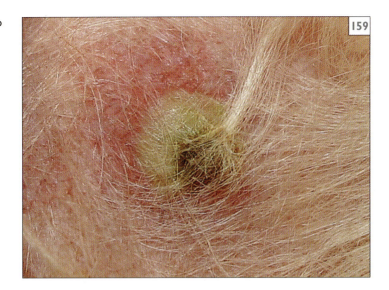

160 Erythematous papules, pustules, and epidermal collarettes in a dog with bacterial folliculitis.

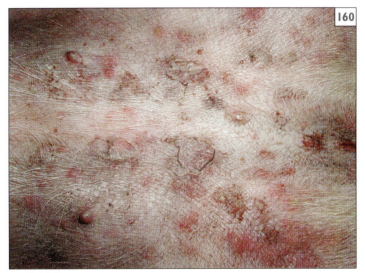

CLINICAL FEATURES

Superficial pyodermas are associated with pruritus, erythema, papules, pustules, epidermal collarettes, and multifocal alopecia (especially obvious in short coated breeds).

Impetigo

Impetigo (**159**) causes non-follicular pustules, with secondary epidermal collarettes and scaling in young animals, particularly if poorly cared for, and in adolescence. Bullous impetigo, characterized by large, flaccid non-follicular pustules, is seen in older animals that are immunosuppressed (e.g. hypothyroidism, hyperadrenocorticism, diabetes mellitus, and chemotherapy). Impetigo is not typically pruritic.

Folliculitis

Folliculitis (**160**) is the most common form of pyoderma. The papules and pustules are small and associated with a hair follicle. Shorthaired dogs often present with patchy tufting of the hairs, which are shed, leaving small oval patches of alopecia and hyperpigmentation with a scaly rim (**161**). Bacterial folliculitis is an uncommon cause of military dermatitis in cats[14].

Superficial spreading pyoderma

Superficial spreading pyoderma (**162**) is characterized by an absence of pustules and large, spreading epidermal collarettes with an erythematous, moist leading edge. Some forms result in large areas of erythema and exfoliation similar to staphylococcal scalded skin syndrome in man and pigs[15].

Mucocutaneous pyoderma

Mucocutaneous pyoderma is seen in German Shepherd Dogs and occasionally in other breeds that develop erythema, exudation, ulceration and crusting of the lips and other mucocutaneous junctions. It can be mistaken for immune-mediated diseases or epitheliotropic lymphoma but, unlike these, responds completely to antibiotic therapy.

DIFFERENTIAL DIAGNOSES

- Demodicosis
- Dermatophytosis
- *Malassezia* dermatitis
- Pemphigus foliaceus (and rare immune-mediated pustular diseases)
- Zinc responsive dermatosis
- Dermatophilosis

Note: Many of these conditions may trigger a secondary pyoderma.

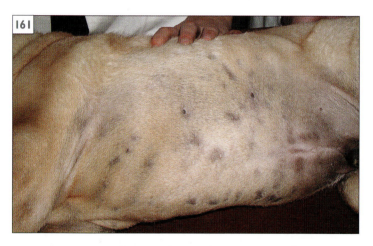

161 Patchy alopecia in a Mastiff with superficial pyoderma.

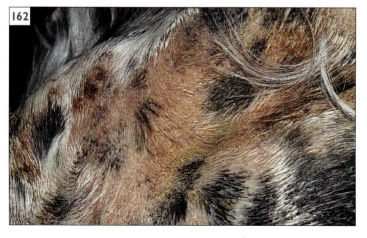

162 Superficial spreading pyoderma in a Cocker Spaniel with a primary keratinization defect.

DIAGNOSIS

The clinical signs are highly suggestive, although not specific. Impression smear, tape-strip, and aspirate cytology may reveal degenerate neutrophils and intracellular cocci (**163, 164**). Diff-Quik-type stains are convenient to use in practice and stain most microorganisms dark blue-purple, but they do not differentiate between gram-positive and gram-negative species. Biopsy and histopathology can also identify infections and help to confirm or rule out underlying conditions. Bacterial culture is not necessary in all cases, as most staphylococci have a predictable antibiotic sensitivity pattern[16], but it should be considered when:

- Cytology reveals rods; antibiotic susceptibility is unpredictable and often limited.

- Empirical antibiotic therapy does not resolve the infection and cytology or culture suggests that staphylococci are involved.
- After multiple antibiotic courses.
- There are non-healing wounds.
- There are postoperative or potentially life-threatening infections.

Samples for culture can be obtained by swabs from the skin or underside of crusts, although these may just reveal non-representative surface contaminants. More representative samples can be obtained by rupturing intact pustules or furuncles, or by biopsy. Wiping the surface with alcohol can reduce contamination but may penetrate superficial lesions and inhibit growth. Formalin fumes can also inhibit bacterial growth.

163, 164 Degenerate neutrophils with extra- and intracellular cocci (**163**) and rods (**164**). (Diff-Quik-stained impression smears, ×1000)

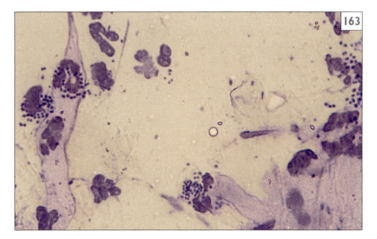

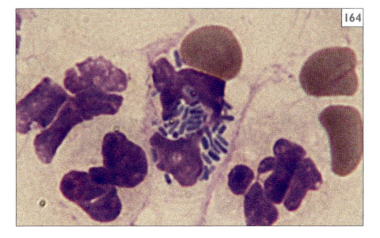

Using local anesthetic at the biopsy site can also inhibit bacterial growth, so it may be better to use a ring block, local nerve block, or general anesthesia.

Culture and antibiotic sensitivity can reveal mixed growths, particularly if enrichment techniques are used. Using cytology to assess relative numbers and intracellular organisms can help identify the most important species. The results will be reported either as Kirby–Bauer disk data (which present the results as resistant, sensitive, or intermediate) or the minimum inhibitory concentration (MIC), which indicates the degree of resistance and helps to calculate an appropriate dose.

MANAGEMENT
Topical therapy
Topical therapy[17,18] softens and removes crusts, ameliorates pain and pruritus, and induces peripheral vasodilation, which promotes healing and antibiotic distribution to the skin. Despite this, topical therapy is rarely effective by itself except in very minor surface infections, although it can be used to prevent recurrence. Treatments should allow a contact time of 5–15 minutes 2–3 times a week initially, tapered to 2–4 times monthly as the condition improves. Microencapsulated and leave-on products deliver the active ingredients more effectively to the skin and have prolonged residual activity (*Table 6*).

Topical antibiotics
Topical antibiotics can be useful in focal lesions, although patients should be carefully checked for more generalized disease. It may also be necessary to treat the ears, mucocutaneous junctions, and feet, as these are likely reservoirs of staphylococcal organisms. Creams and ointments should be massaged in well to maximize uptake and animals prevented from licking the medication off. Gels are an excellent choice; they are rapidly absorbed, are non-occlusive, and do not mat hairs.

Mupirocin 2% has excellent anti-staphylococcal activity combined with good penetration into inflamed skin. It should be applied twice daily for 2–3 weeks then tapered to a maintenance dose. In Europe, however, some countries have restricted its use in animals. Fusidic acid or fusidate is also effective. The veterinary licensed skin preparation also contains betamethasone, but there is an ophthalmic product as well as some human skin products without a glucocorticoid.

Table 6 Useful shampoos

Preparation	Advantages	Other considerations
2.5% benzoyl peroxide	Excellent antibacterial, degreasing, keratolytic, and follicular flushing agent; residual antibacterial activity	May be drying and irritating (can follow with emollient rinse), can bleach dark coats; contact sensitizer and toxic to cats
10% ethyl lactate	Excellent antibacterial and keratoplastic agent	Much less drying; safe in cats
2% miconazole/ 2% chlorhexidine	Excellent antibacterial and antifungal; residual activity	May be drying and irritating (can follow with emollient rinse); safe in cats
3% chlorhexidine	Good antibacterial and antifungal; residual activity	May be drying and irritating; safe in cats
2% sulfur/2% salicylic acid	Antibacterial, antifungal, keratolytic, keratoplastic and antipuritic	Well tolerated in long-term use; safe in cats
Triclosan	Antimicrobial	Well tolerated
Piroctone olamine	Microbial balancing	Non-drying; safe in cats
1% selenium sulfide	Good antifungal, antiparasitic and keratolytic agent	Can be drying and irritating; safe in cats

Systemic antibiotics

It is beyond the scope of this book to provide a complete overview of available antibiotics. The choice will depend on the species, age, and breed of the patient, the target organism, and the type of lesion, as well as the owner's commitment, drug availability, and licensing regulations. Before using systemic antibiotics it is important to ensure that a firm diagnosis of infection using clinical signs, cytology, and culture has been made. Remember also that mild, localized infections may not always need treatment. For example, mild focal pyoderma in an atopic dog will probably resolve once the atopic inflammation is controlled.

General principles in choosing an antibiotic include:

- It should have activity against S. *intermedius*. Most strains produce β-lactamase, conferring resistance to penicillins. Resistance to tetracyclines is also widespread and resistance to macrolides can develop[7,8,16].
- It should reach the skin at an adequate concentration. The ideal is to aim for 8–10 times the MIC at the target tissue. The MIC can be used to calculate an appropriate dose provided that the peak plasma level and tissue concentration are known (often available from the product literature), for example:

MIC	=	0.05 µg/ml
Target tissue concentration (8–10× MIC)	=	0.4 – 0.5 µg/ml
Peak plasma level at 10 mg/kg dose	=	0.3 µg/ml
Skin concentration as a % of plasma	=	80% = 0.24 µg/ml
Dose required	=	20 mg/kg

- The frequency of administration depends on whether the drug is concentration (e.g. fluoroquinolones) or time (e.g. penicillins) dependent. The efficacy of concentration-dependent drugs is reliant on delivering pulses 8–10× MIC once daily. Time-dependent drugs require concentrations above the MIC for at least 50% of the dosing interval; these must be administered every 8–12 hours, depending on the half-life. Compliance with the dosing regime is therefore very important in ensuring clinical efficacy and avoiding resistance.

- Ideally, bactericidal antibiotics should be used, although bacteriostatic (e.g. macrolides and lincosamides) drugs are equally effective provided the immune system is competent.
- Drugs that accumulate in phagocytes (e.g. fluoroquinolones, lincosamides, and macrolides) kill intracellular bacteria and penetrate into inflamed tissues. Pus and necrotic debris can inactivate trimethoprim potentiated sulfonamides (TMPS), macrolides, lincosamides, and aminoglycosides. Fluoroquinolones and rifampin penetrate well into chronically inflamed and fibrosed skin.
- Narrow-spectrum antibiotics (e.g. erythromycin, lincomycin, clindamycin, oxacillin, and cloxacillin) are preferable, as broad-spectrum drugs could upset the gut flora. In practice, however, this is uncommon in dogs and cats and few narrow-spectrum drugs have a veterinary licence.
- Consider any potential interaction with underlying conditions and concurrent treatment, and adverse effects (e.g. sulfonamides in Dobermanns).
- Regular check-ups are necessary to ensure that the infection has resolved before ceasing therapy. Most superficial pyodermas resolve within 2–3 weeks; deep pyodermas may require 4–6 weeks or longer (see *Table 7*).

Methicillin-resistant staphylococci

These are potentially resistant to many antibiotics, but useful drugs include fluoroquinolones, tetracyclines (including doxycycline and minocycline) and rifampin; the MIC must be checked and an effective dose calculated. Individual patients may also need hospitalizing for wound management, joint debridement, etc. Veterinary hospitals should introduce strict infectious disease control polices to prevent and/or contain infection[11,12].

Antibiotic resistance

Antibiotic use inevitably selects for resistance. Macrolides and lincosamides (e.g. lincomycin, erythromycin, clindamycin, and clarithromycin) tend to induce cross-resistance and should not be used for long-term treatment. Rifampin must be administered with a bactericidal antibiotic (except fluoroquinolones) to avoid the rapid development of resistance. Inducible clindamycin resistance is common in MRSA, and repeated courses of broad-spectrum antibiotics are risk factors for the acquisition of MRSA colonization and/or infection.

Good practice to limit antibiotic resistance

The factors that influence prevalence of resistance are listed below:

- Inappropriate case selection
- Inappropriate drug
- Poor compliance
- Low dose
- Infrequent treatment
- Short treatment periods
- Low efficacy

The division of drugs into first-, second- and third-line or tier products can be helpful, although the decision also depends on the type of practice, caseload, host species, target tissue, and type of bacterium (e.g. a first-opinion practice will probably be different from a referral hospital, and respiratory cases from dermatology cases).

First- line drugs could include older antibiotics and/or narrow-spectrum drugs such as simple penicillins, tetracyclines, and sulfonamides, although their use in pyoderma is often restricted by a high frequency of resistance in staphylococci. It is important to remember that these are no less potent than other antibiotics in the appropriate circumstances.

Table 7 Useful antibiotics for superficial pyodermas

Antibiotic	Dosage	Adverse effects
TMPS (also ormetoprim and baquiloprim-potentiated drugs)	15–30 mg/kg p/o q12h	Can cause keratoconjunctivitis sicca, sick euthyroid syndrome, and cutaneous drug reactions (especially in Dobermanns)
Erythromycin*	10–20 mg/kg p/o q8h	Can occasionally cause nausea and vomiting
Lincomycin	15–30 mg/kg p/o q8–12h	
Clindamycin	5.5–33 mg/kg p/o q12h; 11 mg/kg p/o q24h	
Cefalexin	15–30 mg/kg p/o q12–24h	Can occasionally cause vomiting and diarrhea
Cefadroxil	10–20 mg/kg p/o q12h	
Cefpodoxime proxetil	5–10 mg/kg p/o q24h	
Cefovexin	8 mg/kg s/c q14d	
Clavulanate-potentiated amoxicillin	12.5 mg/kg p/o q8–12h; 25 mg/kg p/o q12h	
Oxacillin, cloxacillin*	20 mg/kg p/o q8h	
Enrofloxacin	5–20 mg/kg p/o q24h	Can cause cartilage damage in dogs <12 months of age (18 months in giant breeds), neurologic signs at high doses, and blindness in cats (especially with injectable enrofloxacin). Occasionally cause anorexia, vomiting, and diarrhea
Marbofloxacin	2–5.5 mg/kg p/o q24h	
Difloxacin	5–10 mg/kg p/o q24h	
Orbifloxacin	2.5–7.5 mg/kg p/o q24h	
Rifampin*	5–10 mg/kg p/o q24h	Anorexia, vomiting, diarrhea, hepatopathy, hemolytic anemia, and death

* not licensed for use in animals.

Second-line drugs could include newer products with more extended activity, those that are more important for general human and animal use, and those more prone to resistance (e.g. broad-spectrum β-lactamase-resistant penicillins, cefalosporins, and macrolides). These should be used where culture and sensitivity or good empirical evidence indicates that first-line drugs will be ineffective.

Third-line drugs (fluoroquinlones and human-licensed drugs such as anti-*Pseudomonas* penicillins, ceftazidime, and imipenem) are those that are very important to humans and animals, particularly against multi-drug-resistant gram-negative organisms. They should only be used where culture and sensitivity indicate they are necessary. Drugs vitally important to human health (e.g. vancomycin, teicoplanin) should probably never be used in animals.

Treatment of recurrent pyoderma

Idiopathic recurrent pyoderma is uncommon, but some atopic dogs suffering from recurrent infections benefit from long-term antimicrobial treatment. Antibacterial shampoos (used every 3–14 days depending on the response) can help, and topical antibiotics can be effective on focal lesions. Treatment of mucosal surfaces may reduce mucosal populations and colonization of the skin.

Some animals may require long-term pulse dosing with systemic drugs. A bactericidal antibiotic that is well tolerated should be selected based on culture and sensitivity; good choices are cefalosporins and clavulanate-potentiated amoxicillin. The protocol should be tailored to the individual dog, but general guidelines include:

- If relapses occur more than every two months, treat each infection with a full course.
- If relapses occur less than every two months, use a full dose week on/week off, week on/two weeks off etc. or for 2–3 consecutive days each week (i.e. 'weekend therapy')[19].

Immunostimulants such as staphage lysate and autogenous vaccines[20] may be useful in idiopathic recurrent pyoderma. They are generally given twice weekly for 10–12 weeks, then every 7–30 days for maintenance. Adverse effects are rare, but can include injection site reactions, pyrexia, malaise, and anaphylaxis.

ZOONOTIC INFECTIONS

Most staphylococci are host-adapted (e.g. *S. aureus* is the principal pathogen in humans and *S. intermedius* is the principal pathogen in dogs)[21]. Transmission of organisms between animals and humans has been documented, and may have been underestimated. Recent studies suggest that up to 45% of owners of dogs with pyoderma can be colonized by *S. intermedius*[22] and that approximately 10% of veterinarians attending small animal conferences were colonized by MRSA[23]. MRSA has also been isolated from 12% of veterinary staff and 5% of owners in contact with MRSA-infected animals. In a Canadian study, concurrent human–animal colonization was found in 20% of households with *S. aureus*-positive humans and 67% of *S. intermedius*-positive humans[24]. Simple colonization presents very little risk to healthy humans, but people who are immunocompromised, or have open wounds or implants etc. may be more vulnerable.

KEY POINTS

- An underdiagnosed disease.
- Use appropriate treatment and monitor clinical resolution.
- Do not use steroids unless required by the underlying disease.
- Relapsing pyoderma requires a full work-up; most are secondary to an underlying condition.

Canine acne (chin and muzzle folliculitis and furunculosis)

DEFINITION
Canine acne is a papular and/or pustular dermatosis associated with dilated hyperkeratotic follicles, furunculosis, and para- (peri-)follicular inflammation.

ETIOLOGY AND PATHOGENESIS
The precipitating etiology and pathogenesis are unknown. The follicular plugging and parafollicular inflammation may predispose to follicular rupture. This results in a foreign body reaction and in some cases, eventually, to secondary bacterial infection. The condition resolves spontaneously in many animals when they reach adulthood, although some individuals remain affected for life. In some dogs the lesions may be associated with underlying diseases such as hypothyroidism, atopic dermatitis, adverse food reactions, or lifestyles that result in trauma to the affected skin.

CLINICAL FEATURES
Canine acne occurs most commonly over the chin and lips of young, short-coated breeds of dogs such as the Doberman Pinscher, English Bulldog, Great Dane, Weimaraner, Rottweiler, Boxer, and German Shorthaired Pointer. Lesions consist of follicular papules and/or pustules that may ulcerate and fistulate, draining a serosanguineous to seropurulent material (**165**). Follicles may rupture (furunculosis) and if the accompanying foreign body inflammation is extensive, small fibrous nodules may develop. Animals may suffer no discomfort if the lesions are minimal, although extensively affected areas may be sensitive or painful and mildly pruritic. Affected dogs should be examined carefully for any signs of primary disease.

DIFFERENTIAL DIAGNOSES
- Demodicosis
- Dermatophytosis
- Foreign body reaction
- Mild juvenile cellulitis

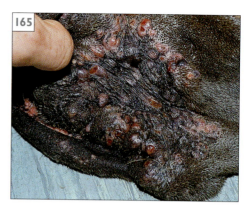

165 Canine acne. Fibrogranulomatous, cystic, and papular lesions due to canine acne.

DIAGNOSIS
The signalment and clinical signs are very suggestive. Skin scrapings should be taken to rule out demodicosis. Bacterial and dermatophyte culture and antibiotic sensitivity testing are indicated in cases that do not respond to empirical treatment. Additional appropriate diagnostics may be necessary for any suspected primary disease.

MANAGEMENT
Affected areas may be cleaned daily with a benzoyl peroxide shampoo or gel to enhance removal of debris from the hair follicle and decrease the number of bacteria on the skin surface. The shampoo should be carefully rinsed from the affected area, as benzoyl peroxide can be irritating in some cases. Mild infections may respond to cleansing and a topical antibacterial such as mupirocin, fusidic acid, or polymyxin B ointment applied twice daily. More severely affected cases may benefit from topical glucocorticoids applied twice daily. Glucocorticoids can help to break down fibrosis and reduce inflammaton, but their use in active infections is controversial. If lesions are extensive, systemic antibiotics for 3–6 weeks would be appropriate (see Superficial pyoderma, p. 146). Underlying diseases should be addressed and lifestyle changes implemented as necessary. A small number of cases require either continuous or episodic treatment for life.

KEY POINT
- Easy to overdiagnose. Do not forget the differential diagnoses.

Pemphigus foliaceus

DEFINITION
Pemphigus foliaceus is an autoimmune disease in which autoantibodies are directed against components of the epidermis, resulting in acantholysis and subcorneal vesicle formation.

ETIOLOGY AND PATHOGENESIS
Autoantibody (IgG) is formed against desmoglein 1(Dsg 1), a component of desmosomes, which are the main intercellular bridges between the keratinocytes and are responsible for cell-to-cell cohesion[1]. The exact pathomechanism leading to cell separation or acantholysis is unknown. However, the binding of autoantibody to Dsg 1 results in activation of intracellular pathways, which ultimately results in loss of cohesion between the keratinocytes. The associated changes result in acantholysis (rounding up of individual keratinocytes) and subsequent pustule formation. These primary lesions are transient owing to the thin canine and feline stratum corneum. A pemphigus foliaceus-like disease can be initiated by drug therapy[2]. If the disease resolves when the drug is discontinued it is called 'pemphigus foliaceus-like drug reaction', and if the disease persists after the drug is discontinued it is called ' drug-induced pemphigus foliaceus'[3]. In dogs, trimethoprim–sulfonamides are generally responsible, but there is a case report with cephalexin[2]. In cats, doxycycline, ampicillin, cimetidine, and methimazole have been implicated[2,3].

CLINICAL FEATURES
Pemphigus foliaceus is the most common form of pemphigus[4–6], and the Bearded Collie, Akita, Chow Chow, Newfoundland, Schipperke, Doberman Pinscher, English Springer Spaniel, Chinese Shar Pei, and Collie are predisposed[3]. Usually a disease of gradual onset, the condition presents as a vesiculobullous or pustular dermatitis with secondary erythema, scale, alopecia, erosion, and prominent crust formation. Epidermal collarettes are common[7]. It is variably pruritic and only rarely is it accompanied by systemic signs in the dog, even though generalized lesions may occur[6,8,9]. Usually, only the skin is affected and lesions on the mucocutaneous junctions and in the oral cavity are rare[8]. In most cases lesions are symmetrical in distribution, usually commencing on the dorsal part of the muzzle[7] (**166**), face, and pinnae (**167**) before

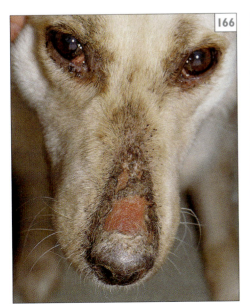
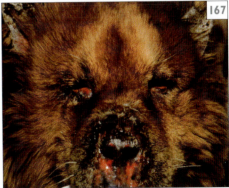

166, 167 Pemphigus foliaceus. Localized lesions on the face of a German Shepherd Dog (**166**); erosions, ulcers, and crusts of the muzzle, eyes, and ears of a dog with pemphigus foliaceus (**167**).

slowly generalizing. In some instances lesions may remain localized to small areas of the body, such as the pinnae (**168**). The footpads may become hyperkeratotic (**169**) and there may be erythema at the margins of the footpads[7]. Occasionally, the epithelium of the pads will slough and, rarely, lesions may be confined to the footpads[6,7,10]. Lesions can also occur in and be confined to the nails of dogs that exhibit subungual or intraungual pustules, causing onychomadesis[11]. Onychoschizia and onychogryphosis were also noted in some nails[11]. Pemphigus foliaceus is less common in cats and lesions tend to be more localized and present on the muzzle, planum nasale, ear pinnae, around the nipples, in the footpads, and in the ungual folds, which often contain a gray-tan caseous material. Malaise, anorexia, and pyrexia may also be noted[12].

DIFFERENTIAL DIAGNOSES
- Demodicosis
- Superficial pyoderma
- Zinc responsive dermatosis
- Dermatophytosis
- Actinic dermatosis
- Epitheliotropic lymphoma
- Drug eruption
- Discoid lupus erythematosus

DIAGNOSIS
Consideration of history and clinical signs and the results of microscopic examination of skin scrapes will generally rule out demodicosis and dermatophytosis. The presence of primary lesions (pustules) is of great significance; a good place to look for them is the concave surface of the pinnae. If pustules are present, the bevel of a 25 gauge needle may be used as a scoop to obtain exudate, which is then smeared onto a slide. Smears made from the underside of a lifted crust can also provide diagnostic information. Microscopic examination of cytologic samples usually reveals large numbers of neutrophils, with variable numbers of rounded keratinocytes (acanthocytes) (**170**) and either minimal or small numbers of bacteria. While acanthocytes are highly suggestive of pemphigus foliaceus, they may be seen in cases of superficial pyoderma and dermatophytosis. In rare cases there may be a positive Nikolsky's sign; lateral digital pressure on the skin produces erosions. Histopathologic examination of biopsy material is diagnostic in some 80% of cases and rules out almost all of the differential diagnoses. Direct immunofluorescence or peroxidase/immunoperoxidase staining may be performed in cases where routine histopathologic examination is not diagnostic.

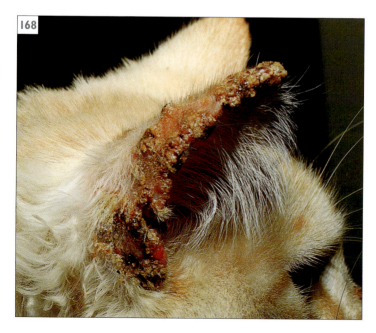

168 Lesions confined to the pinnae of a cat with pemphigus foliaceus.

MANAGEMENT

The management of pemphigus foliaceus encompasses two aims: suppression of clinical signs and maintenance of clinical remission. Suppression of the clinical signs is achieved with immunosuppressive doses of prednisolone. Initial doses (1–2 mg/kg p/o q12h) should be prescribed and if there is no improvement within 10–14 days, the dose should be increased (to 2 mg/kg, or even 3 mg/kg p/o q12h) and steroid-sparing regimes considered[6,13]. Animals should be closely monitored during induction for side-effects, and once remission is achieved the dose should be slowly tapered (to 0.25–1.0 mg/kg p/o q48h). In one study, 42% of dogs could be maintained on alternate-day prednisolone[6]. Methylprednisolone can be used in the same dosage regime as prednisolone (0.8× the dose). Generally, dogs treated with methylprednisolone will evidence fewer side-effects such as polyuria and polydipsia[14]. Some cases may also have a more favorable response to methylprednisolone[14]. The majority of feline cases respond well and are maintained comfortably in clinical remission with prednisolone therapy[6,11]. Some of the dogs that exhibit unacceptable side-effects to prednisolone or methylprednisolone may be controlled on alternate day (or every third day) dexamethasone (0.1 mg/kg or 0.15× the prednisolone dose p/o). However, a significant proportion of dogs will fail to respond to glucocorticoid regimes or exhibit severe side-effects[6], and steroid-sparing regimes or alternative therapy must be considered[3–5].

Azathioprine is the most common agent employed for steroid-sparing or adjunctive treatment in autoimmune conditions[13]. The beneficial effects of azathioprine may not be apparent for 3–5 weeks, and the aim is to use azathioprine alternated with prednisolone at the lowest doses necessary to maintain remission. Doses of 1–2 mg/kg p/o q24h or q48h are usually well tolerated in dogs[6]. Azathioprine is contraindicated in cats. Bone marrow suppression or gastrointestinal side-effects may occur, and animals should be closely monitored with bi-weekly blood counts for the first 8–12 weeks of therapy and, if no abnormalities develop, every six months[13,14]. One author (PJM) routinely starts dogs out on the combination of methylprednisolone (0.5–1.1 mg/kg p/o q12h) and azathioprine (2.2 mg/kg p/o q48h). When controlled, the methylprednisolone dose is reduced to q24h.

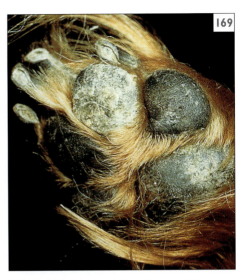

169 Pedal lesions on a dog with pemphigus foliaceus.

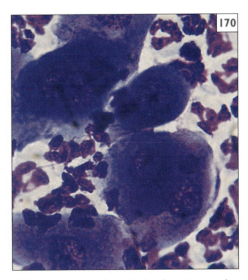

170 Acanthocytes (rounded-up keratinocytes) with clustering neutrophils from a pustule in a case of pemphigus foliaceus.

If control is maintained at this dose for three weeks, it is further reduced to the least amount that will maintain resolution of lesions. The dose should be lowered much more slowly than in atopic dermatitis, as the consequences of a relapse are more severe. One author (TJN) reduces the alternate day dose by 20–25% in weekly steps. Once (and if) this is zero, then the remaining day's dose is slowly reduced to maintenance.

Chlorambucil (0.1–0.2 mg/kg p/o q24–48h) may also be used as a glucocorticoid-sparing drug in both dogs and cats. It can be used as a sole therapy in feline cases that are not responsive to glucocorticoids or where glucocorticoids are not tolerated[14]. Myelosuppression is a potential side-effect and complete blood counts should be performed as described for azathioprine therapy.

Aurothioglucose (gold salt therapy) has also been advocated as a steroid-sparing agent and as an adjunctive agent, and was useful in 23% of canine cases and 40% of feline cases according to one study[6]. Sodium aurothiomalate is administered intramuscularly at an initial dose of 1 mg (dogs <10 kg and cats) or 5 mg (dogs >10 kg). If no side-effects are noted after seven days, the dose is doubled. If no side-effects are observed, treatment is continued with weekly doses (1 mg/kg)[13]. The animals are closely monitored for side-effects; in particular, renal, hematologic, and dermatologic disease. Recently, an oral gold preparation (auranofin) has been described[6]. Dosage is between 0.05 and 0.2 mg/kg q12h, and side-effects appear to be much less frequent than with the parenteral forms of gold therapy.

Other suggested immunosuppressive drugs that are not used routinely include cyclophosphamide (50 mg/m^2 body surface area p/o q48h or 4 consecutive days per week [**Note:** may induce hemorrhagic cystitis]), dapsone (1 mg/kg p/o q12h [**Note:** may induce liver disease and thrombocytopenia]), sulfasalazine (22–44 mg/kg p/o q8h), and tetracycline/niacinamide (dogs <10 kg, 250 mg each p/o q8h; dogs >10 kg, 500 mg p/o q12h) (doxycycline 10 mg/kg p/o q24h may be used instead of tetracycline)[15]. Mycophenolate mofetil (22–39 mg/kg p/o divided q8h) has been used in conjunction with glucocorticoids to successfully manage pemphigus vulgaris in humans[16] and was found to be beneficial in treating a small number of dogs with pemphigus foliaceus. The benefits of ciclosporin (cyclosporine) are debatable, but there is mounting anecdotal evidence that it is not helpful.

A recent study found that concurrent use of antibiotics during the initial treatment phase significantly improved the remission rate and long-term survival[17].

KEY POINT
• Do not underestimate the difficulty in managing this disease. Some cases may be all but refractory.

Canine juvenile cellulitis
(juvenile sterile granulomatous dermatitis and lymphadenitis, juvenile pyoderma, puppy strangles)

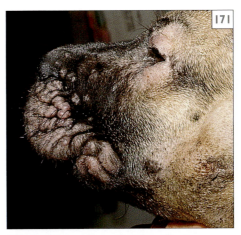

171 Juvenile pyoderma. Facial swelling in a pup.

DEFINITION
Canine juvenile cellulitis is a granulomatous condition of puppies affecting the skin of the face, the pinnae, and the submandibular lymph nodes.

ETIOLOGY AND PATHOGENESIS
The etiology and pathogenesis of this condition are unknown. An immunologic abnormality may be involved, as glucocorticoid therapy results in resolution of lesions. There is some evidence for an hereditary factor, as some breeds, as well as particular lines within a breed, are predisposed[1,2].

CLINICAL FEATURES
The condition develops in puppies from 3–16 weeks of age. It occurs more frequently in Golden Retrievers, Dachshunds, Labrador Retrievers, Lhasa Apsos, and Gordon Setters[1-4]. Puppies are usually febrile, depressed, and anorexic. There is acute swelling of the muzzle, lips, and eyelids (171). Sterile pustules often develop in the skin of these areas as well as on the inner surface of the pinnae. After the pustules rupture, small ulcers, draining tracts, seropurulent exudates, or crusts can develop. Submandibular lymphadenopathy occurs and, occasionally, lymph nodes will abscessate and drain. Nodules over the trunk, preputial, and perineal areas, due to pyogranulomatous panniculitis, as well as sterile suppurative arthritis, have been reported in a small number of cases[2]. Permanent areas of alopecia and scarring may result if the lesions are extensive.

DIFFERENTIAL DIAGNOSES
- Angioedema due to an insect bite reaction or vaccine
- Demodicosis
- Pyoderma
- Pemphigus foliaceus
- Adverse drug reaction

DIAGNOSIS
Signalment and clinical signs are very suggestive. Skin scrapings and cytologic examination of the contents of an intact pustule will help to identify demodicosis or staphylococcal folliculitis, respectively. Bacterial culture of the contents of an intact pustule is important as gram-negative, in addition to gram-positive, bacteria may be secondary pathogens.

MANAGEMENT
Prednisolone (1–2 mg/kg p/o q12h) for 14–21 days, depending on the rate of resolution of the clinical signs. In most cases, significant improvement will be noted during the first 24–48 hours of treatment. Once lesions have resolved, the dosage may be reduced to alternate days to prevent relapse[3]. Warm soaks (twice daily) using aluminum acetate or chlorhexidine solutions can help keep the affected areas clean and prevent the formation of crusts. If a secondary bacterial infection is suspected, systemic bactericidal antibacterial drugs can be used concurrently.

KEY POINT
- These cases require steroid therapy. Be sure to rule out demodicosis.

Diseases characterized by sinus formation

General approach
- These are largely uncommon to rare dermatoses
- The diagnosis depends on biopsy and histopathology
- Biopsy material should also be submitted for microbial culture – aerobic, anaerobic, mycobacterial and/or fungal
- Imaging with contrast may be necessary to detect foreign bodies

Common conditions
- Bite wounds
- Foreign body sinus
- Deep pyoderma
- Anal furunculosis (perianal fistulas)

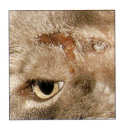
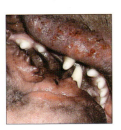
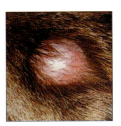
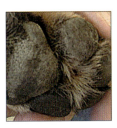

Bite wounds

ETIOLOGY AND PATHOGENESIS

Bite wounds occur following penetration of the skin, which is usually followed by inoculation of oral flora or epidermal flora into the subcutis. The bruising accompanying the wound and the failure of the discharge to drain through the small penetrations facilitate abscess formation. The typical organisms in wounds resulting from dog bites are *Staphylococcus intermedius*, coagulase-negative staphylococci, enterococci, and *Escherichia coli*, whereas in cat bites the usual isolates are *Pasteurella multocida*, *Bacteroides* spp., and β-hemolytic streptococci[1]. Anaerobes such as *Bacillus*, *Clostridium*, and *Corynebacterium* spp. are frequently isolated from bite wound abscesses[1,2]. One report found subcutaneous abscessation and concomitant arthritis in a colony of cats caused by bacterial L-forms[3]. In one study, 65% of bites had positive aerobic cultures, 15% had positive anaerobic cultures, and 33% had negative cultures[2].

CLINICAL FEATURES

In dogs abscesses usually follow bites and these are generally on the limbs, head, and neck. Cats are usually bitten on the head (**172**), distal limb, or tail base. After the bite, the area surrounding the puncture is usually bruised, and there may be serous discharge, crushed or torn tissues, hemorrhage, and crusting. Severe dog bites may cause extensive crushing, damage to deeper tissues and internal organs, and fractures, which may be life threatening. Other complications include lymphangitis and lymphadenitis, septic arthritis, tenosynovitis, osteomyelitis, pneumothorax, pyothorax, and peritonitis[3,4].

Dog bites are often large enough to ensure adequate drainage, so abscessation is unusual. However, the small puncture wounds resulting from cat bites often seal and then present as an abscess after 2–4 days[3] (**173**). Affected animals may be lethargic, inappetent, and in pain. Pyrexia may be noted. A soft, variably painful swelling develops which, if not lanced, bursts. The skin overlying the abscess may be necrotic and may slough. Cats may also develop a cellulitis from bite wounds. Typically, this occurs on a limb and is characterized by subcutaneous swelling, resulting in pain and lameness. Careful examination of the affected area may reveal small crusts covering the puncture tracts.

DIFFERENTIAL DIAGNOSES

- Penetrating foreign body
- Deep pyoderma
- Demodicosis
- Panniculitis
- Feline leprosy and atypical mycobacterial infection
- Nocardiosis
- Dermatophytosis
- Subcutaneous and deep mycoses
- Leishmaniasis
- Cuterebriasis or dracunculiasis
- Neoplasia
- Lymphedema and other causes of peripheral edema

DIAGNOSIS

The clinical signs are usually highly suggestive, although the initial bite wounds may not be immediately obvious in cats. The clinical history is therefore important. Abscessation following bite wounds is usually well documented in dogs. In cats, definitive histories are not common, but consideration of lifestyle and the site of the abscess usually lead to a diagnosis. Cytology will confirm the purulent and infectious nature of the lesions and may guide antibiotic choice, although culture will be necessary to confirm the species and antibiotic sensitivity pattern in mixed infections[3,4]. In one study, no one antibiotic or antibiotic combination was effective against all the cultured bacteria[2].

Recurrent abscess formation demands a thorough work-up to establish the cause. Any underlying immunosuppressive therapy or conditions, metabolic illness (e.g. malnutrition and/or hypoproteinemia), or endocrinopathies should be identified by appropriate investigation and tests. In cats, FeLV and FIV testing is important. Cytologic examination of the discharge, histopathology of infected tissues, bacterial (aerobic and anaerobic), mycobacterial, and fungal culture of the discharge or infected tissues, and fungal or *Leishmania* specific serology or PCR may all be necessary to achieve a diagnosis.

172 Bite wound on the head of a cat.

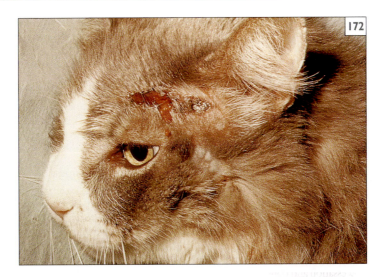

173 Cat bite abscess on the neck.

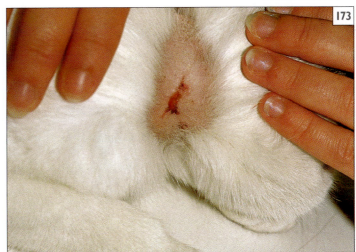

MANAGEMENT

Appropriate management includes preventing and reducing contamination; appropriate antibiotic therapy; removing debris via irrigation and drainage; staged débridement; appropriate wound dressing; and stimulating healing so that an appropriate method of wound closure can be performed[1,4]. Wound management seems to be more important in the successful outcome of bite wound injuries than antibiotic therapy *per se*[1]. Wounds should be kept open, clean, and draining until a bed of healthy granulation tissue has formed to allow secondary wound closure or healing by secondary intention. Broad-spectrum antibacterial agents with anti-anaerobic activity (e.g. amoxicillin) are usually administered. (**Note:** Broad-spectrum, penicillinase-resistant antibacterial agents should be used with dog bites[1].) Treatment of chronic or recurrent infections depends on the underlying diagnosis.

KEY POINTS

- Bite wounds are usually contaminated.
- Contaminating bacteria are variable and may be mixed.
- Failure to respond promptly should be treated seriously.

Foreign body sinus

DEFINITION

Foreign bodies inoculated into the dermis provoke a vigorous inflammatory response that may result in sinus formation.

ETIOLOGY AND PATHOGENESIS

Foreign body granulomas and sinus formation result when the inciting stimulus is not removed by phagocytosis[1]. The list of causal agents is long, but plant awns such as foxtails (*Hordeum jubatum*) in North America and *Hordeum, Stipa,* and *Setaria,* which have a worldwide distribution, are responsible for the majority of lesions (**174**)[2]. Other exogenous foreign bodies include suture material, vaccine adjuvant, pieces of vegetation, insect mouthparts or stings, porcupine quills, and airgun pellets. Endogenous foreign bodies include keratin, displaced hair shafts, free lipid, calcium salts, and urate deposition. The foreign body sinus may get progressively longer as the inoculated agent migrates along tissue planes.

CLINICAL FEATURES

Nodules and a draining sinus are typical (**175**). The most common sites for exogenous foreign body penetrations are the dorsal interdigital regions (**176**) and the anterior aspects of the distal limbs. Local lymphadenopathy is common, but systemic signs are rare unless distant or deep migration (possibly into body cavities) has occurred, resulting in draining tracts. Secondary infection with bacteria, actinomyces or *Nocardia* spp., opportunistic mycobacteria, dermatophytes, and saprophytic fungi may be associated with awn penetration[2]. Initially, only erythema and swelling may be noted. As the foreign body migrates inward and the body mounts an inflammatory response, papules, nodules, abscesses, and draining tracts can develop.

DIFFERENTIAL DIAGNOSES

- Demodicosis
- Panniculitis
- Feline leprosy and atypical mycobacterial infection
- Nocardiosis
- Subcutaneous and deep mycoses
- Cuterebriasis or dracunculiasis
- Acral granuloma
- Neoplasia

DIAGNOSIS

Consideration of the history and clinical signs will narrow the diagnosis down and appropriate laboratory tests will rule out infectious agents. Surgical exploration and contrast radiography may be indicated in cases of deep penetration or migration. Biochemical investigation of renal and hepatic and endocrine function may be indicated if an endogenous foreign body suggests metastatic calcification or urate deposition.

MANAGEMENT

Drainage, plus débridement if indicated, for exogenous foreign bodies[1]. It must be appreciated that pieces of vegetation (particularly grass awns) may migrate from one body cavity to the next, which makes exploration of the tracts a potentially major piece of surgery. Systemic antibacterial treatment is indicated in most cases. Endogenous foreign bodies usually mandate medical management rather than simple surgical removal, although this may play a part.

174 Foxtail.

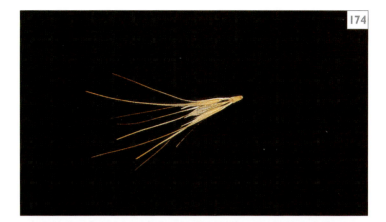

175 Foreign body sinus. Note the swollen, erythematous margins around the tracts.

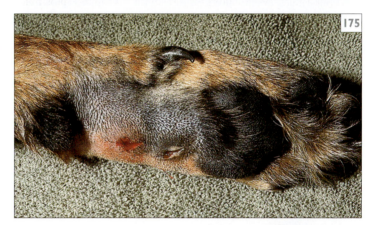

176 Foreign body penetration in the interdigital region due to a foxtail.

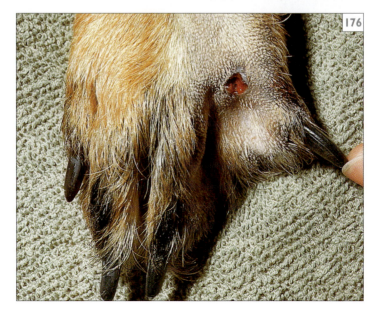

Deep pyoderma

ETIOLOGY AND PATHOGENESIS

Deep pyoderma occurs when infection is present beneath the basement membrane (i.e. in the dermis and/or subcutaneous tissues). It may occur as a consequence of superficial (or pyotraumatic) pyoderma following extension of infection through ruptured follicle walls (furunculosis). However, direct inoculation from contaminated bite wounds or penetrating foreign bodies is the most common etiology, particularly in cats. Some cases are idiopathic, but deep pyoderma, particularly in dogs, should be considered secondary to underlying conditions, especially demodicosis, endocrinopathies, or immunosuppression, until proven otherwise[1-3].

As with the other classifications of pyoderma (see Superficial pyoderma, p. 146), the principal organism recovered from lesions is *Staphylococcus intermedius*, but other staphylococci including *S. schleiferi* and *S. aureus*, some of which may be methicillin resistant, can also be present[4-6]. Less commonly, gram-negative bacteria, particularly *Pseudomonas*, may be isolated[7,8]. Culture and sensitivity are mandatory when investigating deep pyoderma.

CLINICAL FEATURES

The clinical lesions of deep pyoderma are obviously more serious than more superficial infections, and they are usually more painful than pruritic[3]. Clinical signs include erythema, swelling, hemorrhagic bullae, draining sinus tracts, ulceration, crusts, abscesses, and cellulitis (**177, 178**). A number of distinct clinical variants of deep pyoderma are recognized:

- Localized deep folliculitis and furunculosis.
- Nasal pyoderma.
- Foreign body sinus (see p. 164).
- Muzzle furunculosis or canine acne (see p.154).
- Callus pyoderma (see p. 178).
- Interdigital pyoderma or furunculosis ('interdigital cysts').
- Anal furunculosis (see p. 174).
- Bite wounds and subsequent abcessation (see p. 162).
- German Shepherd Dog pyoderma (see p. 98).
- Acral lick dermatitis (see p. 62).

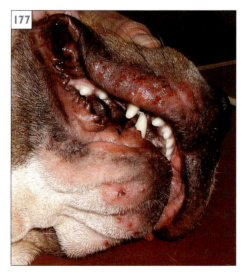

177 Muzzle of a Mastiff-cross with swelling, erythema, hemorrhage, folliculitis, furunculosis, ulcers, sinus tracts, and crusts typical of deep pyoderma.

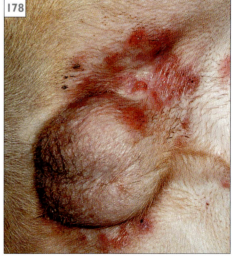

178 Scrotum and groin of the dog in 177.

179 Localized folliculitis and furunculosis on the head of a Golden Retriever.

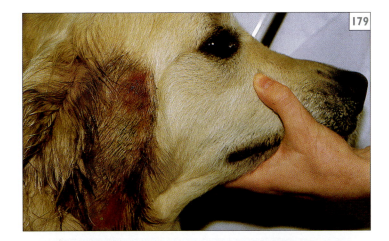

180 Nasal pyoderma. Note the crusting on the nose but the failure of the lesions to affect the nasal planum. This is a key point in trying to differentiate pyoderma from immune-mediated disease.

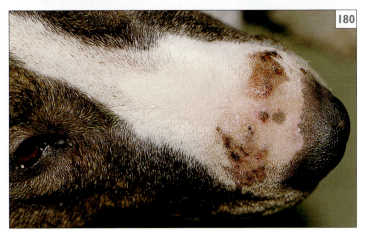

Localized deep folliculitis and furunculosis

This is thought to be a complication of pyotraumatic dermatitis or superficial pyoderma. Affected animals present with a pruritic, exudative, erythematous, thickened patch (**179**). The major differential diagnosis is pyotraumatic dermatitis (see p. 18). Localized deep folliculitis and furunculosis may be differentiated clinically by having a thickened feel and the presence of satellite lesions with draining tracts, which are all uncommon in pyotraumatic dermatitis. Localized deep pyoderma may also follow focal demodicosis, dermatophytosis, and physical or chemical trauma.

Nasal pyoderma

This affects the dorsal muzzle but not the nasal planum. The peracute form presents as inflammatory papules, which rapidly coalesce and progress to an erythematous, eroded, granulomatous, proliferative plaque that is extremely painful. Chronic infections are characterized by crusted papules and occasionally by sinus formation (**180**). These lesions have been traditionally associated with rooting behavior, possibly where trauma drives hairs into the skin, initiating the formation of hair granulomas. Eosinophilic folliculitis and furunculosis have also been associated with arthropod bites and stings (see Bee stings and spider bites, p. 220). Facial dermatophtyosis (see Dermatophytosis, p. 278), especially that caused by *Trichophyton mentagrophytes*, can also result in secondary deep pyoderma.

Interdigital pyoderma

Interdigital pyoderma is a common condition characterized by recurrent furunculosis and draining sinus tracts of the digital and interdigital skin, frequently and mistakenly referred to as 'interdigital cysts' (**181, 182**). Clinically, they resemble small foreign body abscesses. Interdigital pyoderma is most commonly seen in short-haired breeds, where it may be associated with hair granulomas following self- or external trauma. Common underlying conditions include atopic dermatitis and endocrinopathies.

Recently, an apparently immune-mediated, lymphocytic–plasmacytic pododermatitis has been described[9,10]. Clinically, this is very similar to interdigital pyoderma, but it is often much worse, with grossly swollen, very painful feet (**183**). Unlike a true pyoderma, this condition responds poorly to antibiotics, but responds better to treatments such as ciclosporin (cyclosporine) or (less favorably) glucocorticoids.

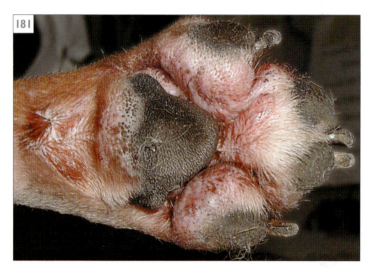

181 Severe erythema, swelling, ulceration, and sinus tracts in a dog with pedal deep pyoderma.

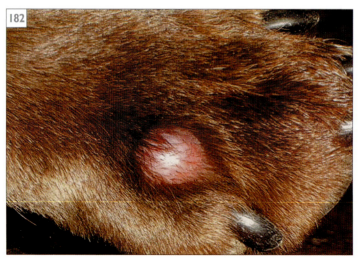

182 Interdigital furunculosis ('cysts') in a Bulldog with atopic dermatitis.

DIFFERENTIAL DIAGNOSES

- Demodicosis
- Deep or superficial fungal infection
- Mycobacterial infection
- Nocardiosis or actinobacillosis
- Immune-mediated disease (e.g. vasculitis, cutaneous or systemic lupus erythematosus, pemphigus foliaceus, pemphigus vulgaris, and sub-epidermal blistering diseases)
- Panniculitis

DIAGNOSIS

A determined search for an underlying disease should be made. Demodicosis should always be considered until ruled out by skin scrapings, hair plucks, or examination of expressed material. Other causes such as hypothyroidism and hyper-adrenocorticism should also be considered. Misuse of glucocorticoids or cytotoxic drugs for the symptomatic control of pruritic dermatoses (e.g. atopic dermatitis), internal disease (e.g. musculoskeletal problems), immune-mediated diseases, and chemotherapy may also contribute. Cytology from intact furuncles or fresh draining sinuses usually reveals pyogranulomatous inflammation with degenerate neutrophils, activated macrophages, lymphocytes, and plasma cells. Bacteria can be scarce, but a thorough search usually reveals intracellular organisms. Histopathology will confirm the clinical suspicion of furunculosis. Free hair fragments and/or primary factors such as *Demodex*, fungal elements, or other microorganisms may be seen on both cytology and histopathology. Bacterial culture and sensitivity testing are mandatory, and fungal or mycobacterial cultures may be necessary in suspicious cases.

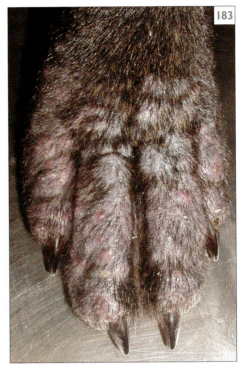

183 Severe erythema, furunculosis, scarring, and alopecia in a Staffordshire Bull Terrier with idiopathic sterile lymphocytic–plasmacytic pododermatitis.

MANAGEMENT

Affected areas should be clipped out to reveal the extent of the lesions, improve access for treatment, and prevent matting. Whole body clips may be necessary with generalized disease in long-haired animals. Whirlpool baths are helpful, if available. Antibacterial shampoos such as benzoyl peroxide and chlorhexidine are useful. Systemic treatment according to sensitivity testing is required until the lesions have resolved. In practice this usually means 8–12 weeks of therapy; there is often a dramatic improvement in the first 2–4 weeks, but full resolution will require prolonged treatment as fibrosed pyogranulomas resolve.

(See Superficial pyoderma, p. 146, for more details of topical and systemic antibacterials.)

The prognosis is generally good if the primary cause is identified and managed. Relapse in idiopathic cases, however, is frequent and will require long-term antibacterial strategies (see Superfical pyoderma, p. 146).

KEY POINTS

- Culture and sensitivity testing are mandatory.
- Search for underlying disease.
- Do not forget demodicosis.

Opportunistic (atypical) mycobacterial infections

ETIOLOGY AND PATHOGENESIS

Opportunistic (previously known as atypical) mycobacterial infections are associated with mostly fast-growing, saprophytic and usually non-pathogenic species including the *Mycobacterium fortuitum/peregrinium* group, *M. chelonae/abscessus*, *M. phlei*, *M. genavese*, *M. simiae*, *M. thermorestible*, *M. xenopi*, *M. smegmatis*, and *M. terrae* complex[1-3]. The association of particular species with certain presentations has become less clear, and recently it has been suggested that the varied presentations of feline cutaneous mycobacterial infections can be associated with a variety of different *Mycobacterium* species and non-mycobacterial organisms[4,5].

These species are ubiquitous in soil, water, and decaying vegetation. Infection usually occurs following traumatic wounds and is particularly common in adipose tissue such as the ventral abdomen and inguinal area[1,3]. Gastrointestinal tract and respiratory infections are very rare. Cats are much more commonly affected than dogs, especially those with an active outdoors lifestyle[1,6]. Although the organisms are found worldwide, infections are more common in subtropical or tropical climates. There does not appear to be any association with immunosuppression.

CLINICAL FEATURES

Most lesions affect the ventral abdomen, flanks, and base of the tail. The most common presentation is panniculitis with multiple punctuate ulcers and draining sinus tracts[1,7]. Other clinical signs include ulcerated and draining nodules, and subcutaneous granulomas (**184**)[2]. The affected areas may be markedly firm on palpation. Pain is variable, but may be severe in some cases. Systemic signs are minimal in the early stages, but there may be depression, pyrexia, lymphadenopathy, anorexia, and weight loss in chronic cases. Wound dehiscence and necrosis, with marked worsening of the lesions, is commonly seen following surgery. Superficial secondary infection of ulcerated tissue is common, but the clinical signs and poor response to antibiotics should indicate that there is an underlying problem.

DIFFERENTIAL DIAGNOSES

- Penetrating foreign body
- Demodicosis
- Panniculitis
- Feline leprosy and other mycobacterial infections
- Nocardiosis
- Infections with resistant bacteria (e.g. MRSA)
- Subcutaneous and deep mycoses
- Cuterebriasis or dracunculiasis
- Neoplasia

DIAGNOSIS

Clinical suspicion may be raised by the chronic history, resistance to systemic antibacterial agents, and failure to demonstrate a foreign body. Cytology of fresh discharge or deep tissue usually reveals pyogranulomatous inflammation. Most practices will not have easy access to Ziehl–Neelsen stains, but these species are frequently acid-fast negative anyway. Activated macrophages often have multiple, tiny, round to oval vacuoles (**185**), which presumably contain the organisms[1,7]. Similar vacuoles can be seen in the amorphous background matrix.

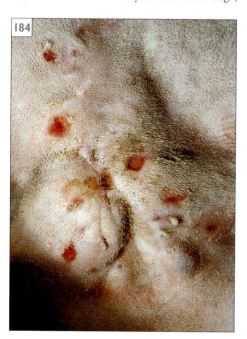

184 Atypical mycobacterial infection. Pyogranulomatous panniculitis in the groins and ventral abdomen due to *Mycobacterium smegmatis*.

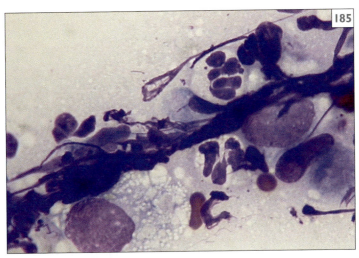

185 Pyogranulomatous inflammation from a cat with an opportunistic mycobacterial infection. The macrophages contain numerous round to oval vacuoles. Similar spaces are also present in the background material. (Diff-Quik-stained impression smear, ×1000)

Biopsy for histopathology is mandatory with this presentation[1,7]. Special stains should be requested, although the organisms are frequently acid-fast negative. Culture and antibiotic sensitivity testing should be performed by specialist mycobacterial laboratories capable of handling and identifying these organisms[3,7,8]. This may take several weeks, although recent advances in PCR techniques may make identification much quicker in the future[4,9].

Affected animals should be screened for systemic disease and possible immunosuppressive factors such as concurrent illness, FeLV, or FIV. These mycobacteria are not normally zoonotic, but veterinary staff and owners should observe hygienic precautions and guard against inoculation into deep tissues.

MANAGEMENT

Fluoroquinolone treatment is appropriate while waiting for confirmation of the diagnosis[1,2,8]. Surgical debulking in combination with systemic antibacterial treatment offers the best chance of success[1,8,10]. If possible, surgery should be delayed until the diagnosis is confirmed and antibiotic sensitivity is known. Surgery should be radical in order to remove as much infected tissue as possible. Surgery, however, is not appropriate in many cases.

Antibacterial treatment should be based on sensitivity testing, as mycobacteria vary in their susceptibility (e.g. *M. smegmatis* is most sensitive, *M. fortuitum* sensitive only to amikacin and fluoroquinolones, and *M. chelonae* is often sensitive only to clarithromycin and amikacin)[3]. Double or triple therapy is often recommended[1–3,8]. Treatment should continue for 6–12 weeks. Potentially effective drugs include: enrofloxacin (5 mg/kg p/o q24h); marbofloxacin (2 mg/kg p/o q24h); rifampicin (10–20 mg/kg p/o q12–24h); clarithromycin (5–10 mg/kg p/o q12–24h); azithromycin (7–15 mg/kg p/o q24h); and doxycycline (5–10 mg/kg p/o q12h).

The prognosis is guarded to poor. Some cases never resolve, whereas others may go into remission only to relapse when therapy is withdrawn. Unsuccessful surgery worsens the prognosis.

KEY POINTS
- More common in some countries than others. Local knowledge is important.
- Recognize the clinical signs, and perform cytology, biopsy, and culture early.

Feline leprosy

DEFINITION

Feline leprosy is a cutaneous infection caused mainly by infection with *Mycobacterium lepraemurium*[1]. However, *Mycobacterium visibilis*[2], *Mycobacterium szulgai*[3], and *Mycobacterium kanasii*[4], as well as a yet unnamed organism, have also been isolated[4].

ETIOLOGY AND PATHOGENESIS

The rat leprosy bacillus *M. lepraemurium* results in a tuberculoid form with sparse to moderate numbers of organisms[5]. In Australia, a lepromatous or organism-rich form of feline leprosy caused by a distinct and unnamed mycobacterial species has been documented[1]. In Canada and California, *M. visibilis* has been isolated from cats with lepromatous leprosy[4]. As lesions are most often noted about the head and neck, it is felt that transmission may occur from bites of rats or other cats[6]. The seasonal nature of cases (most occur during the autumn and winter) and the knowledge that arthropods can transmit mycobacteria have been interpreted as suggestive of an insect vector[7]. The natural host is unknown. The immune status of the cat, and the type of host response to the bacilli, dictates the clinical course and the signs of the disease[6,7].

CLINICAL FEATURES

There are regional differences in the seasonal frequency of feline leprosy, although the occurrence of the disease is worldwide[6,7]. Young adult cats are predisposed[6]. The most frequent sites for lesions to occur are the head, neck, and limbs. Clinical signs vary, with single or multiple cutaneous nodules being apparent (**186**), which may or may not ulcerate[6]. Occasionally, local lymphadenopathy is noted.

DIFFERENTIAL DIAGNOSES

- Penetrating foreign body
- Demodicosis
- Panniculitis
- Nocardiosis
- Subcutaneous and deep mycoses
- Cuterebriasis or dracunculiasis
- Neoplasia

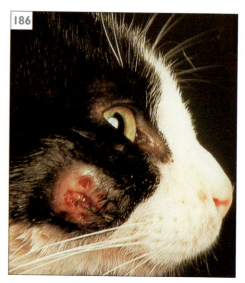

186 Feline leprosy. A discrete, erythematous nodule on the lateral aspect of the face of a cat.

DIAGNOSIS

Diagnosis is made on the basis of histopathologic observation of a granulomatous response in association with the presence of acid-fast bacilli[6], and on culture.

MANAGEMENT

If feasible, surgical removal of the nodules will result in a cure for many cases[8]. When surgery is not an option, clofazimine has been reported as useful in the management of feline leprosy[9]. A course of this antibacterial drug (8 mg/kg p/o q24h for 6 weeks and then twice weekly for 6 weeks, or 2–3 mg/kg p/o q24h for 5–8 months) was reported to induce remission in three cats[9]. Other drugs that have proved successful include rifampin (15 mg/kg p/o q24h) and clarithromycin (5 mg/kg p/o q12h)[9].

KEY POINT

- A rare infection.

Dermoid sinus

ETIOLOGY AND PATHOGENESIS
A dermoid sinus is a persistent congenital connection between the dura and the skin of the dorsal midline. It results from incomplete separation of the ectoderm and the neural tube during embryogenesis[1]. The sinus usually passes from the dura to the skin of the dorsal midline by way of the interarcuate ligaments, but may sometimes pass through a defect in the dorsal arch. Rarely, similar cysts and connections may be seen on the head connecting with the dura via a skull defect. Accumulation of keratinaceous debris and sebum may result in inflammation and secondary bacterial infection[2]. Neurologic signs may accompany inflammation or infection.

CLINICAL FEATURES
There is no sex predisposition, but Rhodesian Ridgebacks are predisposed, with an autosomal dominant mode of inheritance[1,3]. Rarely, other breeds may be affected such as Boxers, Shih Tzus, Bull Terriers, Golden Retrievers, Huskies, Springer Spaniels, and Yorkshire Terriers[2,4–6]. The clinical signs may be minimal; for example, a whorl of hair in the dorsal midline. Sometimes, hairs or even discharge may be apparent emerging from the sinus (**187**). Closed sinus tracts may present as non-painful, soft to fluctuating nodules in the midline. Neurologic signs vary from non-existent to dramatic.

DIFFERENTIAL DIAGNOSES
- Foreign body penetration
- Injection reaction
- Sterile or infected pyogranuloma
- Neoplasia, particularly keratoacanthomas or follicular tumors
- Cysts
- Nevi

DIAGNOSIS
The clinical signs are very suggestive, especially if neurologic signs are present. Radiography and contrast radiography may be necessary to delineate the sinus tract and confirm the diagnosis[2].

MANAGEMENT
Surgical excision of the tract and associated debris is the treatment of choice[2].

KEY POINT
- Pathognomonic presentation in Rhodesian Ridgebacks.

187 Dermoid sinus. A discrete tuft of hair is plainly visible emerging from the sinus in the dorsal midline.

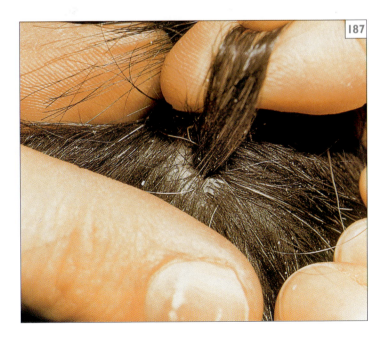

Anal furunculosis
(perianal fistulas)

DEFINITION
Anal furunculosis is characterized by chronic draining sinus tracts involving the perianal and perirectal tissues.

ETIOLOGY AND PATHOGENESIS
The cause of anal furunculosis is unknown. Most affected animals have a broad-based tail and low tail carriage. It has been hypothesized that this reduces anal ventilation and results in a fecal film over the perianal area. This predisposes to infection and abscessation of the circumanal glands and hair follicles in the perianal skin, resulting in fistula formation[1]. Day (1993)[2] has identified infiltration by eosinophils into ductal tissue and aggregates of T lymphocytes within the depths of the tissue, suggesting that complex immunologic processes are at play in these dogs.

CLINICAL FEATURES
The condition is most common in German Shepherd Dogs, but it has also been diagnosed in Irish Setters, Labrador Retrievers, Old English Sheepdogs, Border Collies, and Bulldogs, as well as in an English Setter, a Dandie Dinmont Terrier, and mixed breeds[3,4]. Historically, the most common complaint is tenesmus or straining to defecate. Dyschezia (painful defecation), weight loss, matting of hair surrounding the anus, foul odor, diarrhea, and frequent licking of the anal area may also be noted. The perineum is often very painful and many animals will have to be sedated in order to evaluate adequately the extent of the lesions. On physical examination the perianal area is often covered with a foul-smelling exudate and fecal material. Erythema, as well as varying numbers of shallow ulcers and fistulous tracts, may be present (**188**). In severe cases there may be 360 degree ulceration of the perianal area[5].

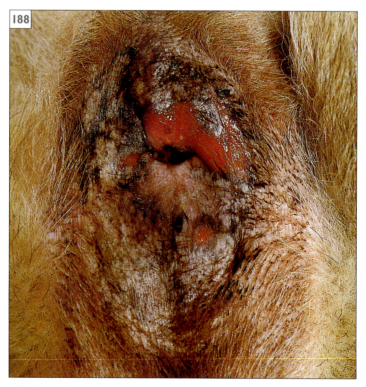

188 Perianal fistulas. Discrete foci of erosion and ulceration are apparent around the anal ring in this German Shepherd Dog.

DIFFERENTIAL DIAGNOSES

- Anal sac disease
- Anal or rectal neoplasia
- Rectal foreign bodies
- Anal pruritus secondary to *Malassezia pachydermatis*, atopic dermatitis, or cutaneous adverse food reaction

DIAGNOSIS

Diagnosis is based on history and clinical findings.

MANAGEMENT

Ciclosporin (cyclosporine) (5 mg/kg p/o q12h) has resulted in clinical improvement in 100% of cases and resolution of lesions in 83–100% of cases[6–9]. Clinical improvement is generally seen in two weeks, but it may take up to 20 weeks for resolution of lesions. Lesions reoccurred in 17–40% of animals after therapy was discontinued. Ketoconazole inhibits hepatic metabolism of ciclosporin by competitively binding to cytochrome P450; it can therefore be used in combination with ciclosporin to lower the ciclosporin dose. In one study ketoconazole (10 mg/kg p/o q24h) in combination with ciclosporin (1 mg/kg p/o q12h for 16 weeks) resulted in resolution of lesions in 93% of the cases[10]. (In some countries the use of both drugs would be off-license.) However, after discontinuing therapy, lesions returned in 50% of the cases. Because of the high rate of recurrence, maintenance dosing individualized for each animal may be necessary. Alternatively, tacrolimus ointment 0.1% applied twice daily may prevent recurrence. However, it is largely ineffective as a sole treatment for initiating remission of lesions.

Because the cost of ciclosporin can be prohibitive for some clients, one author (PJM) has used the following protocol, developed at Michigan State University, successfully in a limited number of cases:

- Diet: dogs are placed on a strict alternative protein/hypoallergenic diet (fish and potato diet [PJM uses a hydrolysed diet]). The dogs are not allowed any treats or snack-type foods containing meat or meat by-products.
- Sulfasalazine is given (1 g p/o q8h for at least four months, or one month after cessation of prednisone therapy). The length of use depends upon the resolution of lesions.
- Prednisone is given (1 mg/kg p/o q24h until resolution of lesions, and then the dose is reduced to 0.5 mg/kg p/o q24h for an additional 6–8 weeks).
- Tacrolimus ointment 0.1% is applied to the affected area twice daily.
- Monthly examinations are performed until a controlled state is reached. The goal is to maintain on the diet plus the tacrolimus ointment, or the diet, tacrolimus ointment, and sulfasalazine.

KEY POINTS

- Pathognomonic presentation.
- More likely to be a situation where the disease is controlled rather than cured.

Metatarsal fistulation of the German Shepherd Dog

DEFINITION

Metatarsal fistulation of the German Shepherd Dog is an uncommon condition whereby draining tracts occur in the skin of the plantar metatarsal area.

ETIOLOGY AND PATHOGENESIS

The pathogenesis of this condition is unknown, but circulating antibodies to types I and II collagen were elevated in some affected dogs[1].

CLINICAL FEATURES

The condition is found in German Shepherd Dogs, crossbreeds of GSDs[2], and occasionally other breeds. Initial lesions consist of a soft swelling in the skin, which progress to well-demarcated single or multiple tracts containing a serosanguineous discharge located on the plantar metatarsal skin surface just proximal to the metatarsal pad. Both hindlimbs are affected and occasionally lesions can occur in the plantar metacarpal skin. Secondary bacterial infection can occur once sinus tracts develop. Affected skin of chronic lesions may become scarred (**189**). Pain is variable, but is mild in most dogs. The condition can be concurrent with lesions of the German Shepherd Dog pyoderma syndrome.

DIFFERENTIAL DIAGNOSES

- Foreign body
- Puncture wound
- Blastomycosis or other subcutaneous mycosis

DIAGNOSIS

Diagnosis is based on history, clinical findings, and ruling out other differentials.

MANAGEMENT

Topical application of 0.1% tacrolimus ointment twice daily in combination with 500 mg of tetracycline (or 10 mg/kg doxycycline q24h) and 500 mg of niacinamide orally three times daily is beneficial in many cases. Alternatively, prednisolone (1.1–2.2 mg/kg p/o q24h) may be used and then tapered for maintenance. Topical glucocorticoids may also be beneficial as adjunct therapy. Although the authors have no experience of using ciclosporin (cyclosporine) to treat this condition, it is speculated that its use at a dose of 5 mg/kg orally once daily may be of benefit. However, one author (TJN) has seen the condition develop in atopic German Shepherd Dogs managed with 5 mg/kg ciclosporin once daily to every other day.

KEY POINT

- Be aware that this is a condition that is generally controlled but not cured.

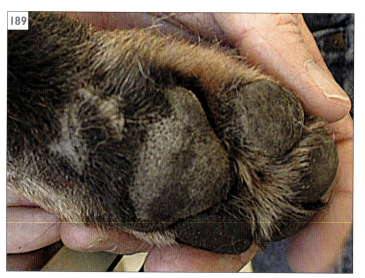

189 Scarred tracts in a German Shepherd Dog with metatarsal fistulation.

Diseases characterized by crust and scale

General approach
- Crust and scale are common, but are secondary and often non-specific lesions
- Crusts are dried exudates; scales are accumulated keratinocytes
- Carefully evaluate the history and clinical signs to narrow the differential diagnosis
- It is helpful to initially consider groups of differential diagnoses before focusing on individual conditions (e.g. ectoparasites; hypersensitivity; infections; endocrine, metabolic, or nutritional; immune-mediated; congenital or hereditary; miscellaneous)

Common conditions
- Callus formation
- Actinic dermatosis
- Feline acne
- Sebaceous adenitis
- Idiopathic (primary) keratinization defect (seborrhea)
- Vitamin A responsive dermatosis
- Leishmaniasis

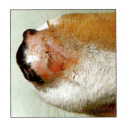
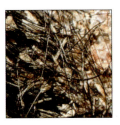
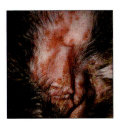
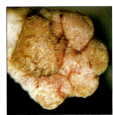

Callus formation

ETIOLOGY AND PATHOGENESIS

A callus is a defined area of hyperkeratosis, which is sometimes lichenified and typically occurs over bony pressure points. The hyperkeratosis and thickening of the skin are due to irritation resulting from frictional contact with a hard surface on the exterior of the skin and pressure from an underlying bony prominence.

CLINICAL FEATURES

Callus development occurs more frequently in large, shorthaired breeds that sleep on hard surfaces such as concrete, wood, brick, or rock. Lesions usually develop on the lateral aspect of the elbows or hocks (**190**). They may also develop on the sternum of deep-chested dogs or dogs with short limbs in which the sternum may continually contact objects such as stairs. Calluses appear as focal areas of alopecia, hyperkeratosis, and lichenification with a light gray surface. Entrapment of hair and/or sebum in a callus may result in a foreign body reaction with draining tracts and secondary infection (**191**). Fissuring and secondary infection can be painful. Calluses may erode, ulcerate, and form non-healing wounds in dogs with underlying disorders such as hyperadrenocorticism. Calluses with underlying subcutaneous hygromas may present as fluctuant, mobile masses.

DIFFERENTIAL DIAGNOSES
- Demodicosis
- Neoplasia
- Dermatophytosis
- Deep pyoderma
- Zinc responsive dermatosis

DIAGNOSIS

Diagnosis is generally based on the history and clinical features. Further investigation for underlying causes may be necessary in cases of non-antibiotic responsive infections or non-healing wounds.

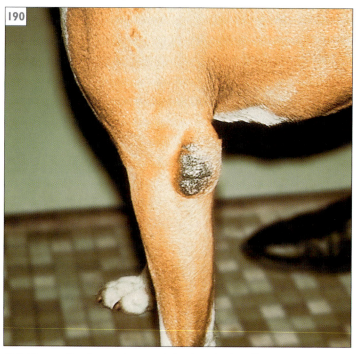

190 Elbow callus. Large, pigmented, deeply convoluted lesions on the lateral aspect of elbows are typical of callus.

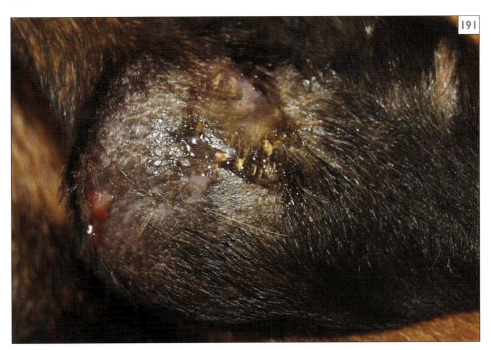

191 Infected callus on a dog's hock.

MANAGEMENT

The animal's sleeping habits should be modified so that it rests on soft bedding material such as foam rubber padding. Custom or home-made clothing with pads over the affected pressure points are also useful. Callus size may be reduced by daily application of a preparation containing 6.6% salicylic acid, 5% sodium lactate, and 5% urea, which promotes desquamation of the stratum corneum. Twice daily treatment with flucinolone acetonide in dimethyl sulfoxide hastens the process by reducing inflammation and decreasing basal cell turnover rates. Care must be exercised to avoid overdoing treatment and creating an erosion or ulcer. Calluses and subcutaneous hygromas should not be surgically removed, as this frequently results in a non-healing wound.

If infection is present, systemic treatment with bactericidal antibacterial agents is indicated based on culture and sensitivity testing. Treatment should be continued until the lesions have resolved. For deep infections associated with hair granulomas and fibrosis this may take many weeks.

KEY POINT

• Management is a key issue in the control of this problem.

Actinic dermatosis

ETIOLOGY AND PATHOGENESIS

Actinic dermatosis is skin damage resulting from prolonged exposure to ultraviolet (UV) light. UV light is divided into UV-A (320–400 nm) and UV-B (290–320 nm)[1,2]. UV-A penetrates into the deep dermis, while UV-B penetrates only to the upper dermis. Exposure to UV light results, progressively, in erythema, heat, edema, pain, and pruritus[1,2]. Chronic actinic damage results in inflammatory, locally proliferative lesions and, possibly, tumor induction[1,2]. Chronic exposure to UV-B results in a progressive decrease in epidermal Langerhans cell numbers[1,3]. Reduced immune surveillance may result in local oncogenic changes escaping detection, facilitating the development of neoplasia, especially squamous cell carcinoma and hemangioma/sarcoma[4].

CLINICAL FEATURES

Both dogs and cats are affected. Lesions are most common in countries with high levels of sunlight. Actinic lesions develop in lightly pigmented, lightly haired, or alopecic areas of the body such as the face, lower flanks, and ventrum[1]. Any depigmented and/or alopecic skin (e.g. secondary to scarring, endocrine or immune-mediated disease) will also be vulnerable[2]. The tips of the pinnae, above the hairline, are particularly susceptible (**192**), especially in white-haired cats[5]. There is local thickening and a fine scale develops. Scarring, curling, and cutaneous horns of the distal pinnae may be noted[1,2]. Eventually, an ulcerative, invasive, and variably proliferative squamous cell carcinoma develops[4,5].

In light-colored dogs the most common site of actinic radiation damage is the rostral face, immediately caudal to the planum nasale (**193**). There is erythema, fine scale, and progressive alopecia. There may be loss of pigmentation and scarring. In dogs that habitually sleep in the sun, lesions may develop on the lower flank, ventrum, scrotum, and limbs[1,2]. Many cases become secondarily infected with *Staphylococcus intermedius*. Chronic actinic damage can result in alopecia, lichenification, hyperpigmentation (often macular), loss of elasticity, and wrinkling of the skin[2,3].

DIFFERENTIAL DIAGNOSES

- Demodicosis
- Dermatophytosis
- Cutaneous lupus erythematosus
- Superficial pyoderma
- Pemphigus foliaceus or erythematosus
- Dermatomyositis
- Uveodermatologic syndrome
- Drug eruption
- Cutaneous neoplasia

DIAGNOSIS

Local knowledge of climate and breeds at risk will greatly aid diagnosis. Observation that lightly pigmented skin is affected whereas adjacent pigmented skin is unaffected is very suggestive of an actinic dermatosis. Microscopic examination of skin scrapings will allow demodicosis to be ruled out. Fungal culture will allow dermatophytosis to be ruled out. Biopsy samples will reveal changes consistent with actinic dermatitis (e.g. superficial dermal fibrosis and follicular keratosis)[1,2].

MANAGEMENT

Elimination of secondary pyoderma is important[2]. Sun avoidance measures may be helpful, although they are difficult to institute for free-roaming cats[2]. Local sun protection may be achieved with heavy T-shirts (fitted over the trunk) or PABA sun-blocking cream. Items such as hats and goggles can be adapted for suitable dogs. Tattooing is not usually effective, as the pigment sits beneath the epidermis; indelible marker pens can be used on the skin surface, but there is little evidence that they protect against UV-A and UV-B. In cats with pinnal lesions the distal pinnae may be amputated to below the hair line as a preventive measure. Topical glucocorticoids may help ameliorate acute erythematous lesions, but they should not be used routinely as skin thinning and local immunosuppression may facilitate actinic damage and neoplastic transformation[2]. Imiquimod has been of some benefit in humans[6].

KEY POINT

- Treat actinic dermatosis seriously. Neoplastic transformation may occur.

192, 193 Actinic dermatitis. Pinnal lesions in a cat (**192**) and facial lesions in a dog (**193**).

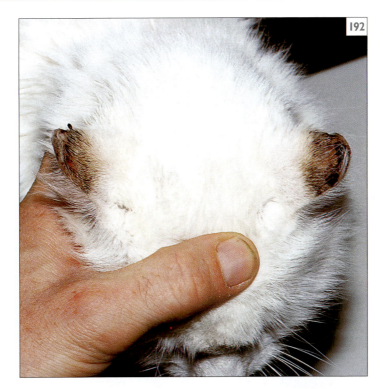

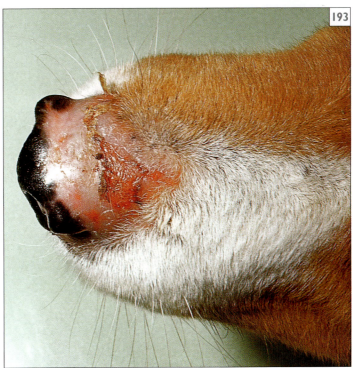

Sebaceous adenitis

ETIOLOGY AND PATHOGENESIS

Sebaceous adenitis is an uncommon disease characterized by loss of sebaceous glands, scaling, and alopecia. The etiology and pathogenesis are unknown. In Standard Poodles the disease is hereditary and appears to be an autosomal recessive[1,2]. There may also be a hereditary predisposition in Akitas[3] and Hovawarts[4]. Theories include an autoimmune response to sebaceous gland antigens or a primary structural defect of the sebaceous gland or its duct, which allows the leakage of sebum into the dermis where it provokes a foreign body reaction[2,3]. During the early stages there is a mild perifolliculitis, which develops into a nodular granulomatous inflammatory reaction around the sebaceous glands. End-stage follicles exhibit a lack of sebaceous glands and parafollicular fibrosis, with keratin plugging of the follicular infundibulum. It is not known if there is a causal relationship between the sebaceous gland changes and the abnormal follicular keratinization, or whether these are simply coexisting features of a common inheritable process[2,3]. Alopecia associated with sebaceous gland adenitis is thought to be a consequence of the parafollicular fibrosis interfering with stem cells of the follicle.

CLINICAL FEATURES

Sebaceous gland adenitis occurs in young adult to middle-aged dogs, with no sex predilection. There is a breed predilection for Standard Poodles, Akitas, Hungarian Vizslas, and Samoyeds, but it is also seen in a wide variety of other breeds[1-3]. The clinical appearance, distribution, and severity of lesions vary from breed to breed, and from animal to animal within a breed.

In Standard Poodles the first signs of clinical disease generally appear in young adult to middle-aged animals, with 90% of affected animals 1.5–5 years of age[1,2]. Lesions first start on the top of the neck, head, back, or ears. Initially, they appear as scaling and thinning of the hair, focal areas of alopecia, and discoloration of the coat (**194**). There are usually prominent follicular casts; tightly adherent follicular debris around the base of the hair shaft (**195**). As the condition progresses, more areas of skin become involved with severe scaling characterized by tightly adherent silver-white scales incorporating small tufts of matted hair. Alopecia becomes more severe as the condition advances (**196**). Secondary bacterial folliculitis commonly results in inflammation and pruritus. Samoyeds have lesions similar to Standard Poodles, except that the scale tends to build up into plaque-like lesions.

Akitas exhibit similar clinical signs to Standard Poodles, but often have a more extensive alopecia, seborrhea, and superficial bacterial folliculitis or deep bacterial folliculitis and furunculosis. They may also manifest systemic signs of malaise, fever, and weight loss, especially if there is a severe secondary infection[2,3].

Hungarian Vizslas and other short-coated breeds have clinical signs that are characterized by multifocal annular and serpiginous areas of alopecia and fine white scaling that occur progressively over the head, ears, and trunk[2]. The scaling may be the most prominent sign in Springer Spaniels.

Sebaceous adenitis is also seen in cats and rabbits, although there are clinical and histopathologic differences from the canine condition[5,6]. In cats it may play a role in some cases of feline acne[7].

DIFFERENTIAL DIAGNOSES

- Vitamin A responsive dermatitis
- Primary keratinization defects
- Leishmaniasis
- Dermatophytosis
- Demodicosis
- Superficial pyoderma
- Zinc responsive dermatosis
- Endocrinopathies
- Color-dilution alopecia
- Follicular dysplasia
- Pemphigus foliaceus
- Epitheliotropic lymphoma

DIAGNOSIS

Hair plucks reveal the typical profuse follicular casts. These are often macroscopically visible and matt the hairs together. Histopathology reveals a multifocal inflammatory infiltrate of histiocytes, lymphocytes, neutrophils, and plasma cells around the sebaceous glands and other adnexal structures in early disease[2-4,8,9]. Advanced cases have moderate acanthosis, hyperkeratosis, follicular hyperkeratosis, and an absence of sebaceous glands. Multiple biopsies are frequently necessary to observe the diagnostic pathology.

194 Scaling, alopecia, and coat discoloration in a West Highland White Terrier with sebaceous adenitis and secondary pyoderma.

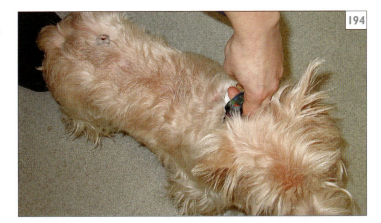

195 Severe scaling and numerous follicular casts in a Bernese Mountain Dog with sebaceous adenitis.

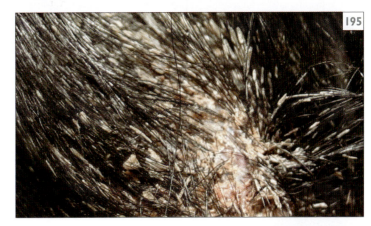

196 Sebaceous adenitis. Note the patchy alopecia and scale.

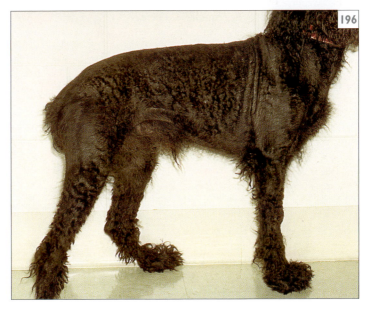

MANAGEMENT

The prognosis is fair to guarded, as therapy is palliative and response to various medications is variable. Early or mild cases may be helped by keratolytic shampoos, emollient rinses, and omega-3 and omega-6 essential fatty acid dietary supplements[2,4,9]. More severe or advanced cases may be helped by spraying or rinsing daily or every 2–3 days with a mixture of 50–75% propylene glycol in water. This helps soften and loosen scale before bathing. Emollient soaks and rinses such as coconut oil in water can help moisturize the skin and coat.

The synthetic retinoid isotretinoin or acitretin (1–3 mg/kg p/o q12–24h to remission and then taper to maintenance) can result in improvement in some cases[2,4]. These drugs are generally well tolerated, but adverse effects can include keratoconjunctivitis sicca, gastrointestinal tract upsets, hepatopathy, musculoskeletal pain, and hyperostosis. They are also potent teratogens and should not be used in breeding animals or handled by women of child bearing age unless on oral contraception. Hungarian Vizslas and possibly Springer Spaniels have a better response to isotretinoin than other breeds. Retinoids are expensive, and vitamin A (see Vitamin A responsive dermatosis, p. 185) may be an effective and cheaper alternative in some dogs.

Ciclosporin (cyclosporine) (5 mg/kg p/o q12–24h) (see Canine atopic dermatitis, p. 20) has been reported to help some animals that have not been responsive to the retinoids[2,8]. There is a recent report of a beneficial response to topical ciclosporin[10] diluted to 10 mg/ml in water; however, ciclosporin is not absorbed topically so it is unclear whether it has an anti-inflammatory action or acts as an emollient. The anagen inducing activity of ciclosporin may help resolve the alopecia. Ciclosporin was also reported to be effective in a cat with sebaceous adenitis[5].

The use of systemic glucocorticoids (e.g. prednisolone) at anti-inflammatory doses (0.5–1.0 mg/kg p/o q12–24h) may be of value in early cases[2,4]. However, glucocorticoids are of less value once the follicular damage has occurred and the inflammatory reaction has ameliorated.

As sebaceous adenitis in Standard Poodles is a genetic disease, its prevalence can be decreased by identifying and not breeding animals who are carriers or who are affected with the disease. To assist owners and breeders in identification of both normal and affected animals, the Sebaceous Adenitis Registry for Standard Poodles has been established. Current information about this can be obtained by contacting the Institute for Genetic Disease Control, P.O. Box 222, Davis, CA 95617, USA.

KEY POINTS
- Diagnosis is only made by histopathologic examination of multiple (at least three, preferably five) biopsy samples.
- Management involves considerable effort, and good client communication is imperative.

Vitamin A responsive dermatosis

ETIOLOGY AND PATHOGENESIS

Vitamin A responsive dermatosis is a rare dermatosis characterized by epidermal hyperkeratosis with markedly disproportionate follicular hyperkeratosis. The etiology is not known. Retinoic acid is essential for a wide range of cell and tissue functions, but its cutaneous role is particularly directed towards keratinocyte proliferation and differentiation by regulating the expression of keratins[1,2]. Even though the clinical signs resolve with vitamin A supplementation, there is no evidence that affected animals are deficient in vitamin A[1-3].

CLINICAL FEATURES

The dermatosis is almost entirely confined to Cocker Spaniels[1,2]. The clinical signs usually begin at between two and five years of age, and clinical signs get progressively more severe. The scaling typically involves prominent, frond-like follicular casts and multifocal, frond-like, erythematous, crusted plaques, particularly on the lateral thorax and ventrum (**197**). Affected animals are often pruritic and have malodorous skin, especially if there are secondary bacterial or *Malassezia* infections[1-3].

DIFFERENTIAL DIAGNOSES

- Scabies
- Demodicosis
- Flea allergic dermatosis
- Atopic dermatitis
- Cutaneous adverse food reaction
- Primary idiopathic keratinization defect (seborrhea)
- Sebaceous adenitis
- Icthyosis

DIAGNOSIS

The clinical signs and history are highly suggestive. Histopathology will help confirm the presence of a follicular oriented keratinization defect, but response to therapy is necessary to differentiate this condition from other keratinization disorders. Recently, however, it has become clear that some keratinization defects traditionally treated with synthetic retinoids can also respond to vitamin A. Cytology can be helpful in identifying secondary infections.

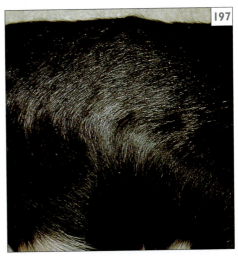

197 Vitamin A responsive dermatosis. Alopecia and focal accumulations of scale are typical of this condition.

MANAGEMENT

The prognosis is generally good. Treatment with 10,000 IU (maximum 800–1000 IU/kg/day) vitamin A in food once daily usually resolves the clinical signs in 4–6 weeks[1-3]. Appropriate keratolytic and/or antimicrobial treatment will aid clinical resolution. Once in remission, affected dogs can be maintained with daily (or less frequently if possible) vitamin A supplementation. At these doses vitamin A is very well tolerated[1,2,4], but potential adverse effects include hepatopathy, hyperostosis, and keratoconjunctivitis sicca.

KEY POINT

- An uncommon dermatosis ultimately diagnosed by response to vitamin A.

Feline acne

DEFINITION

Feline acne is a multifactorial skin disease characterized by comedo formation on the chin and lips.

ETIOLOGY AND PATHOGENESIS

Feline acne may be idiopathic or the condition may develop due to multiple factors that result in a localized keratinization defect of hair follicles and hyperplasia of the sebaceous glands. Diseases and conditions that may predispose to the development of acne include demodicosis, dermatophytosis, virus infections (FeLV or FIV and upper respiratory viruses), irritant contact dermatitis, atopic dermatitis, and stress from moving to a new location or other causes[1]. The hair follicles become distended with lipid and keratinous debris, resulting in the classic comedones (blackheads) of acne. If these follicles rupture and release keratin and sebaceous material into the dermis, a foreign body reaction with inflammation will develop. Many bacteria are often found in the follicular plugs and their presence can lead to infection and further inflammation.

CLINICAL FEATURES

Feline acne can occur in cats of any age and there is no breed or sex predisposition[2]. Lesions generally occur on the lower lips, the chin, and, occasionally, the upper lips. Comedones, especially around the lateral commissures of the mouth and the lower lip, are the predominant findings (**198, 199**). Initially, these lesions are not pruritic, but they may be noticed by the owner. If the condition progresses, erythematous crusted papules, folliculitis, and furunculosis may develop, which can result in pruritus and scarring. Alopecia, erythema, and swelling of the chin is seen in severe cases[1,2]. In Persian cats the lesions may affect the face as well as the chin. Excoriations from scratching may occur in cases with severe inflammation. When secondary bacterial infections are present, *Pasteurella multocida*, β-hemolytic streptococci, and coagulase-positive *Staphylococcus* spp. have been isolated[1].

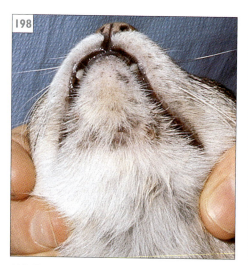

198 Feline acne. Characteristic appearance of multiple comedones on the rostral aspect of the mandible.

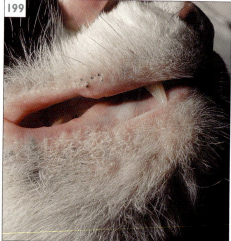

199 Feline acne. Comedones on the upper lip.

DIFFERENTIAL DIAGNOSES

- Contact dermatitis
- Eosinophilic granuloma
- Pyoderma
- *Malassezia* dermatitis
- Dermatophytosis
- Demodicosis
- Trauma
- Dietary intolerance
- Atopic dermatitis

DIAGNOSIS

The history and clinical signs are characteristic. Microscopic examination of skin scrapings and impression smears of follicular plugs, dermatophyte culture, virus isolation, and bacterial culture and sensitivity will rule out infectious causes. Histopathologic examination of biopsy samples will confirm the diagnosis.

MANAGEMENT

Clients should be forewarned that feline acne is a condition that generally is not cured, but just controlled with periodic or continuous treatment. If there is an underlying predisposing condition (e.g. demodicosis or dermatophytosis), it should be addressed with specific treatment.

Treatment for idiopathic feline acne will vary with the type and severity of lesions. Small numbers of asymptomatic comedones may not require any treatment. Larger numbers of comedones with seborrhea and some swelling of the chin will benefit from the antibacterial and follicular flushing actions of alternate day or twice-weekly benzoyl peroxide gel or shampoo. Benzoyl peroxide may be irritating to some cats and should be discontinued if erythema develops; this is less likely to happen if the concentration is kept to 3% or less[1]. Cats cannot detoxify benzoyl products as readily as humans or dogs, but toxicity is unlikely if the products are used in small quantities on small areas, treated skin is rinsed, and cats are prevented from ingesting the products as much as possible. Alternative shampoos would be those containing ethyl lactate, sulfur–salicylic acid, and chlorhexidine. A product containing phytosphingosine, which is antibacterial and decreases sebaceous secretions when applied weekly, is also beneficial.

If bacteria are found on impression smears, topical antibacterial preparations containing mupirocin, fusidic acid, or polymixin B may be helpful. If bacterial folliculitis or furunculosis is present, systemic antibiotics (e.g. clavulanated amoxicillin or cefalosporins) for 2–6 weeks would be appropriate. The comedolytic activity of topical vitamin A products (0.05% retinoic acid cream), applied daily at first and then on alternate days or twice weekly, has been beneficial in some cases[1]. This product may also cause irritation and its use should be monitored closely.

If there is severe inflammation resulting from a foreign body reaction to keratin and sebum of ruptured hair follicles, a course of systemic corticosteroids (prednisone, prednisolone, or methylprednisolone [1–2 mg/kg p/o q24h for 10–14 days]) is indicated. Isotretinoin (2 mg/kg p/o q24h) has been advocated for the treatment and control of refractory cases[1]. It acts by decreasing the activity of sebaceous glands and normalizing keratinization within hair follicles; therapeutic benefits have been observed in 30% of treated cases. Clinical response should occur within one month[1]. Once improvement is seen, the isotretinoin dose may be reduced to twice weekly for control. Side-effects of its use in cats include conjunctivitis, periocular crusting, vomiting, and diarrhea[1]. Monthly laboratory screenings are suggested when it is used over prolonged periods[1]. (**Note:** Isotretinoin is extremely teratogenic and appropriate caution should be observed for both animals and humans.) As the commercial availability of this drug is limited, the alternative would be acitretin (0.5–2 mg/kg p/o q24h).

KEY POINT

- Although apparently pathognomonic, the clinical signs may also reflect demodicosis or dermatophytosis. All cases should be subjected to skin scrapings and fungal culture.

Idiopathic (primary) keratinization defect
(seborrhea)

ETIOLOGY AND PATHOGENESIS
Idiopathic (primary) keratinization defect or seborrhea in Cocker Spaniels is a common, possibly familial, dermatosis associated with abnormal basal epidermal cell kinetics. Compared with normal dogs, basal epidermal cells in affected dogs undergo accelerated cellular proliferation and turnover[1-3]. There is an increase in the number of actively dividing basal cells, a shortened cell cycle, and a decreased transit time to the stratum corneum (7–8 days compared with 21–23 days). Hair follicles and sebaceous glands are similarly affected. This results in marked scaling, greasiness, and alopecia. The disrupted epidermal barrier and altered cutaneous micro-environment predispose to secondary pyoderma and *Malassezia* dermatitis. Similar conditions are recognized in other Spaniels, especially English Springers, and, less commonly, in other breeds[4].

CLINICAL FEATURES
Most animals display abnormal keratinization from an early age. The clinical signs vary in severity and extent, but tend to worsen with time. Mildly affected dogs exhibit adherent, greasy scales around the nipples, lip folds, and external ear canals (**200**, **201**). More severely affected animals have more severe and generalized lesions

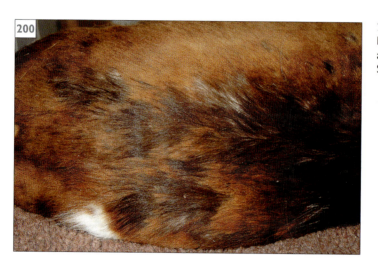

200 Primary keratinization defect in an English Springer Spaniel.

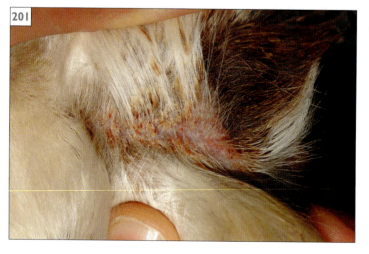

201 Same dog as in **200**; severe scaling.

in skin folds, ventral neck, ventral body, medial limbs, trunk, and feet. Severely affected dogs are malodorous, greasy, alopecic, and pruritic, with a papular scaling and, occasionally, crusting dermatosis (**202, 203**). Chronic or recurrent, and often severe, otitis externa is common.

DIFFERENTIAL DIAGNOSES

- Dietary, especially essential fatty acid, deficiency
- Ectoparasite infestation
- Atopic dermatitis
- Cutaneous adverse food reaction
- Sebaceous adenitis
- Vitamin A responsive dermatosis
- Pyoderma

- *Malassezia* infection
- Dermatophytosis
- Leishmaniasis
- Pemphigus foliaceus
- Epitheliotropic lymphoma
- Endocrinopathies
- Superficial necrolytic dermatitis (metabolic epidermal necrosis or hepatocutaneous syndrome)
- Allergic or irritant contact dermatitis to shampoos etc.

Some of these conditions may be concurrent (especially parasites and hypersensitivities) or may be secondary keratinization defects (e.g. pyoderma and *Malassezia*).

202, 203 Primary keratinization defect in a Cocker Spaniel with severe erythema, alopecia, scaling, and superficial spreading pyoderma.

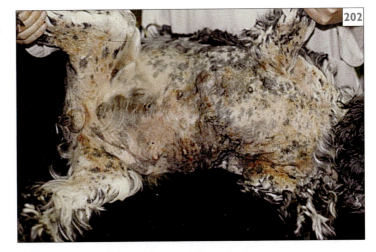

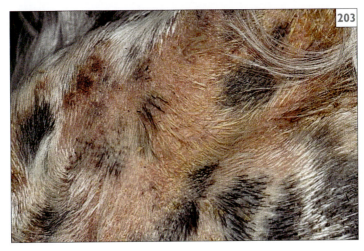

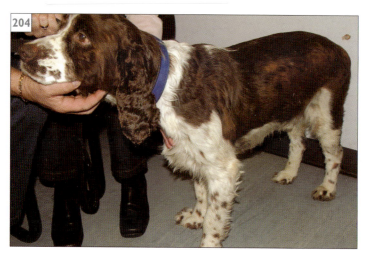

204, 205 Same dog as in 200; good response to treatment with essential fatty acids, keratolytic and emollient shampoos, and vitamin A.

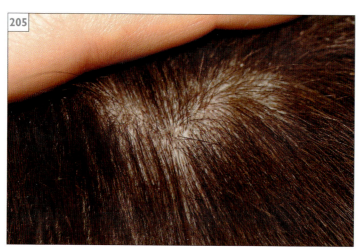

DIAGNOSIS

The breed, history and clinical signs are highly suggestive. Nevertheless, secondary scaling is much more common than primary keratinization disorders and other underlying conditions should be ruled out[4-6]. The history should reveal management factors, bathing, and diets that could be involved. Skin scrapes, tape strips, and trial therapy will eliminate ectoparasites. Secondary bacterial and *Malassezia* dermatitis and/or otitis can be identified on cytology and should be treated appropriately. Elimination diet trials are indicated where significant erythema and pruritus remain after ectoparasite and antimicrobial treatment. It can be difficult to assess the contribution of atopic dermatitis as this is a diagnosis of exclusion, allergen specific tests are not diagnostic, and the two conditions may be concurrent. It is therefore important to evaluate carefully the history, clinical signs, and response to anti-inflammatory therapy (see Canine atopic dermatitis, p. 20). Routine hematology, biochemistry, urinalysis, basal thyroid tests, and dynamic tests may be necessary if an endocrinopathy or metabolic disease is suspected. Investigation of the latter may necessitate liver function tests, radiography, and ultrasonography. Biopsy and histopathology are supportive but nonspecific, although they can help to eliminate some of the differential diagnoses.

MANAGEMENT

If a primary cause cannot be identified and controlled, lifelong therapy is necessary. Management must be tailored to the individual depending on the response to therapy, adverse effects, owner's commitment, and financial resources. It is very important to maintain rigorous flea control and treat secondary skin and ear infections promptly[4–6].

Topical therapy

Topical therapy can be very effective, is generally safe, and is traditionally the mainstay of treatment[7]. It does, however, require an amenable patient, adequate facilities, and a committed owner, and is not therefore suitable in every case. Topical therapy should be keratolytic (to soften and remove existing scale) and keratoplastic (suppress basal cell turnover and excessive keratinization), and degreasing or moisturizing to help restore the epidermal barrier and reduce transepidermal water loss (see *Table 8*). The relative importance of these factors varies with each case. Treatment may require a combination of products, which are best selected by trial and error.

Topical therapy should be instituted 2–3 times weekly with a 10–15 minute contact time. Once in remission the frequency can be reduced. It may also be possible to switch to less aggressive products and/or reduce the number of different products employed.

Systemic therapy

Systemic therapy can be used in cases where topical therapy is ineffective or inappropriate. Essential fatty acid supplementation can be helpful in restoring normal epidermal barrier function[4]. Synthetic retinoids (e.g. isotretinoin or acitretinoin [1–2 mg/kg q24h, reducing to 1 mg/kg q48h for maintenance]; see Sebaceous adenitis, p. 182) can be effective in suppressing the accelerated cellular kinetics and associated keratinization defects[5,6]. Vitamin A (10,000 IU q24h, maximum 800–1000 IU/kg q24h (see Vitamin A responsive dermatosis, p. 185) can also be effective and is cheaper and better tolerated than synthetic retinoids (**204, 205**). This blurs the distinction between what is vitamin A responsive dermatosis and primary keratinization defect in Cocker Spaniels.

Table 8 Topical therapies

Keratolytics

Sulfur and salicylic acid (synergistic; also antimicrobial and antipruritic)

Selenium sulfide (also antimicrobial and antiparasitic; degreasing but drying and irritating)

Benzoyl peroxide (also antimicrobial; degreasing but drying, irritating and bleaching)

Tar (less commonly available; degreasing but drying, irritating, staining and potentially carcinogenic)

Propylene glycol (very effective and well tolerated; mixed 50:50 with water and sprayed on as a soak; may need degreasing afterwards)

Urea (well tolerated)

Free fatty acids (well tolerated and moisturizing)

Keratoplastics

Sulfur and salicylic acid

Selenium sulfide

Tar

Ethyl lactate (well tolerated; also antimicrobial)

Sodium or ammonium lactate

Moisturizing

Linoleic acid and free fatty acids

Lanolin

Mineral and vegetable oils

Vitamin E

Colloidal oatmeal

Propylene glycol

Urea

Sodium or ammonium lactate

KEY POINTS

- Common, but Cocker Spaniels can have other conditions.
- The prognosis is good, but treatment can be complex and involved.
- Avoid systemic glucocorticoids wherever possible.

Nasal and digital hyperkeratosis

DEFINITION
Nasal hyperkeratosis is associated with excessive amounts of horny tissue confined to the planum nasale. Digital hyperkeratosis presents similarly and affects the footpads.

ETIOLOGY AND PATHOGENESIS
Hyperkeratosis occurs as a consequence of increased production of, or retention of, keratinized tissue. This abnormal keratinization may be the result of an inborn error of metabolism, as occurs in ichthyosis. Familial footpad hyperkeratosis has been reported in Dogues de Bordeaux[1].

Nasal and digital hyperkeratosis may occur in the same individual. Canine distemper virus infection may result in nasodigital hyperkeratosis, but this disease is seen less frequently nowadays. Systemic disease, such as pemphigus foliaceus and dietary deficiency, in particular, zinc, may also result in pedal, nasal, or nasodigital hyperkeratosis. Spontaneous idiopathic disease, particularly of the older dog, is the most common clinical presentation.

CLINICAL FEATURES
Nasal hyperkeratosis is confined to the planum nasale and presents as a variably thickened, fissured accumulation of dry, horny tissue (**206**). Pedal hyperkeratosis is more variable in presentation (**207, 208**). Frond-like proliferations of keratin may occur in both locations. Areas of hyperkeratosis may fissure, leading to secondary bacterial or *Malassezia* infection. In old dogs with idiopathic disease, the periphery of the footpads is more severely affected and this pattern of hyperkeratosis is also seen in metabolic epidermal necrosis, although in the latter condition there are usually lesions elsewhere in addition to signs of systemic disease. Pemphigus foliaceus may result in footpad hyperkeratosis, and in some cases the pedal lesion may be the only sign of disease[2].

DIFFERENTIAL DIAGNOSES
- Canine distemper virus infection
- Pemphigus foliaceus
- Zinc responsive dermatosis
- Superficial necrolytic dermatitis (metabolic epidermal necrosis/hepatocutaneous syndrome)
- Ichthyosis

DIAGNOSIS
Consideration of the vaccinal history, and the risks of exposure to the virus, is particularly important *vis-à-vis* a diagnosis of canine distemper virus infection. Dietary history will raise suspicions of absolute or relative zinc deficiency, and consideration of the clinical signs and history will suggest the presence, or otherwise, of systemic disease. Ichthyosis is congenital. Histopathologic examination of biopsy samples is the most useful diagnostic tool.

MANAGEMENT
If a specific disease can be identified, it should be managed accordingly. The management of idiopathic disease can be difficult because of the nature of the lesions and the tendency of the animal to lick topically applied agents. Local application of keratolytic and keratoplastic agents, such as preparations containing 60% salicylic acid, 5% urea, and 5% sodium lactate, may be of value, as may application of petroleum jelly[3]. Topical application of 50% propylene glycol may also be useful in more severe cases[1]. Topical tretinoin gel can also be of value in severe cases[4]. The fissures in the hyperkeratotic tissue may become infected, and in these cases systemic glucocorticoid, antibacterial, or antiyeast treatment will be necessary. One author (PJM) has found the application of a solution containing flucinolone acetonide in 60% dimethylsulfoxide to the affected areas twice daily to be beneficial in many cases.

There are anecdotal reports that the retinoid tazarotene (0.1% gel applied topically q24h until improvement of lesions and then 2–3 times weekly for control) is beneficial for the treatment of this condition. One author (PJM) has used it successfully in the treatment of two cases. The drug is teratogenic and may be irritating if applied to normal skin.

KEY POINT
- A frustrating disease to manage.

206 Nasal hyperkeratosis in a Cocker Spaniel.

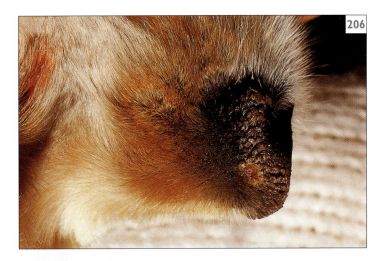

207, 208 Digital hyperkeratosis.

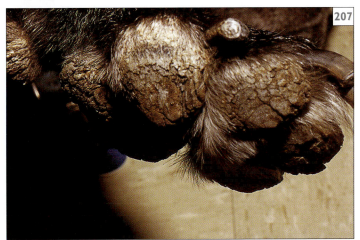

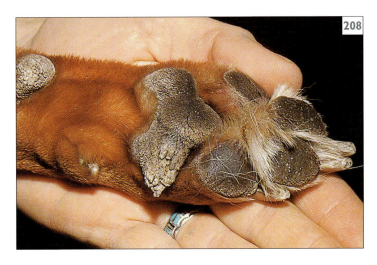

Erythema multiforme complex

ETIOLOGY AND PATHOGENESIS

Erythema multiforme (EM) complex is a group of rare, immune-mediated dermatoses with varied clinical signs. The classification of the complex is controversial, but it has been sub-divided into the progressively more severe variants EM minor, EM major, Stevens–Johnson syndrome (SJS), SJS–toxic epidermal necrolysis (TEN) overlap syndrome, and TEN[1].

The pathogenesis is not completely under-stood, but it is thought to represent a specific immune-mediated assault on keratinocytes causing widespread, confluent keratinocyte apop-tosis and epidermal necrosis[2]. Lesions are associ-ated with the deposition of immunoglobulin and complement, up-regulation of adhesion and other pro-inflammatory molecules on keratino-cytes, and recruitment of cytotoxic CD8+ T cells[3–5].

EM minor and EM major are most commonly idiopathic or associated with infections (especially canine distemper virus) and neoplasia, whereas SJS, SJS–TEN overlap, and TEN are more commonly associated with drug eruptions[1].

CLINICAL FEATURES

EM minor and EM major typically have a chronic, insidious history, whereas SJS and TEN have an acute onset and are two of the few genuine dermatologic emergencies. EM typically presents with variable erythematous macules, papules, plaques, wheals, scaling, and crusts, often arranged in annular, arcuate, or polycyclic shapes (**209–211**)[1]. There may be some mucosal involvement in EM major (**212**), but blistering and ulceration are uncommon. The polycyclic lesions are uncommon in SJS and TEN, which are characterized by extensive erythematous to purpuric macules or patches and mucosal involve-ment. There is usually blistering, necrosis, and ulceration in up to 10% (SJS) (**213**), 10–30% (overlap), or >30% (TEN) of the skin (**214**)[1]. Severely affected dogs can be in considerable pain, pyrexic, depressed, and dehydrated.

DIFFERENTIAL DIAGNOSES

- Superficial and deep pyoderma
- Superficial and deep mycoses
- Demodicosis
- Pemphigus foliaceus and vulgaris

- Bullous pemphigoid
- Drug eruption (**Note:** Remember that drug reactions can trigger lesions of the EM complex)
- Systemic lupus erythematosus
- Epitheliotropic lymphoma
- Thermal or chemical burns

DIAGNOSIS

The history and clinical signs are highly sugges-tive, and the diagnosis can be confirmed by histopathology of early lesions. Histopathology, however, does not differentiate between the various forms of EM, and a final diagnosis relies on careful evaluation of the clinical signs and history[1,5].

MANAGEMENT

EM can be a challenging condition to manage. The prognosis is better if the inciting cause can be identified and removed. Some cases of EM can resolve spontaneously or wax and wane. The role of glucocorticoids is controversial; most cases do not seem to respond to prednisolone, but dexamethasone (0.05 mg/kg p/o q24h) may be more effective. There are anecdotal reports of successful therapy with ciclosporin (cyclosporine) (5 mg/kg p/o q24h) or pentoxifylline (10–15 mg/kg q8–12h). Long-term maintenance treat-ment may be necessary in idiopathic cases.

Severe cases with widespread ulceration should receive intravenous fluid therapy to combat dehydration and shock. The ulcers should be cleaned and protected with silver sulfa-diazine cream, with activated silver and other protective dressings to encourage healing and prevent infection. Consideration should also be given to analgesia and antibiotics to prevent sepsis, although this must be weighed against the risk of potentiating a drug reaction. Intravenous therapy with human immunoglobulin (0.5–1.5 g/kg i/v over 6–12 hours) has been helpful in a few cases of SJS and TEN in dogs and cats[6,7].

KEY POINTS

- EM minor and EM major are most likely to be idiopathic or post infection.
- SJS, overlap, and TEN are most likely to be caused by a drug eruption.
- Severe ulceration warrants intravenous fluids, intensive care, and wound management.

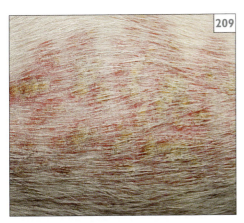

209 Arcuate erythema, crusting, and erosions on the ventral abdomen of a dog with erythema multiforme complex.

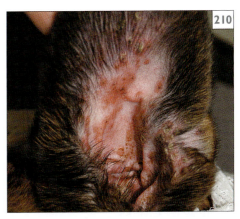

210 Irregular erythema, pustules, and crusts on the medial pinna of a dog with erythema multiforme complex.

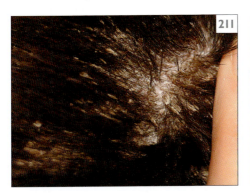

211 Severe scaling and follicular casts in a dog with generalized erythema multiforme complex.

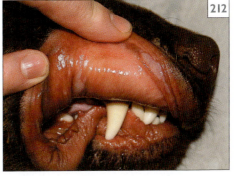

212 Oral plaques and erosions in canine erythema multiforme complex (same dog as **211**).

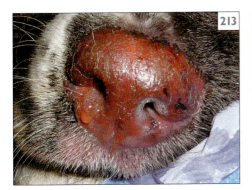

213 Complete sloughing of the nasal epidermis in canine Stevens–Johnson syndrome triggered by trimethoprim-sulfonamide (same dog as in **116**, p. 107).

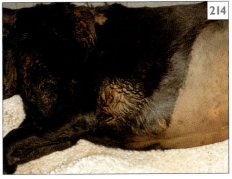

214 Full thickness skin necrosis and jaundice in a dog with toxic epidermal necrolysis and hepatic necrosis following administration of amoxicillin and carprofen.

Canine ear margin seborrhea

DEFINITION

Canine ear margin seborrhea is a syndrome resulting in scaling and, in some cases, alopecia on the margins of the pinnae.

ETIOLOGY AND PATHOGENESIS

The pathogenesis of canine ear margin seborrhea is thought to be an idiopathic cornification abnormality, but it may be secondary to other diseases[1].

CLINICAL FEATURES

Lesions are seen in animals with pendulous pinnae, especially Dachshunds, Springer Spaniels, and Cocker Spaniels. Initially, excessive adherent keratin accumulation is noted on the pinnal margins. In some cases the accumulations may be waxy or greasy and follicular casts may be present. Focal areas of alopecia may develop along the ear margins. If a thick layer of keratin debris accumulates, it may dry, resulting in fissures. Removal of thick keratin may result in an area of ulceration. The lesions are only occasionally pruritic.

DIFFERENTIAL DIAGNOSES

- Atopic dermatitis (the scaling and alopecia of the ear margins often develop in German Shepherd Dogs and, less often, in Cocker and Springer Spaniels secondary to atopic dermatitis)
- Early vasculitis (vasculitis will eventually have complete ear tip or focal areas of tissue necrosis)
- Sarcoptic mange (usually much more pruritic)
- Frostbite

DIAGNOSIS

Diagnosis is based on clinical findings and ruling out other differentials. Dermatohistopathology can provide supporting evidence. However, biopsy of the ear margin can be associated with considerable hemorrhage and a lesion that is slow to heal due to head shaking. One author (TJN) prefers taking narrow full thickness wedges and closing the wound with a double layer suture pattern, closing the the dorsal and ventral skin separately, thus avoiding the cartilage.

MANAGEMENT

The ear margins should be shampooed daily with a shampoo containing salicylic acid or similar keratolytic agent. Topical glucocorticoids such as fluocinolone acetonide 0.1% in 60% dimethylsulfoxide, dexamethasone solution 4%, or betamethasone valerate cream 0.1% should be applied twice daily.

KEY POINT

- Be aware that this is a condition that is generally controlled but not cured.

Exfoliative cutaneous lupus erythematosus of the German Shorthaired Pointer

DEFINITION
This is a rare, breed specific, scaling exfoliative dermatitis[1,2].

ETIOLOGY AND PATHOGENESIS
The pathogenesis of this condition is unknown, but there is circumstantial evidence that it is hereditary[3]. Recent work has demonstrated both humoral and cell-mediated immune responses directed against basal epithelial cells that resemble an exfoliative form of cutaneous lupus erythematosus in man[4].

CLINICAL FEATURES
Lesions are first noticed in animals when they are between five and eight months of age and initially consist of scaling and thinning of the hair over the face, ears, and back (**215, 216**). The condition often becomes generalized and lesions may be most prominent on the muzzle, pinnae, hocks, scrotum, and pressure points[2,3]. Affected skin has tightly adherent scale with fronds of keratin surrounding hair shafts. Scale builds up, resulting in crusts. Secondary bacterial and *Malassezia* infections can occur. Papules, pustules, and erythema of the axillae, scrotum, and interdigital areas and erythema on the concave aspect of the pinna have been reported in a small number of cases[3]. Pruritus is generally minimal and pain variable. Pyrexia, lethargy, and peripheral lymphadenopathy may be observed[3]. In some cases the condition can wax and wane.

DIFFERENTIAL DIAGNOSES
- Sebaceous adenitis
- Primary idiopathic keratinization defect (seborrhea)
- Ichthyosis
- Demodicosis
- Dermatophytosis
- Follicular dysplasia

DIAGNOSIS
Diagnosis is based on history, clinical findings, and supporting histopathology.

MANAGEMENT
There are anecdotal reports of response to immunosuppressive doses of corticosteroids and azathioprine, but these are inconsistent and most cases are refractory to treatments tried to date.

KEY POINT
- A scaling crusting dermatosis of young German Shorthaired Pointers that is refractory to treatment.

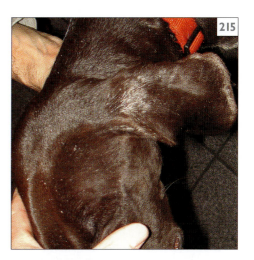

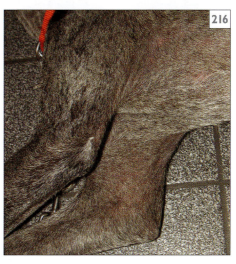

215, 216 Scaling over the head and ears (**215**) and forelimb and trunk (**216**) of a dog with exfoliative cutaneous lupus erythematosus of German Shorthaired Pointers.

Leishmaniasis

ETIOLOGY AND PATHOGENESIS

Canine leishmaniasis is a serious systemic disease with a diverse clinical presentation resulting from an infection by diphasic *Leishmania* protozoa. There are at least 30 species in five groups: *L. donovani*, *L. major*, *L. tropica*, *L. aethiopica*, and *L. mexicana*. *L. infantum* (*L. donovani* complex) are primarily responsible for canine cutaneous leishmaniasis and human visceral and cutaneous leishmaniasis in the Mediterranean basin (Spain, Portugal, France, Italy, Greece, and northern Africa), southern Russia, India, China, and eastern Africa[1–3]. In Central and South America *L. infantum* is responsible for visceral lesions, with *L. braziliensis* and *L. tropicana* responsible for cutaneous and mucocutaneous lesions[4,5]. Isolated outbreaks have also been reported in Oklahoma, Ohio, and Texas[6]. A form endemic to Fox Hounds has been reported from the eastern US and south-eastern Canada[6].

Leishmania are transmitted by blood feeding sandflies (*Phlebotomus* spp. in Europe and Asia; *Lutzomyia* in the Americas)[2,5]. Dogs are the main vertebrate hosts, although rats and foxes are minor hosts. Female flies feeding on infected hosts ingest amastigotes. These multiply and become flagellated promastigotes in the gut of the sandfly. The promastigotes migrate to the esophagus and pharynx of the insect, attracted by chemotaxic substances in the fly's crop. When a fly feeds on another vertebrate host, promastigotes that have become lodged in the proboscis are transferred. Most promastigotes are killed in the host, but the survivors are phagocytosed by macrophages and dendritic cells. These become non-flagellated amastigotes within 2–5 days and start to multiply. Infected cells eventually burst, releasing free amastigotes to infect adjacent cells. Free and cell-associated organisms disseminate to bone marrow, skin, liver, pancreas, kidneys, adrenal glands, digestive tract, eyes, testes, bone, and joints. The onset of clinical signs can vary from one month to seven years[5,7–9]. It is likely that there are alternative modes of transmission, as cases have been seen in areas without sandflies. Transmission by direct contact, blood transfusions, and placenta has been reported in humans.

The organisms induce local pyogranulomatous inflammatory responses. TH1 dominant responses, characterized by IFNγ and IL-2, activate macrophages to kill intracellular organisms. Cell-mediated immunity is therefore associated with resistance to infection. In contrast, TH2 responses with increased IL-4 are associated with induction of humoral responses, high antibody titers, persistent infection, and clinical signs[7,10–12]. The Ibizan Hound, a breed from endemic areas that is nevertheless rarely affected, has predominantly cell-mediated immune responses to *Leishmania*[13]. Sandfly saliva can also enhance TH2 and inhibit TH1 responses in the host, which therefore favors *Leishmania* infection.

Chronic dermal inflammation and cutaneous parasite loads are directly related to the severity of clinical disease in New World canine visceral leishmaniasis[14]. The parasite causes tissue damage through two pathogenic mechanisms:
- Non-suppurative granulomas, responsible for skin, hepatic, enteric, and osseous lesions.
- Circulating immune complexes that lodge in the blood vessels, renal glomeruli, and joints, resulting in vasculitis, glomerulonephritis, ocular lesions, and lameness.

CLINICAL FEATURES

Canine leishmaniasis is an insidious, slowly progressive, multi-systemic condition. The time course of infection is very variable; exposure to infected bites may result in no infection, a rapid establishment of a patent infection within two months, a prolonged sub-patent infection (4–22 months) before progression to overt clinical signs, or a transient sub-patent period followed by 10–21 months of apparent *Leishmania*-negative status before progression[8]. The clinical signs are very varied between individual dogs. Leishmaniasis is rare in cats, but isolated cases with localized papular to nodular, erosive and crusting lesions have been reported. Cats can act as reservoir hosts for Old World leishmaniasis, transmitting viable organisms to sandflies[15].

Cutaneous lesions (**217, 218**) affect up to 80% of infected dogs. These include:
- Localized or generalized exfoliative dermatitis with characteristic small, adherent silvery-white scales (56%).
- Nasodigital hyperkeratosis.
- Ulcerations, especially pressure points, extremities (40%), and mucocutaneous junctions (5.7%).
- Onychogryphosis (24%), onychorrhexis, and paronychia.

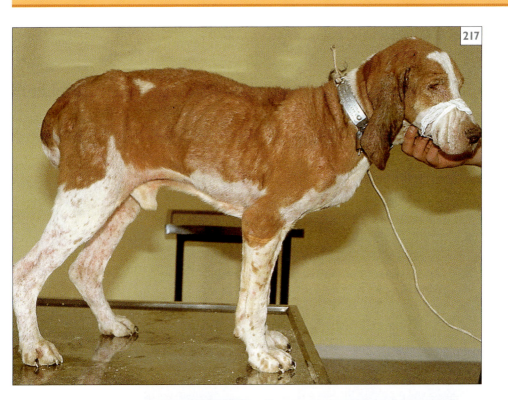

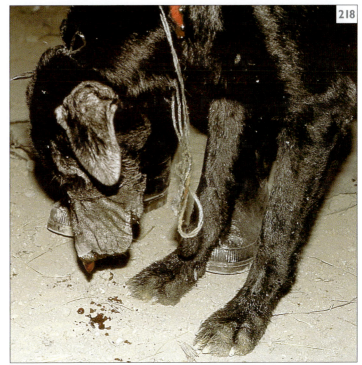

217, 218 Canine leishmaniasis. Emaciation is common (**217**). Hyperkeratosis and systemic disease are also features of leishmaniasis. Note the epistaxis in this dog (**218**).

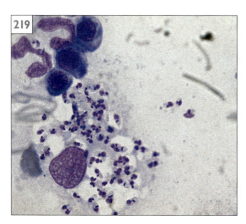

219 *Leishmania* organisms in a lymph node aspirate.

- Focal alopecia predominately on the head and pinnae or periocular.
- Dry and dull hair coat.
- Sterile pustular dermatitis, especially ventral.
- Diffuse erythema and erythematous plaques.
- Nasal depigmentation, erosion, and crusting.
- Nodules and papules of the skin and mucocutaneous junctions (6%).
- Secondary pyoderma (25%) and demodicosis (due to poor cell-mediated immune responses).

Systemic signs (**217, 218**) can be very varied and include:
- Generalized lymphadenopathy (70%).
- Anemia and pale mucous membranes (50–70%).
- Polydipsia, polyuria, glomerulonephritis (20%), and renal failure (30%). Sixty per cent of dogs with renal failure will die.
- Hepatic and splenic enlargement (50%). Also hepatitis, jaundice, and ascites.
- Exercise intolerance, weight loss, muscle wasting, and pyrexia (30–40%).
- Uveitis, keratitis, conjunctivitis, and other ocular disease (16%).
- Epistaxis, melena, and other coagulopathies (10%).
- Lameness, polyarthritis, polymyositis, or osteomyelitis.
- Meningitis.
- Anorexia, vomiting, and diarrhea.
- Sneezing and coughing.

DIFFERENTIAL DIAGNOSES
- Pemphigus foliaceus
- Systemic lupus erythematosus
- Sebaceous adenitis
- Zinc responsive dermatitis
- Bacterial folliculitis
- Dermatophytosis
- Demodicosis
- Superficial necrolytic dermatitis
- Epitheliotropic lymphoma

Due to the very varied clinical presentation, *Leishmania* should also be considered in many other cases, especially in, or if there has been travel to, endemic areas.

DIAGNOSIS
Clinical examination and the knowledge that the affected animal lives in or has come from an area where leishmaniasis is prevalent will raise clinical suspicion. Most cases have a non-regenerative, normochromic, normocytic anemia, hypergammaglobulinemia, hypoalbuminemia, and low albumin:globulin ratio and proteinuria, with a protein:creatinine ratio of >1. ANA tests are positive in roughly 50% of cases.

Organisms can be detected on cytology (**219**) of scrapes from superficial lesions or aspirates from lymph nodes (30%), bone marrow (50%), or spleen. Cytology may be more sensitive than serology in early cases.

Histopathologic inflammatory patterns are very variable and often non-specific. Most cases have orthokeratotic hyperkeratosis with mononuclear inflammatory infiltrates, which may be perifollicular, perivascular, interstitial to diffuse, nodular, interface, pustular, or mixed. Vasculitis, ischemia, and necrosis may also be present. Organisms can be seen in about 50% of cases with Giemsa stains.

PCR is highly sensitive and widely used, although contamination and false-positive results can be seen. False-negative PCR is also seen, as organisms may not be present in all tissues. Bone marrow and tissue samples are near 100% sensitive, but PCR on blood, lymph node, and CSF is less sensitive.

Leishmania specific IgG serology is usually highly sensitive, but positive serology is associated with infection and not necessarily disease. It is therefore less useful in endemic areas, where most dogs will be infected, but only a minority will develop clinical signs. Titers remain high for prolonged periods after infection and successful treatment, although the response to individual antigens is variable[16]. An indirect immunofluorescent antibody test (IFAT) to detect whole organisms is 98–99% sensitive and high titers are associated with clinically affected dogs or infected dogs that will develop clinical signs. ELISA tests detect a variety of antigens and are approximately 90% sensitive.

Definitive diagnosis relies on demonstrating organisms in affected tissues, although this is not possible in all cases. Therefore, diagnosis is often based on compatible clinical signs together with supportive evidence from a range of other tests. In one study of 160 dogs diagnosed with leishmaniasis, approximately 42% were positive by PCR, 46% by IFAT, and 19% by lymph node aspirate cytology[17].

MANAGEMENT

Dogs should only be treated if the health legislation of the country concerned permits therapy, as euthanasia is necessary in some countries. It is also important to determine if the patient's condition will allow a reasonable chance of successful treatment, as renal failure is a poor prognostic indicator. It is important to remember that parasite burdens may remain after treatment, permitting possible relapse or transmission. Effective treatment with meglumine antimonate and allopurinol (see below), however, has been shown to reduce or eliminate cutaneous parasite burdens, decreasing the likelihood of *Leishmania* transmission[18].

A recent review[19] concluded that there was good evidence to recommend the use of a combination of meglumine antimonate (50–75 mg/kg s/c q12h) and allopurinol (10–20 mg/kg p/o q12h). Animals should be treated until there is clinical remission and normal serum protein electrophoresis (SPE). Treatment is then continued with allopurinol for at least a further 12 months. Treatment can then stop if the animal is in clinical remission and if hematology, biochemistry, urinalysis and protein:creatinine ratio, SPE, serology (IFAT), and PCR are all normal. Two negative PCRs six months apart are needed to demonstrate a parasitologic cure. Therapy with meglumine antimonate should be restarted if clinical signs recur.

Meglumine antimonate inhibits glycolysis and is parasiticidal. Adverse effects include asthenia, pain at the injection site (myositis is common if given intramuscularly), and nephrotoxicity. Allopurinol interferes with *Leishmania* replication and does not kill the organisms. It should not be used alone and has no protective effect. ACE inhibitors and dietary management are recommended in cases with glomerulonephritis and/or renal failure. Dogs in renal failure should only receive allopurinol until renal function has improved.

There is fair evidence for the use of aminosidine (5 mg/kg p/o q12h for 3–4 weeks), but relapses are common. Aminosidine interferes with protein synthesis and is parasiticidal. It is synergistic with meglumine antimonate, and it can be nephrotoxic and ototoxic.

There is as yet insufficient evidence to recommend the use of amphotericin B, ketoconazole, metronidazole, enrofloxacin, marbofloxacin, buparvaquone, spiramycin, and miltefosine, although these agents may be effective in some cases. The efficacy of amphotericin B (0.5–0.8 mg/kg i/v twice weekly to a cumulative dose of 6–16 mg/kg) is limited by severe adverse effects including nephrotoxicity, vasculitis, and anemia. Liposome encapsulated formulations (3 mg/kg i/v for 4 days repeated at day 10 to a cumulative dose of 12–18 mg/kg) are better tolerated[20]. Metronidazole and ketoconazole may be synergistic with meglumine antimonate.

Protection against sandfly bites is very important in endemic areas. Deltamethrin-impregnated collars and washes, and permethrin spot-on products are useful[21,22].

The first vaccine against canine visceral leishmaniasis (Leishmune®) was recently licensed in Brazil. This has been shown to be effective in the prevention of and blocking transmission of canine visceral leishmaniasis, although the efficacy is not complete[23,24].

KEY POINTS

- A disease that is difficult to diagnose and to treat.
- Potentially zoonotic.

Canine distemper

DEFINITION

Canine distemper is a systemic viral condition that may cause skin lesions in addition to those in internal organs.

ETIOLOGY AND PATHOGENESIS

The causal agent is a paramyxovirus, which is transmitted in infected droplets and aerosol from infected animals. Viral multiplication occurs in lymphoid tissue before dissemination to other tissues.

CLINICAL FEATURES

The prominent clinical signs of this condition are systemic illness associated with the respiratory, gastrointestinal, and central nervous systems. Some dogs may develop an erythematous papulopustular dermatitis on the ventral abdomen during this acute stage. Nasal and footpad hyperkeratosis may develop in some animals. Due to this hyperkeratosis, the footpads become progressively harder, flattened, and smooth (**220**). If the animal recovers from the disease, the footpad lesions will generally resolve, while the nasal hyperkeratosis remains.

DIFFERENTIAL DIAGNOSES

- Idiopathic nasal digital hyperkeratosis
- Pemphigus foliaceus
- Vitamin A responsive dermatosis
- Zinc responsive dermatosis
- Lethal acrodermatitis of Bull Terriers
- Superficial necrolytic dermatitis

DIAGNOSIS

Diagnosis of canine distemper is based on history and clinical findings. As the clinical signs of canine distemper can be quite vague and varied, the changes in the pads may serve as a diagnostic aid. Serologic tests are available, but they do not differentiate between infected and vaccinated animals. Rising titers can help confirm the diagnosis. Histopathology and/or virus isolation from infected tissues are/is diagnostic.

MANAGEMENT

No specific treatment, other than supportive care, is available.

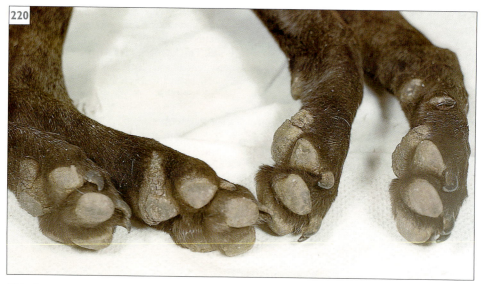

220 Canine distemper virus infection. Digital hyperkeratosis of all the footpads.

Cutaneous horn

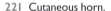

DEFINITION
Cutaneous horns are localized, benign out-growths of horny tissue with the appearance of small horns.

ETIOLOGY AND PATHOGENESIS
Cutaneous horn is a descriptive term and the lesions may be associated with viral papillomas, actinic keratoses, Bowenoid in situ carcinoma, invasive squamous cell carcinoma, and infundibular keratinizing acanthoma[1]. Multiple cutaneous horns have been reported in the cat associated with FeLV infection[2,3].

CLINICAL FEATURES
Cutaneous horns are localized and non-pruritic (**221**). Multiple lesions may be seen in some individuals. In animals with long coats the horns may not be immediately apparent and it is not until they are groomed that the lesions are noticed. In cats, cutaneous horns may affect the footpads[2,3]. There is no breed, age, or sex incidence. The horn may be 3–5 cm (1.2–2.0 in) in length, firm to the touch, and not easily removed from the underlying skin. If pulled off, cutaneous horns tend to regrow.

DIFFERENTIAL DIAGNOSES
- Papilloma
- Crusted, ulcerative neoplasms
- Infundibular keratinizing acanthoma

DIAGNOSIS
To determine the specific etiology, biopsies should be taken or the lesion surgically removed and submitted for histopathologic evaluation. Affected cats should be screened for FeLV infection.

MANAGEMENT
Surgical excision is generally curative, although this depends on the specific etiology of the lesion. Therefore, the horn and underlying tissue should be submitted for histopathologic examination in an attempt to identify any underlying cause. Cutaneous horns of the footpads of FeLV-positive cats will often reoccur after surgery[3].

KEY POINT
- Cutaneous horn is a clinical term associated with several etiologies.

221 Cutaneous horn.

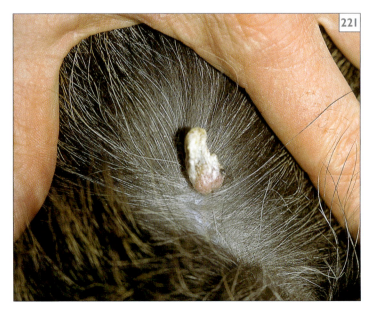

Zinc responsive dermatosis

ETIOLOGY AND PATHOGENESIS

Zinc responsive dermatosis in dogs occurs due to an impaired ability to absorb zinc from the gut (type 1) or a relative or absolute deficiency of zinc in the diet (type 2)[1,2]. Naturally occurring zinc deficiency has not been reported in cats.

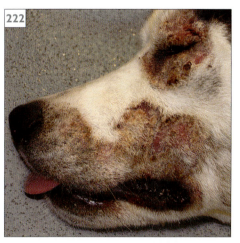

222 Zinc responsive dermatosis in a Siberian Husky.

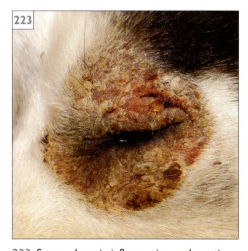

223 Severe alopecia, inflammation, and crusting around the eye.

Type 1 disease is most frequently seen in Siberian Huskies and Alaskan Malamutes (possibly due to autosomal recessive inheritance), although it has been recognized in other breeds[1,3]. These animals appear unable to absorb adequate zinc, even when fed a nutritionally balanced diet. Lethal acrodermatitis in Bull Terriers (see p. 206) is thought to involve a congenital, autosomal dominant inability to utilize zinc[4,5].

Type 2 disease, due to an absolute dietary zinc deficiency, is rare in animals fed high-quality, commercially-prepared diets[1,2]. More commonly, there is a relative deficiency due to interaction with other dietary components or an inability to utilize dietary zinc. Absorption of zinc from the gut is inhibited by iron, copper, and calcium, which compete with zinc for absorption[1,2]. Intestinal phytate and inorganic phosphate bind zinc and hinder absorption. This is most likely to be seen in rapidly growing animals, particularly giant breeds, fed inadequate diets or diets in which nutritional antagonism occurs, particularly due to high phytate content or oversupplementation with calcium.

CLINICAL FEATURES

There is no sex predisposition, although clinical lesions may be associated with or exacerbated by estrus, pregnancy, and lactation in intact females. Most cases of type 1 disease are seen between 1 and 3 years of age, although there is a wide age range of up to 11 years at first presentation[1]. Type 2 is normally seen in young, growing dogs fed home-prepared diets, although it can be seen in older animals depending on the dietary history.

Cutaneous lesions include well-demarcated, symmetrical areas of scaling, crusting, and erythema predominantly around the mouth and other mucocutaneous junctions, the eyes, and pressure points (**222–224**). Pruritus is variable, but it may be severe[3]. Affected skin may fissure and ulcerate, which is often painful[1]. Secondary pyoderma is common[6]. The coat is generally dull and harsh and may exhibit multifocal hypopigmentation. Other clinical signs include lymphadenopathy (especially if there is fissuring, inflammation, and/or pyoderma), poor wound healing, anestrus, infertility, inappetence (possibly due to altered taste and/or smell), failure to thrive, and weight loss.

224 Hyperkeratosis of the footpads.

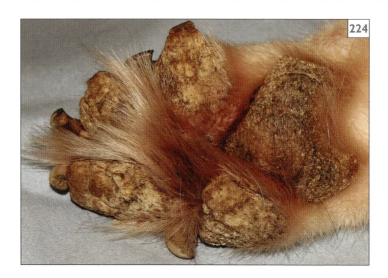

DIFFERENTIAL DIAGNOSES
- Superficial pyoderma
- *Malassezia* dermatitis
- Demodicosis
- Dermatophytosis
- Pemphigus foliaceus
- Superficial necrolytic dermatitis (migratory necrolytic erythema or hepatocutaneous syndrome)

DIAGNOSIS
The history (particularly the breed and diet) and clinical signs are highly suggestive[1]. Cytology reveals numerous nucleated keratinocytes consistent with widespread parakeratosis, with or without bacteria and neutrophils consistent with secondary pyoderma. Histopathology will confirm acanthosis with diffuse parakeratosis. Parakeratosis, however, may be focal or minimal in some cases[2]. Low zinc levels in plasma or hair are supportive, but there is a wide overlap with normal dogs and false-negative results due to zinc contamination from reagents and equipment are common[7]. Final confirmation of the diagnosis relies on response to treatment[1,2].

MANAGEMENT
The prognosis is generally good. Therapy involves correction of any dietary factors and zinc supplementation with starting doses of 1–3 mg/kg/day elemental zinc[1–3]. Higher doses may be necessary in some dogs[2,3]. Zinc sulfate can cause vomiting and diarrhea, so zinc gluconate or methionine are often preferred. There is a better response to higher doses, especially initially, but these may be less well tolerated. Animals that do not respond to oral medication may benefit from zinc sulfate given intramuscularly or slow intravenously (weekly doses to a maximum of 600 mg/month)[2], although this can be painful and irritating to surrounding tissues. The most common cause of treatment failure is to base the dose on the zinc compound and not the elemental zinc content. There is anecdotal evidence that treatment with essential fatty acids (EFAs) and prednisolone may speed the clinical response, although it is unclear whether this is associated with enhanced uptake or utilization of zinc or amelioration of cutaneous inflammation[8]. Retinoids may be of help in severe cases[2]. There is some rationale to feeding zinc and EFA supplemented diets. Antibiotics may be necessary to control secondary infections. Zinc supplementation may be required for life in type 1 disease, whereas it should be possible to maintain affected animals on a nutritionally balanced diet once the clinical signs have resolved in type 2 disease.

KEY POINTS
- Rare condition.
- May occur in dogs on a commercially prepared diet given calcium and/or cereal supplements.
- Calculate dose on elemental zinc.

Lethal acrodermatitis of Bull Terriers

DEFINITION
Lethal acrodermatitis of Bull Terriers is an hereditary, congenital disease of white Bull Terriers, resulting in erythematous crusting lesions predominating on the face and feet.

ETIOLOGY AND PATHOGENESIS
The syndrome is an inherited autosomal recessive metabolic disease that is thought to be due to defects in absorption and metabolism of zinc and copper[1,2].

CLINICAL FEATURES
Lesions are first noted in animals when they are about eight weeks of age[1]. Initially, erythema and papules are seen over the feet, muzzle, bridge of the nose, elbows, hocks, pinnae, periorbital areas, and skin surrounding mucocutaneous junctions (**225**)[1,3]. Affected skin becomes ulcerated and covered with crusts. Secondary infection with bacteria and/or *Malassezia* is common. A severe hyperkeratosis develops over the footpads, which splay out (**226**)[1,3]. As the keratin dries it may crack, develop fissures, or exfoliate. Affected animals have difficulty walking or cannot walk at all. Paronychia may be seen along with dystrophic nails[1]. The hard palate is abnormally arched and can become impacted with food. Along with the skin lesions, growth retardation, abnormal behavior, diarrhea, and bronchopneumonia may be observed[1].

DIFFERENTIAL DIAGNOSES
- Generic dog food dermatitis and other nutritional deficiencies
- Zinc responsive dermatitis
- Pemphigus foliaceus
- Dermatophytosis
- Demodectic mange in the early stage of the disease
- Superficial necrolytic dermatitis (metabolic epidermal necrosis/hepatocutaneous syndrome)

DIAGNOSIS
Diagnosis is based on history, clinical findings, and ruling out other differentials. Histopathology can be helpful in identifying characteristic changes, although these are similar to those of zinc responsive dermatosis and superficial necrolytic dermatitis.

MANAGEMENT
Supportive care and treatment for secondary bacterial or yeast infection. The prognosis is very poor, with a reported mean survival time of seven months and few animals living beyond 18 months[1,3].

KEY POINT
- Condition of young white Bull Terriers that is generally fatal.

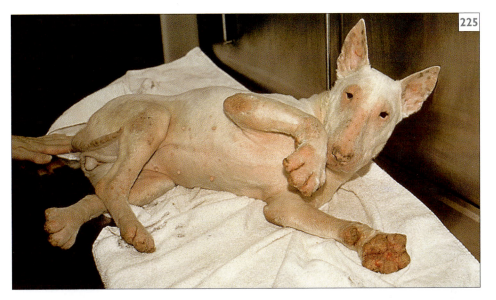

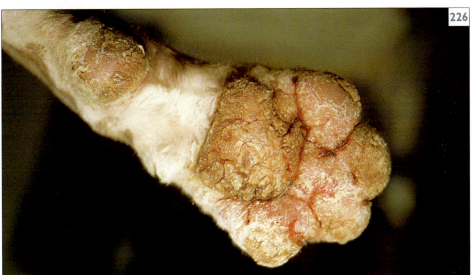

225, 226 Stunting (**225**) and chronic pododermatitis (**226**) in a Bull Terrier with lethal acrodermatitis. (Photos courtesy HW Richardson)

Facial dermatitis of Persian and Himalayan cats

DEFINITION
Facial dermatitis of Persian and Himalayan cats is characterized by the accumulation of dark waxy debris around the eyes, facial folds and chin.

ETIOLOGY AND PATHOGENESIS
The pathogenesis of this condition is unknown, but the waxy debris is thought to originate from the sebaceous glands[1].

CLINICAL FEATURES
Lesions are characterized by the accumulation of a black, waxy, tightly adherent material that mats the hair of the chin, perioral, and periocular facial fold areas (**227**). Affected areas may have varying degrees of erythema, which may be associated with pruritus when it becomes severe[1]. A bilateral erythematous otitis with accumulation of black waxy debris is seen in many cases[1]. *Malassezia* and bacteria are frequently found in impression smears from affected areas and submandibular lymphadenopathy may develop in some cats[1].

The age of onset varies from ten months to six years[1]. Persian and Himalayan cats are predisposed but one author (PJM) has observed the condition in a domestic shorthair cat.

DIFFERENTIAL DIAGNOSES
• Demodicosis
• Feline acne

DIAGNOSIS
Diagnosis is based on history and clinical findings.

MANAGEMENT
Systemic corticosteroids have been associated with partial response in some cats[1]. Ketoconazole (10 mg/kg p/o q24h) has also resulted in partial response in some cats with *Malassezia* infection[1]. There are anecdotal reports of ciclosporin (cyclosporine) (5–7 mg/kg p/o q24h) being beneficial in some cats. Topical application of phytosphingosine, which controls sebum production, warrants a trial.

KEY POINT
• Be aware that there is no consistently successful treatment for this condition.

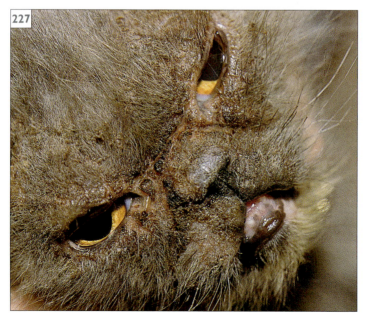

227 Persian cat suffering from facial dermatitis, with severe lesions affecting the rostral chin and face.

Spiculosis

DEFINITION
Spiculosis is a rare condition of Kerry Blue Terriers, characterized by pruritus and hard brittle spicules protruding from hair follicles.

ETIOLOGY AND PATHOGENESIS
The pathogenesis of spiculosis is unknown. It is possible that the condition is congenital, with six months to one year needed for expression of the clinical disease. Cells of the hair bulb show premature keratinization that results in an amorphous keratinized mass, which is shaped by the outer root sheath and follicular wall into a spicule[1].

CLINICAL FEATURES
Spiculosis is a disease of young intact male Kerry Blue Terriers. It is characterized by hard brittle spicules that are 1.0–2.5 mm in diameter and 0.5–3.0 cm in length (**228, 229**). In the reported cases, onset of lesions occurred spontaneously at between six months and one year of age[1]. Lesions may be found on any haired area of the body, but they are found most frequently over the lateral aspect of the hocks. Affected animals may be asymptomatic or may lick and chew excessively at the involved areas. Licking or chewing of affected areas can be excessive to the point that the animals develop acral lick granulomas[1].

DIFFERENTIAL DIAGNOSES
Spiculosis is highly distinctive clinically. The only time confusion could arise is if secondary acral lick granulomas are present.

DIAGNOSIS
Diagnosis is based on history and clinical findings.

MANAGEMENT
Isotretinoin (1 mg/kg p/o q24h) resulted in complete remission in two reported cases and marked improvement in one[1]. As the commercial availability of this drug is limited, the alternative would be acitretin (0.5–2.0 mg/kg p/o q24h).

KEY POINT
• A breed specific condition characterized by hard spicules protruding from the skin.

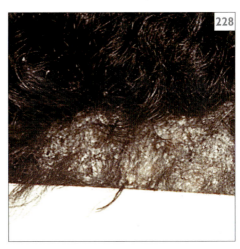

228 Spicule protruding from a papule of a Kerry Blue Terrier with spiculosis.

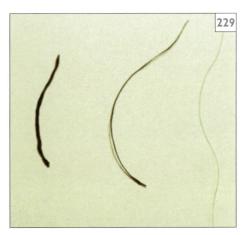

229 Spicules of varying sizes (left and center) and normal hair (right) from a dog with spiculosis.

CHAPTER 7

Pigmentary abnormalities

General approach

- Difficult to diagnose with certainty – use biopsy and histopathology
- Treatment is difficult
- Depigmentation is often permanent – affected skin may need sun protection

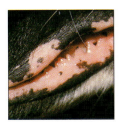
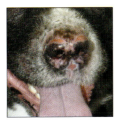
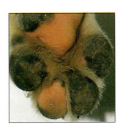
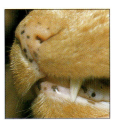

Vitiligo

DEFINITION

Vitiligo is an acquired disorder characterized by selective destruction of melanocytes in skin and hair matrix cells; this results in leucoderma (depigmentation of skin) and leucotrichia (depigmentation of hair).

ETIOLOGY AND PATHOGENESIS

Vitiligo is thought to result from an aberration of immune surveillance, which allows the development of antimelanocytic antibodies. These antibodies have been demonstrated in dogs and cats with vitiligo, but not in normal animals[1]. Additional theories in humans revolve around the possibility that either there is a neurochemical mediator that destroys melanocytes or inhibits melanin production, or there is an intermediate metabolite in melanin synthesis that causes melanocyte destruction[2].

CLINICAL FEATURES

There is a marked breed predisposition for vitiligo in the Belgian Tervuren. Other dogs that appear to be at increased risk include the German Shepherd Dog, Rottweiler, and Doberman Pinscher. It has also been diagnosed in various other breeds and has been reported in Siamese cats[1,3]. Vitiligo generally appears in young adulthood as asymptomatic macules on the planum nasale, lips, muzzle, buccal mucosa (**230**), and footpads. Leucoderma and, in some cases, leucotrichia (**231**) occur in affected areas[4]. Progression of lesions is variable, with lesions in some animals repigmenting, while others have permanent depigmentation[4]. Idiopathic depigmentation of the nose can develop and may be a form of vitiligo. Lay terms for this are 'Dudley nose' and 'snow nose'. There appears to be a predisposition for this in the Golden Retriever, Yellow Labrador Retriever, and Arctic breeds such as the Siberian Husky and Alaskan Malamute[3]. Apart from the pigment changes, the underlying skin is normal with no evident signs of inflammation. Animals do not seem to be affected by the lesions. Sudden onset depigmentation of the skin in older animals can be an early sign of epitheliotropic lymphoma and should be investigated. Depigmentation is also seen as a (post-) inflammatory change in many immune-mediated dermatoses, particularly lupus erythematosus, and with leishmaniasis.

DIFFERENTIAL DIAGNOSES

- Canine uveodermatologic syndrome
- Cutaneous lupus erythematosus
- Dermatomyositis
- Systemic lupus erythematosus

DIAGNOSIS

Diagnosis is based on history, physical examination, and microscopic examination of skin biopsy samples.

MANAGEMENT

There is no treatment that has been shown to be of benefit, although the disease is largely only cosmetic. However, depigmented skin may need sun protection (see Actinic dermatosis, p. 180).

KEY POINT

- Vitiligo is quite common – client education is important.

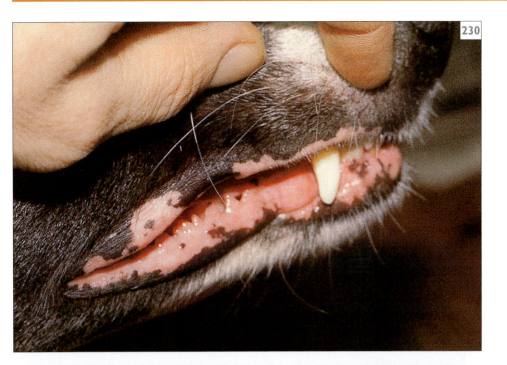

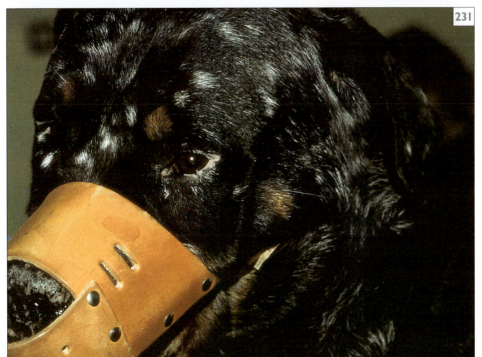

230, 231 Vitiligo. Loss of pigment on the lips of a Border Collie (230); patchy leucotrichia on the head of a Rottweiler (231).

Canine uveodermatologic syndrome

(Vogt–Koyanagi–Harada-like [VKH] syndrome)

DEFINITION

Canine uveodermatologic syndrome is a rare canine condition that is believed to be an immune-mediated antimelanocyte disease resulting in ocular, dermal, and hair abnormalities[1–4].

ETIOLOGY AND PATHOGENESIS

Although the underlying mechanism of immuno-regulatory dysfunction has not been elucidated, it is known in humans that a type IV or cell-mediated hypersensitivity exists against melanin and melanocytes[1,3]. Distinct subpopulations of cytotoxic T lymphocytes with activity against melanocytes have been identified[3]. Similar mechanisms have been proposed for dogs[1–3]. In addition, circulating antimelanocytic antibodies have been detected in both man and dogs[1,4].

CLINICAL FEATURES

Breeds at risk include Akitas, Samoyeds, Siberian Huskies, Alaskan Malamutes, Chow Chows, and their related crossbreeds[1,3]. The syndrome has also been diagnosed in the Shiba Inu, Shetland Sheepdog, German Shepherd Dog, Old English Sheepdog, Irish Setter, and Dachshund. Ocular signs generally precede skin changes and consist initially of bilateral uveitis to severe panuveitis. Later, retinal detachment, posterior synechiae with secondary glaucoma, and cataracts may develop. Skin and hair abnormalities consist of leukoderma and leukotrichia that often involve the eyelids, nasal planum, lips, scrotum, vulva, pads of the feet, and scrotal and vulvar areas (**232, 233**). Variable degrees of erythema, ulceration, and crusting may occur in the depigmented areas[1,3]. Depigmentation, erythema, and erosions may occur in the oral cavity[5]. Pain or pruritus may be a feature and lymphadenopathy is common[1]. Initial onset of lesions has been noted in animals ranging from 13 months to six years of age[3]. In contrast to humans, neurologic signs are uncommon in dogs.

DIFFERENTIAL DIAGNOSES

- Cutaneous lupus erythematosus
- Systemic lupus erythematosus
- Pemphigus foliaceus
- Pemphigus erythematosus
- Epitheliotropic lymphoma
- Vitiligo
- Dermatomyositis
- Leishmaniasis

DIAGNOSIS

Diagnosis is based on history, ophthalmic examination, physical examination, and histopathologic examination of skin biopsy samples.

MANAGEMENT

Topical or subconjunctival corticosteroids and topical cycloplegics are beneficial in patients with anterior uveitis[3]. Prednisolone, methylprednisolone, or prednisone (0.5–2.0 mg/kg p/o q12h) is usually required to resolve the uveitis and dermatologic lesions. After resolution of lesions, the dose can be tapered, although long-term therapy is often required to maintain remission. Azathioprine (2 mg/kg p/o q24–48h) with tapering after clinical resolution (to 0.5 mg/kg p/o q24–48h) may allow for a reduction of the corticosteroid dose. In some patients it may be possible to discontinue the corticosteroids and rely on azathioprine alone[3]. Systemic administration of ciclosporin (cyclosporine) has been used in man for the treatment of refractory cases and may be another treatment option for the dog[6]. One author (TJN) has found combinations of topical tacrolimus and systemic ciclosporin useful.

KEY POINT

- This condition requires aggressive treatment and demands definitive diagnosis.

232, 233 Canine uveodermatologic syndrome. Loss of pigment on the nasal planum and nose, with lesions affecting the eyes (**232**) and on the footpads (**233**).

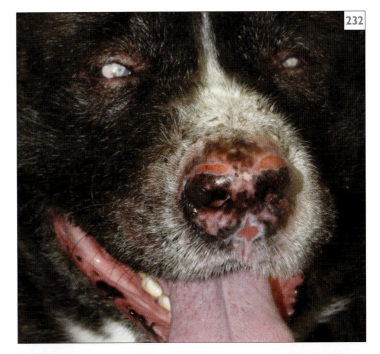

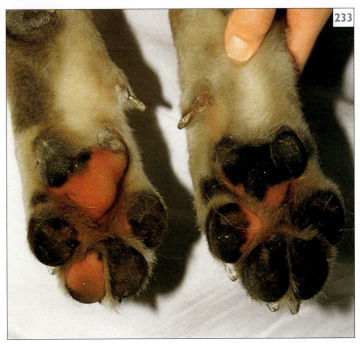

Lentigo and lentiginosis profusa

ETIOLOGY AND PATHOGENESIS

A lentigo (plural lentigines) is a brown-black, circular hyperpigmented macule or patch. They are associated with increased numbers of melanocytes at the dermo-epidermal junction, but without evidence of focal proliferation or invasive behavior[1–3]. The etiology is not known, although papillomavirus infection has been postulated in dogs[4,5]. While there is a biochemical relationship established between inflammatory reactions and postinflammatory hyperpigmentation, there is no suggestion that lentigines have a similar etiology. Hereditary autosomal dominant lentiginosis profusa has been reported in Pugs, and Miniature Schnauzers may also be predisposed[1,5,6]. Lentigo is common in orange and tortoiseshell cats[2].

CLINICAL FEATURES

In Pugs, macules were first noted between one and four years of age. The lesions were discrete, well-demarcated, slightly raised and non-pruritic, and mostly found on the distal limbs, although lesser numbers were present on the proximal limbs and trunk. The macules gradually enlarge to approximately 10 mm (0.4 in) in diameter and then remain static. With time, the density of coloration faded. In cats the lesions are first noted on the lips (**234**), and most affected animals are under a year old. In most cases the lentigines coalesce and spread locally to affect the mucous membranes, eyelids, and nasal planum, but are otherwise non-symptomatic. There is one case recorded of an adult silver shorthair cat that developed non-pruritic generalized lesions[7].

DIFFERENTIAL DIAGNOSES

- Superficial pyoderma
- Demodicosis
- Pigmented neoplasia
- Post-inflammatory hyperpigmentation

DIAGNOSIS

The clinical appearance of these lesions is highly suggestive and is usually sufficient to make a diagnosis. Histopathologic examination of biopsy samples will allow a definitive diagnosis. This is of most use to rule out melanoma.

MANAGEMENT

These are purely cosmetic lesions that do not require therapy. Neoplastic progression has not been reported in cats, but malignant transformation of canine lentiginosis profusa into squamous cell carcinoma is possible[5,6].

KEY POINTS

- Reassure owners that these are benign lesions.
- Monitor multiple lesions in dogs for malignant transformation.

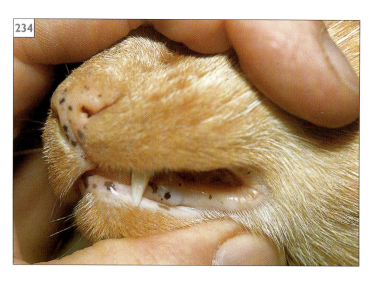

234 Lentigines on the lower lip of a cat.

Environmental dermatoses

General approach

- These diseases are often acute, but animals may be presented with chronic clinical signs or complications
- The diagnosis is easy if the inciting cause is obvious
- Take a careful history and do a thorough clinical examination if it is not

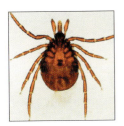
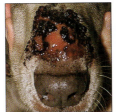
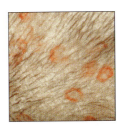
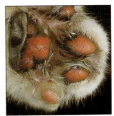

Tick infestation

ETIOLOGY AND PATHOGENESIS

Based on taxonomic classifications, ticks are generally divided into two Classes: hard (ixodic) and soft (argasid). Most clinical problems are due to infestations with ixodic ticks. Several species are capable of infesting dogs and cats including *Rhipicephalus sanguineus* (brown dog tick or kennel tick, found worldwide) (**235**), *Dermacentor variabilis* (American dog tick, wood tick), *D. andersoni* (Rocky Mountain wood tick), *D. occidentalis* (Pacific or West Coast tick), *D. reticularis* (found in Europe) (**236**), *Amblyomma maculatum* (Gulf Coast tick), *A. americanum* (Lone Star tick), *Ixodes dammini* (deer tick), *I. scapularis* (black-legged tick), *I. pacificus* (found in California and Oregon), *I. hexagonus* (hedgehog tick, found in Europe), and *I. ricinus* (castor bean tick, found in Europe) (**237**)[1–5].

Both Classes pass through four stages[1–3]: egg, larva (seed tick), nymph, and adult. The larvae, nymphs, and adults of both sexes feed on blood and lymph. Adult females become engorged after feeding. In general, the ixodic ticks are three-host ticks with the larva and nymph stages primarily feeding on small rodents. *R. sanguineus* is a three-host tick that can complete its life cycle on dogs.

Ticks can transmit a variety of microbial diseases[2,4–6]:

- *R. sanguineus*: *Babesia gibsoni, Coxiella burnetii, Ehrlichia canis, Hepatozoan canis, Pasteurella tularensis.*
- *D. andersoni*: *B. canis, C. burnetti,* Rocky Mountain spotted fever.
- *D. variabilis*: *P. tularensis,* Rocky Mountain spotted fever.
- *A. americanum*: Rocky Mountain spotted fever.
- *A. maculatum*: *Leptospira pomona.*
- *I. dammini, pacificus,* and *ricinus*: *Borrelia burgdorferi* (Lyme disease).

The only argasid tick of clinical importance in dogs and cats is the spinous ear tick *Otobius megnini*, which is found worldwide in warm, moist climates. This is a one-host tick, with only the larva and nymph stages parasitic[3].

Risk factors for tick infestation vary with species and geographical location, but generally include an outdoor lifestyle, thick vegetation, and a warm, humid season[3,7,8].

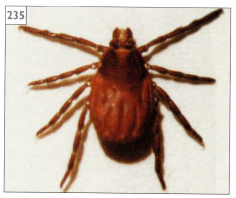

235 *Rhipicephalus* species tick. (Photo courtesy Merial Animal Health)

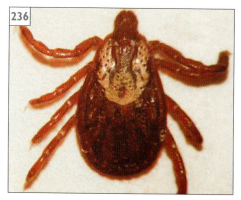

236 *Dermacentor* species tick. (Photo courtesy Merial Animal Health)

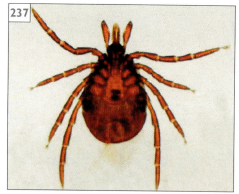

237 *Ixodes* species tick. (Photo courtesy Merial Animal Health)

238 Tick infestation. Two ticks, not yet engorged, on the neck of a cat.

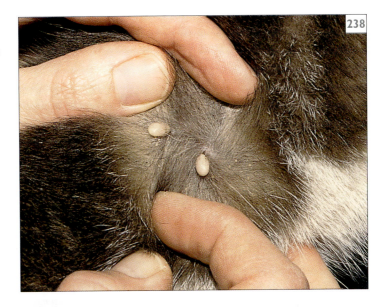

238

239 A tick, and an erythematous reaction to it, on the neck of a cat.

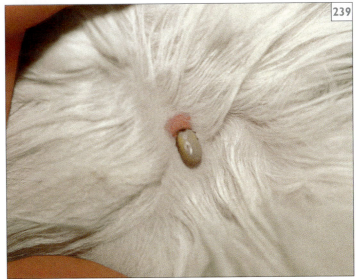

239

CLINICAL FEATURES

Ticks of various stages of the life cycle may be seen attached to the skin (**238**). Erythema associated with mild pruritus may be present in the skin adjacent to the attached tick (**239**). Crusting and a small nodule may develop at the site where a tick was removed. This is mostly due to an immunologically-mediated inflammatory reaction to the tick saliva rather than because the head of the tick or mouthparts have been left in the skin. Otitis externa may result from the irritation of large numbers of spinous ear ticks in the canal. Tick paralysis (an ascending flaccid lower motor neuron paralysis) may occur due to a neurotoxin in the saliva of engorging females of several species of ixodic ticks, particularly those of the genus *Dermacentor*.

DIAGNOSIS

Observation of ticks during physical or otic examination confirms the diagnosis.

MANAGEMENT

Ticks can be removed by grasping them with proprietary tick removal devices, forceps, or gloved fingers and applying slow traction until they are pulled free[9]. Twisting the tick may help release the mouthparts. In some cases a small amount of skin will be pulled off and still be attached to the tick mouthparts. Permethrin dips, sprays, or concentrated drops may be applied to dogs if there is a heavy infestation and will provide protection against reinfestation. Fipronil, deltamethrin, moxidectin, and amitraz-containing products will also protect against infestation[1–3,10–12]. They do not necessarily prevent attachment, but ticks die and drop off within 12–24 hours. Disease transmission usually requires at least 24–48 hours attachment[6]. Because of cat grooming patterns, tick infestations are less common in cats. The principles of control are similar to those in dogs, except that many pyrethroid-containing products for use in dogs are toxic to cats.

The premises need to be treated with an effective acaricidal product if *R. sanguineus* is responsible for the infestation. This is because the entire life cycle of this tick can be completed on the dog, which results in large numbers of all life stages in the animal's immediate surroundings.

KEY POINTS

- Ticks are vectors for a number of infectious diseases.
- Live ticks may be seen for 12–24 hours on treated animals.

Bee stings and spider bites

ETIOLOGY AND PATHOGENESIS

The stings of bees and other Hymenoptera contain phospholipases, hyaluronidases, and bradykinin-like mediators, which induce local vasodilation and pain[1]. Spiders, caterpillars, and other insects may cause localized reactions either through implantation of spicules or through bites that introduce a variety of necro- and neurotoxins into the skin[2–4].

CLINICAL FEATURES

Most reactions to insect and arthropod toxins are localized and are characterized by erythema, edema, and transient pain[1]. In cats, sudden, soft, regional edema of the distal forelimb is a common reaction to stings, presumably a consequence of the cat playing with the insect. In dogs, edema and angioedema of the eyelids and muzzle are most common (**240**). Occasionally, the urticaria may be generalized and severe, and fatal, systemic anaphylactic reactions have been reported[1,5,6]. Peracute nasal and facial dermatitis in dogs associated with eosinophilic folliculitis and furunculosis[7,8], may be a reaction to insect stings as well as mosquito bites (see p. 222) (**241**). Occasionally, arthropod bites or stings result in nodular granulomatous dermatitis[9]. Fire ant stings result in non-follicular pustules with a neutrophilic interstitial dermatitis and collagen degeneration[2].

Spider bites are inherently more dangerous, with those from the most dangerous species (e.g. Black Widow spiders [*Latrodectus* spp.], the Brown Recluse spider [*Loxosceles reclusa*], and theraphosid [Old World tarantula] spiders) resulting in severe localized to regional vasculitis and tissue necrosis, and systemic reactions including paralysis, widespread vasculitis, cardiac and respiratory failure, and death[3,4]. Australian theraphosid spider venom is highly toxic to dogs and bites are invariably rapidly fatal[10]. New World tarantula spiders rarely bite, but they possess highly irritant and urticarial hairs. Bites from Sydney Funnel Web spiders (*Atrax robustus*), in contrast, while deadly to humans, do not appear to harm cats and dogs.

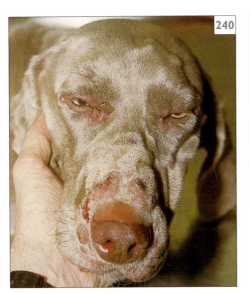

240 Urticaria. Symmetrical swelling of the face following a sting from a bee.

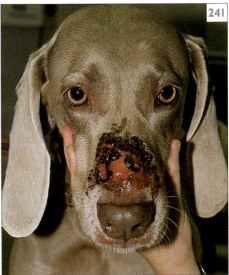

241 Peracute eosinophilic furunculosis following stings from a bee.

DIFFERENTIAL DIAGNOSES (of localized reactions)

- Nasal pyoderma
- Urticaria and angioedema
- Mosquito bite dermatitis
- Eosinophilic furunculosis
- Sterile or infectious nodular pyogranuloma
- Cutaneous histiocytosis
- Dermatophytosis
- Immune-mediated dermatoses and drug eruption

DIAGNOSIS

A clinical history of a peracute onset following the bite or sting eliminates most of the differential diagnoses. Often, however, the insect or spider is not seen and a bite or sting is inferred rather than documented. Cytology or histopathology is necessary to differentiate nasal pyoderma from eosinophilic furunculosis. Hypersensitivity to Hymenoptera venom can be demonstrated by intradermal tests or IgE specific serology[1]. Reactions to other insects such as cockroaches, ants, biting flies, wasps, and moths are reported much less frequently and are often regarded as clinically irrelevant or cross-reactions[11]. The clinical relevance of reactions and efficacy of allergen specific immunotherapy are highly controversial.

MANAGEMENT

Systemic glucocorticoids, at anti-inflammatory doses, are indicated once the diagnosis is established[7,8]. Systemic antihistamines may be of value in cases characterized by edema and urticaria. Intravenous fluids, antihistamines, adrenalin/epinephrine, bronchodilators, and oxygen may be necessary in severe cases[1,5,6]. Local bathing with wet dressings may be of value in cases of peracute nasal eosinophilic furunculosis. Sedation may be indicated to prevent the dog causing severe self-trauma. The owner should be warned that some loss of hair and scarring may occur in severely affected animals. More severely affected animals will require appropriate supportive therapy and wound management. Immediate treatment for spider bites is similar to that for snake bites, and includes tight bandaging and compression, splinting of limbs, and keeping the patient calm and quiet (with careful use of sedation if necessary). If the species of spider can be identified, antivenom (e.g. for Black Widow spiders) may be available, although treatment protocols are not validated for dogs and could trigger anaphylaxis.

KEY POINT

- Treat peracute eosinophilic folliculitis aggressively.

Fly and mosquito bite dermatosis

DEFINITION
A papular or papulocrustous reaction to the bites of flies and mosquitoes.

ETIOLOGY AND PATHOGENESIS
Fly bite dermatitis is usually caused by the stable fly *Stomoxys calcitrans* and is considered to be a non-specific reaction to the pain and injury caused by the bite. Similarly, the clinical signs of insect bite dermatosis in dogs are thought to be caused by bites of the mosquito, bush fly, sand fly, or buffalo fly. Other biting insects may also be involved. In contrast to canine dermatosis, feline mosquito bite hypersensitivity is caused by a type 1 reaction to substances within saliva that are injected into the skin when the mosquito bites.

CLINICAL FEATURES
Fly bite dermatitis is a crusting, pruritic dermatosis that affects the tips of the pinnae of dogs during the summer months. In Rough Collies, Shetland Sheepdogs, and other breeds in which the tips of the pinnae bend over, the bites occur on the fold, whereas in those breeds with erect ears the lesions occur at the tips of the pinnae. Lesions consist of erythema, hair loss, and hemorrhagic crusting resulting from oozing of blood and serum. Insect bite dermatitis is most commonly seen in short-coated dogs such as Weimaraners, Doberman Pinschers, German Shorthaired Pointers, and Bull Terriers which are kept outdoors, especially in warm climates. Papules and crusted papules are followed by focal alopecia (**242**). The lesions are usually confined to the dorsal and lateral surfaces of the trunk and upper limbs. Buffalo gnat bites will result in circular 1 cm (0.4 in) areas of erythema on the non-haired areas of the ventral abdomen (**243**). Fly and mosquito bites may trigger eosinophilic folliculitis and furunculosis in some dogs.

Feline mosquito bite hypersensitivity (**244**) affects cats of any breed during the summer months in warm climates[1,2]. Typically, there is papular eruption on the outer and inner aspects of the pinnae and on the nose. Erosions, crusting, scaling, and, sometimes, depigmentation may follow. Cats often exhibit a mild pyrexia. Hyperkeratosis of all the pads of all four feet, preceded by swelling, tenderness, erythema, and, sometimes, fissuring may be seen. There is peripheral lymphadenopathy. Rarely, the condition will be accompanied by a corneal eosinophilic granuloma.

DIFFERENTIAL DIAGNOSES
- Squamous cell carcinoma
- Scabies
- Superficial pyoderma
- Demodicosis
- Urticaria
- Pemphigus foliaceus
- Feline eosinophilic granuloma complex
- Notoedric mange
- Pemphigus erythematosus
- Systemic lupus erythematosus
- Atopic dermatitis

DIAGNOSIS
The seasonal and environmental nature of the dermatosis means that many individuals are affected year after year. A history of exposure is often known, particularly for fly bite dermatosis of the pinnae. Microscopic examination of skin scrapes will eliminate *Demodex canis* from the differential of insect bite dermatitis. Superficial pyoderma is characterized by papules, pustules, and epidermal collarettes. The combination of the clinical signs described for the cat is pathognomonic.

MANAGEMENT
Ideally, these dermatoses are managed by preventing animals being exposed to the insects, although in reality it is often impossible to enforce. *S. calcitrans* may be deterred by the use of insect repellents such as DEET; however, DEET should not be used in cats because of toxicity concerns. Water based pyrethrins used according to the manufacturer's recommendation also have repellent activity. Flies and mosquitoes may be excluded from closed areas by fine mesh. Most cases resolve spontaneously when exposure to the insects is prevented, although in some instances it may be necessary to use systemic glucocorticoids to induce remission.

KEY POINT
- Control of the condition is difficult unless management changes are invoked.

242 Insect bite dermatitis. Patchy alopecia on the flanks of a Wire-haired Pointer.

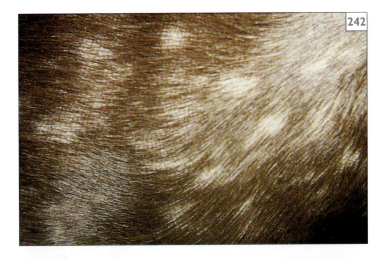

243 Erythematous target lesions due to gnat bites.

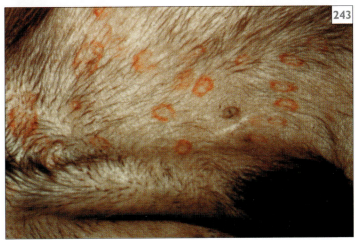

244 Feline mosquito bite hypersensitivity. (Photo courtesy K Mason)

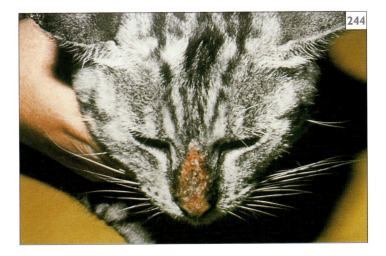

Myiasis

DEFINITION
Myiasis is infestation by fly larvae that feed on necrotic or living tissue of the host.

ETIOLOGY AND PATHOGENESIS
Lesions are generally associated with larvae of flies that produce facultative myiasis in contaminated skin wounds. Typically, they are from the genera *Musca*, *Calliphora*, *Phaenicia*, *Lucilia*, *Phormia*, and *Sarcophaga*[1]. They go through four developmental stages: egg, larva, pupa, and adult. For facultative myiasis to develop in a warm-blooded animal, there must be a factor such as traumatized skin, ocular discharge, neglected wound, or fecal soiling to attract the female fly to deposit eggs. Primary flies (*Lucilia*, *Phormia*, and some *Calliphora*) lay eggs in such sites; their larval stages can move independently over the surface of a wound, ingesting secretions, exudate, dead cells, and debris, but not live tissue. However, they can induce irritation, injure cells, and provoke exudation. Secondary flies (*Calliphora*, *Chrysomyia*, and *Sarcophaga*) are attracted to the damaged tissue. Their larvae can attack both dead and living tissue, extending and enlarging the lesions. Under controlled circumstances sterile maggots from primary species have been used in wound care very effectively. Obligatory myiasis is due to the screw-worm fly *Cochliomyia hominivorax*[1]. This fly is dependent on fresh wounds as a site for larval development. The larvae can liquefy and devour viable tissues, thereby enlarging the wound. They occur infrequently in North America, but are of major importance in Central and South America[1].

CLINICAL FEATURES
Affected animals often have predisposing factors such as matting of the hair coat or a thick coat, which hinders drying of the skin, resulting in maceration, necrotic tissue from wounds or neoplasia, urine or fecal soiling of the hair coat, fold dermatitis, or ocular discharge. Larvae can be found under the matted hair or in the wounds. They produce punched-out lesions in the tissues and may tunnel in diseased tissues, producing cavities (**245**). There is usually a foul odor.

DIAGNOSIS
Diagnosis is based on clinical findings of maggot infested wounds.

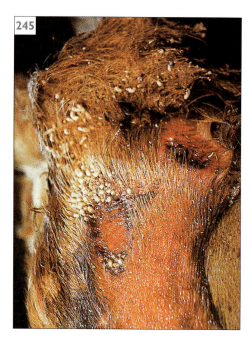

245 Myiasis. Focal, punched-out ulcers are often found in these cases when the overlying matted hair and crust are removed.

MANAGEMENT
Hair and mats should be clipped from infested areas. The area can be flushed with either Burrow's solution or a dilute chlorhexidine solution to clean debris and larvae from the wound. Flushing around deeply imbedded larvae may cause them to float free. If not, they will have to be removed with a forceps. Necrotic tissue, if present, should be removed and the wound dressed with silver sulfadiazine to control infection. Appropriate treatment should be administered for any systemic signs. Antibiotics are frequently necessary to control secondary infection. The client should be informed that the animal's wounds should be kept clean and, if possible, the animal housed in a fly-free environment until healing occurs. They should also be made aware of predisposing conditions so that steps can be taken to prevent recurrence.

KEY POINT
• Look for the underlying cause in these cases.

Dermatoses caused by body fluids

DEFINITION
Dermatoses caused by chronic exposure to urine, feces, saliva, or tears.

ETIOLOGY AND PATHOGENESIS
Chronic exposure to any bodily fluid results in surface maceration, erythema, secondary infection, and alopecia. Common examples are facial fold inflammation in Persian cats and lip fold dermatitis in Spaniels.

CLINICAL FEATURES
These dermatoses are usually focal, with little tendency to spread. The lesions usually extend from the source of the discharge and follow local skin folds (**246, 247**). The affected areas are erythematous, alopecic, moist, and often malodorous. Secondary infection is common. Pruritus is variable.

DIFFERENTIAL DIAGNOSES
- Intertrigo (body fold dermatitis)
- Demodicosis
- *Malassezia* dermatitis (which can also be a complication of body fold dermatitis)
- Bacterial overgrowth syndrome
- Mucocutaneous candidiasis
- Immune-mediated ulcerating diseases
- Metabolic epidermal necrosis (superficial necrolytic dermatitis, hepatocutaneous syndrome)

Note: *Malassezia* dermatitis, bacterial overgrowth syndrome, and intertrigo can all be complications of dermatoses involving body fluids.

DIAGNOSIS
Breed association and clinical site will allow recognition of fold dermatitis. Microscopic examination of skin scrapes and tape strips will demonstrate ectoparasites, yeasts, and bacteria. Care should be taken to rule out systemic disease, as not all cases are entirely anatomic.

MANAGEMENT
The management of these diseases is directed towards attending to the underlying cause of the discharge and symptomatic treatment of the dermatosis. Once the cause of the discharge is effectively treated, the dermatologic lesions resolve and further treatment is not necessary. Topical or, occasionally, systemic antimicrobials may be used to control secondary infection. In debilitated animals the onset of urine scald may be delayed if petrolatum is applied to the areas of skin adjacent to the urogenital orifices. Placing the animals on mesh floors may help. Unfortunately, some of the underlying conditions are difficult to treat definitively and long-term symptomatic treatment may be indicated.

KEY POINT
- Identification of the underlying cause is mandatory.

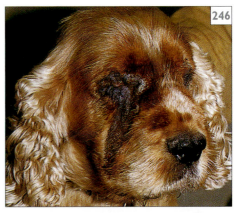

246 Epiphora secondary to hypothyroidism has resulted in periocular alopecia and hyperpigmentation in this Spaniel.

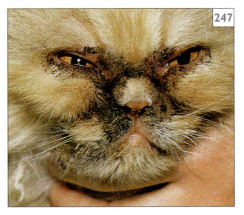

247 Facial fold dermatitis in a Persian cat following chronic epiphora.

Burns

DEFINITION

Burns are tissue damage resulting from thermal or chemical insult.

ETIOLOGY AND PATHOGENESIS

Direct heat burns result from contact with a hot object or substance. The most common direct heat burn is the 'clipper burn', which results from a hot clipper blade contacting the skin. Less frequently, direct heat burns develop from situations such as cats walking over hot stove burners, contact with hot exhaust parts of cars and wood or coal heaters, poor supervision of paralytic animals on heating pads, hot liquids spilled on animals, and malfunction of hair-drying equipment. Flame burns may result from fires in homes or automobile accidents. Electrical burns may be seen in and around the oral cavity when a young dog chews an electrical cord. The severity of a burn is related to the maximum temperature the tissue attains and the duration of the overheating. These in turn are dependent on such variables as the temperature and mass of the burning agent; the mass, specific heat, and thermal conductivity of the burned body; the temperature of the environment in which

post-burn cooling takes place; and the amount of heat convection in the surrounding medium. Body tissues, of which water is the main component, are characterized by high specific heat (which means that a large amount of heat is required to raise the temperature of tissue) and low thermal conductivity (which means the heat will be slow to dissipate). The clinical relevance of this is that the duration of tissue overheating extends beyond the contact time with the burning agent. Therefore, immediate cooling of the burned area can shorten the duration of tissue overheating, thereby decreasing tissue damage. Minimal overheating of tissue causes clinically inapparent, reversible cell damage. Further overheating will produce foci of irreversibly damaged cells scattered among reversibly damaged and non-injured cells. Finally, when a critical threshold is exceeded, necrosis of the entire tissue occurs. Because transition from healthy skin to necrotic skin is gradual, regeneration of skin defects proceeds from partly damaged rather than healthy tissue, and this results in a longer healing time when compared with mechanical injuries of the same depth. Severe burns may also result in shock as well as hemostatic, liver, kidney, respiratory, and immunologic disorders[1,2].

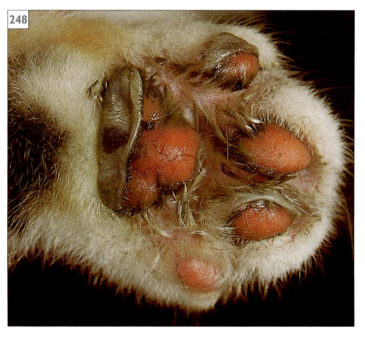

248 Slough of the skin over the pad secondary to scald.

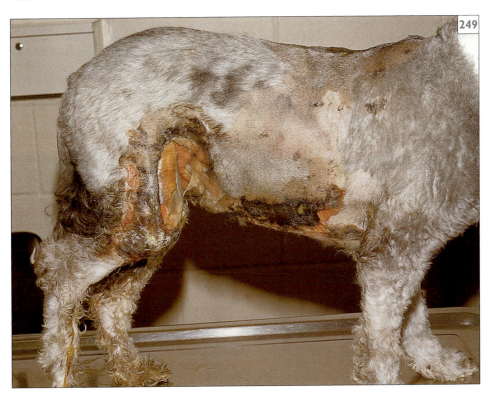

249 Extensive burns in a dog 13 days after the injury occurred.

CLINICAL FEATURES

The clinical appearance of a burn will vary depending on the etiology and severity of the burn. The human classification of burns is not appropriate for dogs and cats, as the skin of dogs and cats is thinner and does not blister as easily. Burns in these species are best classified as either partial thickness or full thickness. Partial-thickness burns are characterized by incomplete destruction of the skin; they are distinguished clinically by erythema, local edema, occasional small vesicles, evidence of persistent capillary circulation, and partial sensation to touch (**248**). Full-thickness burns are characterized by complete destruction of all elements of the skin including adnexa and nerves. Clinically, they are distinguished by lack of superficial blood flow, insensitivity to touch, and easy epilation of hair. It may take 10–14 days before the skin shows a color change and separation of necrotic skin begins (**249**).

DIAGNOSIS

Diagnosis is based on history and clinical features.

MANAGEMENT

Minor burns

Standard principles for the treatment of small traumatic lesions of the skin may be applied to minor burns, as experimental studies in animals and clinical studies in humans have not demonstrated a particular treatment for minor burns that has distinct advantages[3].

Severe burns

Clients should be encouraged to apply ice-water packs (ice and water in a plastic sack) to the burn site if it has occurred within two hours and the animal will permit this action. Exposed tissue may be gently overlaid or loosely wrapped with old towels, pillow cases, or strips of sheets. Owners should be instructed to spend minimal time on these endeavors, as they are not as critical as veterinary management of possible shock. On initial examination, airways should be examined to be sure they are patent and significant hemorrhage should be controlled. Evaluation and, if necessary, treatment for shock should then be instituted according to standard principles[4]. Cooling the affected areas is appropriate if the burn occurred within the past two hours. Cooling reduces pain, depth of the burn wound, edema, and mortality. If appropriate, the skin should be cooled by compresses or immersion in water (3–17°C/37.4–62.6°F) for approximately 30 minutes[5].

Cleaning and débridement are important. Hair should be clipped (with care to avoid any further damage to the skin, especially partially damaged areas) from all of the affected areas and other contamination and debris should be rinsed off by flushing with saline or washing with antibacterial cleanser. All tissue that is devitalized (determined by a change in the color of tissue, lack of sensation to touch, lack of capillary circulation, and easy epilation of hair) should be excised as it serves as a good growth medium for bacteria. Final confirmation of the extent of burn wounds may not be completely possible until about ten days post burn, when separation of normal and necrotic tissue becomes obvious.

Immersion of the affected areas in a whirlpool bath for 15–20 minutes twice daily is effective for the removal of exudate and helpful for the loosening and removal of necrotic tissue. Topical antibacterial treatment is useful. Silver sulfadiazine cream is an effective and practical antibacterial drug for topical therapy. Besides having antibacterial properties, it is non-irritating to exposed tissues, may promote healing, has no systemic side-effects, and is easily applied to the wound, which is then bandaged with loose mesh gauze. Dressings are changed twice daily. During changes, necessary débridement should be performed and old medications along with any exudate are removed by irrigation with saline or immersion in a whirlpool bath.

Use of biological and synthetic dressings and skin grafts should be considered. Biological dressings, such as specially prepared pig skin and synthetic dressings made of either silicone polymers, polyurethane, or polyvinyl chloride polymers provide benefit by maintaining a water layer on the surface of the wound that aids re-epithelialization, clears surface bacteria, and minimizes fibrosis, inflammation, heat loss, and pain[2]. They are most effective when infection and eschar are minimal. Because the skin of dogs and cats is very elastic and has loose subcutaneous tissue, skin defects can often be closed by direct apposition or one of several reconstructive techniques making use of skin flaps. If the defect is too large for direct apposition or a skin flap, a free autogenous graft of either full or partial thickness may be used.

Systemic antibacterial treatment in the management of burn wounds is questionable. Studies in animals and human burn patients show that systemic antibiotic therapy does not favorably influence mortality rates, fever, or rate of healing[3]. Their use should be limited to confirmed cases of bacterial septicemia and selection should be determined by sensitivity tests.

KEY POINT

- Animals with extensive burns will require intensive therapy over a long period of time. Clients must be warned of this fact.

Frostbite

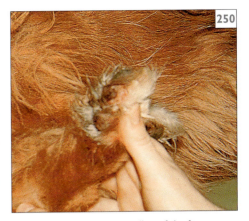

250 Frostbite. Note the pallor of the feet.

DEFINITION

Frostbite is tissue damage that results from freezing.

ETIOLOGY AND PATHOGENESIS

Frostbite occurs with prolonged exposure to freezing temperatures and is more likely to occur if the animal is also exposed to windy conditions or if there is wetting of a body area. The pathogenesis involves direct cold injury to the cell, indirect cold injury by formation of ice crystals, and impaired circulation with hypoxia.

CLINICAL FEATURES

Lesions typically occur in areas where the hair coat is sparse. In cats the tips of the ears, the tail, and the footpads are most commonly affected, while in dogs it is more often the scrotum and footpads (**250**). Cats with mild frostbite may be asymptomatic, with the only noticeable feature being a delayed lightening of hair color on the tips of the ears and curling of the pinnae. Affected skin can be erythematous, tender, or painful and may exfoliate during healing. More severely damaged tissue in the acute phase is cool to the touch, pale, and numb. With thawing, the affected areas become erythematous, painful, edematous and, eventually, may develop either scaling or necrosis.

DIFFERENTIAL DIAGNOSES

- Vasculitis
- Squamous cell carcinoma
- Disseminated intravascular coagulation
- Cold agglutinin disease
- Cryoglobulinemia
- Ischemic necrosis associated with toxins

DIAGNOSIS

Diagnosis is based on history and clinical findings.

MANAGEMENT

Mild cases of frostbite may not require any treatment or only the application of a bland ointment. If there is deep freezing of tissues, the case should be handled in such a way as to avoid thawing and refreezing as this greatly increases tissue damage. Initial treatment should consist of rapid thawing in warm water (38–44°C/100.4–111.2°F)[1]. After warming, the patient should be carefully monitored to ensure that self-mutilation does not occur. Irreversibly damaged tissue demarcates in 7–14 days. Further therapeutic management of necrotic tissue and the resulting defect parallels that of thermal injury.

KEY POINT

- Careful management of severe cases is necessary if further tissue damage is to be avoided.

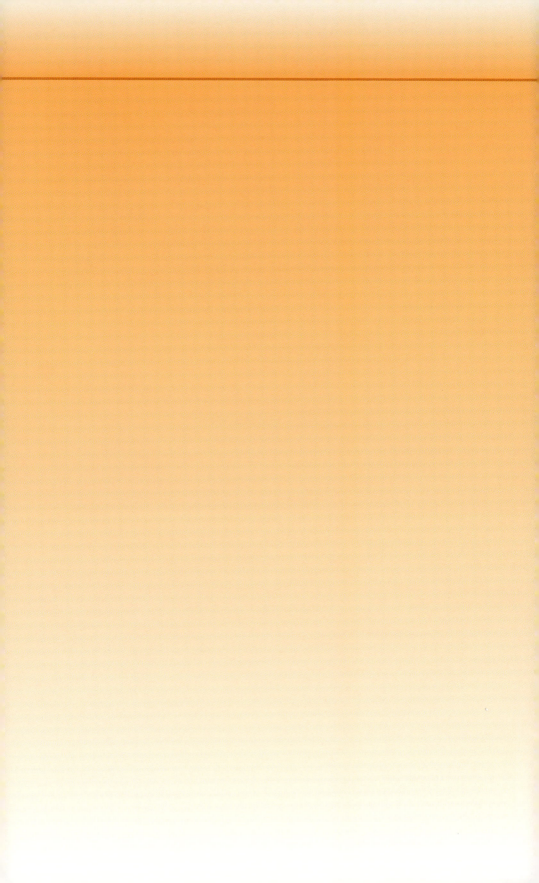

Endocrine dermatoses

General approach

- Not all animals with symmetrical, diffuse, or generalized alopecia have an endocrinopathy
- Many endocrinopathies look the same – take a careful history and do a thorough clinical examination to pick up subtle clues to the diagnosis
- Interpret the results of screening and endocrine tests carefully – do not rely on a single abnormal result for diagnosis
- Biopsy and histopathology are often non-specific – use as a last resort

Common conditions

- Hypothyroidism
- Hyperadrenocorticism
- Sertoli cell tumor
- Alopecia X

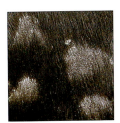
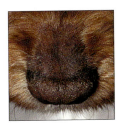
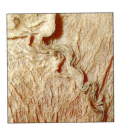
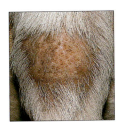

Hypothyroidism

DEFINITION
Hypothyroidism is a clinical syndrome associated with a failure of the thyroid glands to produce and release thyroid hormones[1,2]. It is classified as primary, secondary, or tertiary if the abnormality affects the thyroid gland, pituitary gland, or hypothalamus, respectively. Thyroid hormone is necessary for the initiation of the anagen (growth) phase of the hair cycle and normal metabolism of the skin.

THYROID PHYSIOLOGY
Thyrotropin-releasing hormone (TRH), produced by and released from the hypothalamus, stimulates the synthesis and release of thyrotropin (TSH) from the pituitary adenohypophysis. TSH stimulates the production and release of thyroid hormones from the thyroid gland. Negative feedback from circulating thyroid hormones regulates TSH and TRH release[1,2].

In a healthy animal all 3,5,3',5'tetraiodothyronine (thyroxine, T4) is produced by the thyroid gland, but only 20% of the 3,5,3'triiodothyronine (T3) and 5% of 3,3',5 triiodothyronine (reverse T3, rT3) are of thyroid origin, with the majority derived from de-iodination of T4 in peripheral tissues. T4 is a pro-hormone, T3 the major metabolically active thyroid hormone, and rT3 metabolically inactive[1,2].

Circulating levels of T4 and T3 may be lowered due to non-thyroidal illness or euthyroid sick syndrome (including renal failure, liver disease, diabetes mellitus, hyperadrenocorticism, systemic infection, pyoderma, and demodicosis), and drugs (e.g. glucocorticoids, phenobarbital, clomipramine, NSAIDs, radiograph contrast agents, and amiodarone)[1-3]. The low thyroid hormone levels are thought to be a normal adaptation and do not reflect thyroid dysfunction, although prolonged courses of sulfonamides may result in clinical hypothyroidism[4].

ETIOLOGY AND PATHOGENESIS
In dogs, >90% of clinical cases of hypothyroidism are caused by primary destruction of the thyroid gland[1,2]. Lymphocytic thyroiditis and idiopathic thyroid necrosis and atrophy are cited as the two main causes of acquired primary hypothyroidism. However, some cases of the latter could be end-stage thyroiditis. Lymphocytic thyroiditis is thought to be an autoimmune disorder involving cell-mediated destruction of the thyroid gland. Thyroglobulin autoantibodies (TGAAs) can be detected prior to or in the earlier stages of the disease, but they may be undetectable in end-stage disease with thyroid atrophy. Secondary (i.e. loss of TSH) and tertiary hypothyroidism (i.e. loss of TRH) are rare in dogs[5].

Predisposed breeds include Labrador Retrievers, Golden Retrievers, Dobermanns, Bearded Collies, Borzois, and Beagles[6]. In some of these breeds there is an association with the DLA-DQA1*00101 allele[7]. It is therefore likely that there is a genetic predisposition and affected dogs should not be bred from. Congenital hypothyroidism with goiter is an autosomal recessive trait in Toy Fox Terriers[8]. A genetic screening test is in use to eradicate this trait.

Hypothyroidism is very rare in cats, but naturally occurring congenital cases in kittens and iatrogenic cases after surgical or radioactive treatment for hyperthyroidism may be seen[9].

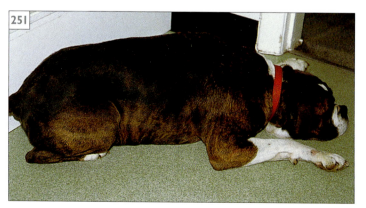

251–253
Hypothyroidism. Lethargy, dullness, and alopecia in a Boxer (**251**); symmetrical alopecia in an Airedale (**252**); alopecia on the flank (**253**).

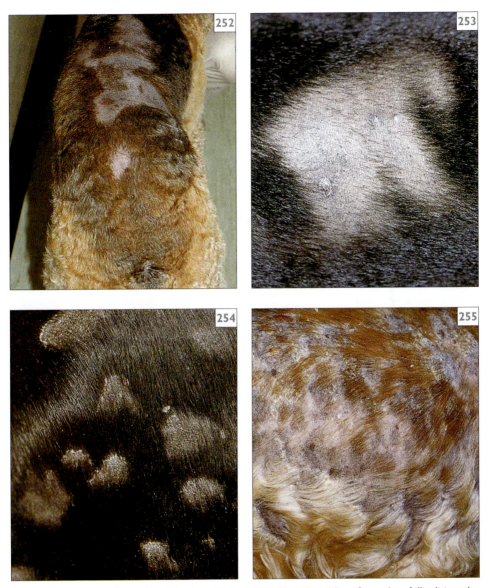

254 Hypothyroidism. Secondary infection with minimal inflammation.

255 Hypothyroidism. Secondary folliculitis and associated patchy alopecia.

CLINICAL FEATURES

The clinical signs of canine hypothyroidism are extremely variable and may include both systemic signs and dermatologic signs[1,2,6]. Bilaterally symmetrical truncal alopecia with thickened, hyperpigmented and cool skin (myxedema) is classical (**251–253**), but is unusual except in advanced cases. Common dermatologic problems include a dry, brittle, lackluster coat, seborrhea, scaling, post-clipping alopecia, hyperpigmentation, and recurrent secondary infections (**254, 255**). In others, alopecia may be restricted

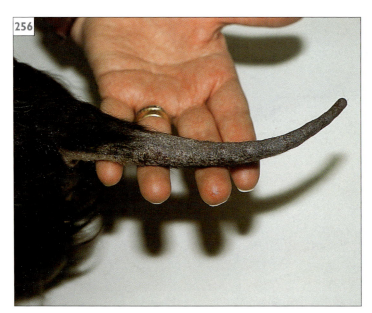

256 Hypothyroidism. Alopecic tail.

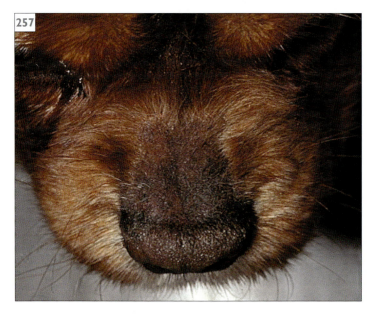

257 Hypothyroidism. Focal alopecia of the dorsal nose in a Cavalier King Charles Spaniel.

to the tail and dorsal nose (**256, 257**). Some dogs have abnormally retained hair (hypertrichosis) instead of alopecia. Clinical hypothyroidism is rarely seen in dogs under two years old. Congenital hypothyroidism is a rare condition that is also associated with disproportionate dwarfism, dental abnormalities, and cretinism. Hypothyroidism can also be a component of pituitary dwarfism. The clinical signs of hypothyroidism are listed below:

- Common signs: thin poor quality coat; alopecia (including post-clipping alopecia); scaling; secondary infections; demodicosis; lethargy; and weight gain.
- Uncommon signs: neuromuscular disease; cretinism; ocular disorders; bradycardia; facial myxedema ('tragic face'); hypothermia ('heat-seeking'); and ceruminous otitis externa.

DIFFERENTIAL DIAGNOSES

- Hyperadrenocorticism
- Alopecia 'X'/alopecia of follicular arrest
- Sex hormone disorders including Sertoli cell tumor
- Sebaceous adenitis
- Color-dilution alopecia
- Seasonal flank alopecia
- Telogen effluvium/anagen defluxion
- Pattern baldness
- Dermatophytosis
- Demodicosis
- Superficial pyoderma

Hypothyroidism may be the underlying cause for some of these conditions in older dogs (e.g. superficial pyoderma, demodicosis, and dermatophytosis). Hypothyroidism can occasionally complicate chronic hyperadrenocorticism if pituitary tumors result in thyrotroph loss (secondary hypothyroidism) or damage to the hypothalamus (tertiary hypothyroidism)[5].

DIAGNOSIS

Routine tests are non-specific[6]: mild, non-regenerative anemia (25–30%); raised fasting plasma lipids (35–50%) and cholesterol (35–75%); mild to moderate elevation of AP and ALT (20–30%); raised creatinine kinase (10–20%).

Basal total T4 (tT4) is not by itself a reliable test to confirm hypothyroidism because tT4 is commonly lowered by various drugs and non-thyroidal illnesses[1,6,10,11]. Free T4 (fT4), which is maintained at the expense of total T4, is less affected by drugs and concurrent disease[12], but nevertheless should not be solely relied on for diagnosis. In one study, fT4 measured by equilibrium dialysis more accurately differentiated hypothyroid, sick euthyroid, and healthy dogs than radioimmunoassay[12]. Free or total T3 is no more informative than T4, and is rarely used in diagnosis.

Endogenous canine TSH assays are now available and can be combined with tT4 or fT4. Values are elevated in 80–85% of animals with primary hypothyroidism[10,11]. It is possible that false-negative tests represent pituitary thyrotroph exhaustion in more chronic cases or concurrent non-thyroidal illness. Elevated TSH levels can also be seen in some dogs with non-thyroidal illness or receiving sulfonamides. TSH levels can also vary by up to 43.6% between dogs and by up to 13.6% in individual dogs[13].

Therapeutic trials with l-thyroxine can be used to confirm the diagnosis where test results are inconclusive or unavailable[1,11,14]. Trial therapy must be undertaken carefully as the metabolic effects of thyroxine can result in non-specific hair growth and clinical improvement. The outcome measures must be clearly established before treatment, with assessments at one, two, and three months.

Stimulation tests using recombinant human TSH (rhTSH) were recently evaluated and found reliably to distinguish hypothyroid and euthyroid dogs. Administration of 75 µg/dog intravenously resulted in a significant rise in tT4 (≥2.5 µg/dl and at least 1.5× basal T4) after six hours in normal animals or animals with non-thyroidal illness; this was not seen in hypothyroid dogs[15]. rhTSH is now available from some laboratories, although it is important to follow their protocol carefully. TRH stimulation tests are much less reliable as T4 levels fail to increase in a significant proportion of euthyroid animals, although they can be used to differentiate primary and secondary hypothyroidism. TRH also causes moderate to severe adverse effects arising from stimulation of the autonomic nervous system in many dogs[1,11].

TGAAs are present in up to 36% of cases of lymphocytic thyroiditis. In one study, 43% of hypothyroid dogs with normal TSH levels had TGAAs[16]. They can also be present in a small number of normal dogs, most, but not all, of whom will go on to develop hypothyroidism.

TGAA, T4, and TSH levels have therefore been used to screen animals in breeds predisposed to hypothyroidism. Anti-T3 and T4 antibodies are seen in some dogs. They are of little diagnostic significance, but can interfere with some tests, leading to spuriously high T3 and T4 levels.

Recent studies have shown that ultrasonographic abnormalities (including decreased echogenicity, heterogeneity, irregular capsule, irregular lobe shape, and decreased thyroid volume) had a sensitivity of 94% for primary hypothyroidism[17]. One study of 30 dogs showed that there was no overlap of $99^{m}TcO_4^-$ uptake between dogs with primary hypothyroidism and non-thyroidal illness[18].

MANAGEMENT

Therapy involves lifelong administration of levothyroxine (l-thyroxine). The initial dose is 0.02 mg/kg or 0.5 mg/m² body surface area p/o twice daily[1,14]. Dosing on the basis of body surface area minimizes underdosing of small dogs and overdosing of large dogs. The dose should be adjusted following the results of pre- and 4–6 hour post-thyroxine dosing T4 levels[14]. Pre-treatment T4 should be near the lower end of the normal range and the post-treatment sample should be near the upper end. T4 testing and dose adjustments should be performed at one, two, and three months, and then every 3–6 months or as necessary in the long term. It is possible to switch most animals to once daily medication once the clinical signs have resolved. In one study dogs were maintained on mean doses of 0.026 mg/kg once daily[14]. Signs of overdose are uncommon, but include anxiety, restlessness, polyphagia, weight loss, and tachycardia. It may be necessary to use appropriate systemic and/or topical treatment to control secondary infections or demodicosis initially.

KEY POINTS
- A common, but overdiagnosed clinical syndrome.
- Diagnosis can be difficult in some cases.
- The prognosis is good.

Hyperadrenocorticism

ETIOLOGY AND PATHOGENESIS

Hyperadrenocorticism (HAC or Cushing's disease) results from prolonged exposure to elevated serum cortisol concentrations, which may be spontaneous or iatrogenic. Most cases (80–85%) of spontaneous HAC in dogs are pituitary dependent (PDH): functional adenomas of the anterior pituitary secrete adrenocorticotropic hormone (ACTH), resulting in adrenocortical hyperplasia. Fifteen to twenty per cent of cases are due to adrenal neoplasia, although this figure may be slightly higher in larger breed dogs[1]. HAC is rare in cats, although iatrogenic and spontaneous cases with a similar proportion of PDH and adrenal tumors to dogs are seen[2].

There is no breed, age, or sex predisposition to iatrogenic HAC. Most cases result from long-term, high-dose administration of glucocorticoid either orally or by depot injection. The risk of inducing iatrogenic HAC is dose and duration related and may be minimized by administering oral prednisone (or prednisolone or methylprednisolone) on an alternate day basis[1], although there is wide individual variation in steroid tolerance. Rarely, cases have been seen following topical administration (**258**)[1].

CLINICAL FEATURES

Animals of any age may be affected, but there is a steadily increasing risk with age up to 7–9 years old[1,2]. There appears to be no sex predisposition to HAC, but females are predisposed to adrenal neoplasia. Any breed may be affected, but Terriers in particular are predisposed to HAC, Dachshunds to adrenal tumors, and Boxers to pituitary neoplasia[1].

Dogs with HAC may exhibit a number of clinical signs[3]. Commonly noted clinical signs are polyuria/polydipsia (PU/PD), a pendulous abdomen, hepatomegaly, polyphagia, weight gain, lethargy, muscular weakness and atrophy, lordosis (ventral bowing of the spine) (**259**), anestrus, pendulous prepuce and testicular atrophy, panting, neurologic deficits (which can be associated with pressure from a pituitary macroadenoma), and insulin-resistant diabetes mellitus[1,3]. Dermatologic signs include:

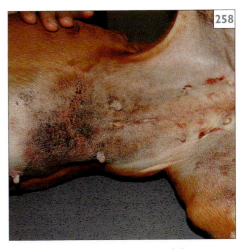

258 Localized changes to the skin following long-term topical administration of betamethasone to an atopic Boxer.

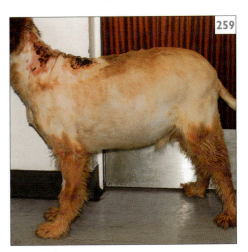

259 Canine hyperadrenocorticism with truncal alopecia, pot-belly, lordosis, and calcinosis cutis.

- Dull, dry, faded coat that is easily epilated.
- Post-clipping alopecia.
- Symmetrical to generalized, complete to diffuse non-inflammatory alopecia, particularly of the trunk, but sparing the head and distal limbs (**259**).

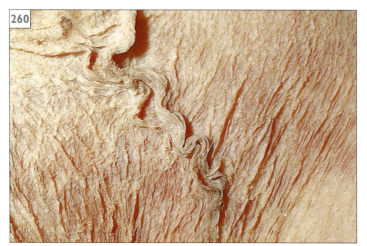

260 Hyperadreno-corticism in dogs. Prominent abdominal veins and tenting due to loss of dermal tissue and thinning of the epidermis.

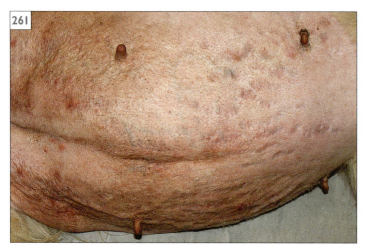

261 Pot belly, alopecia, and cutaneous atrophy with comedones, prominent blood vessels, hemorrhage, bruising, and 'stretch marks'.

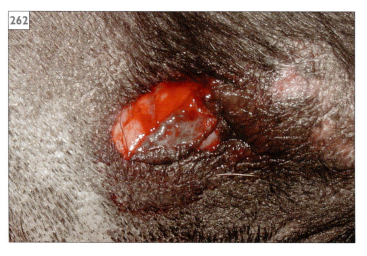

262 Fragile skin and non-healing over the elbow.

263 Calcinosis cutis, ulceration, secondary infection, and crusting.

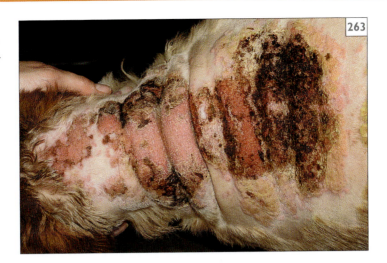

- Mild to moderate scaling.
- Cutaneous atrophy, prominent blood vessels, loss of elasticity, and wrinkling, especially on the abdomen (**260, 261**).
- Comedones (**261**).
- Easily bruised skin and poor wound healing (**262**).
- Calcinosis cutis (**263**).
- Increased susceptibility to pyoderma (especially bullous impetigo), *Malassezia* dermatitis, dermatophytosis, and demodicosis.

Dogs may present with any combination of clinical signs that can develop in any order. This can make the diagnosis difficult. Dogs with secondary infections and calcinosis cutis may be pruritic. Conversely, animals with pre-existing inflammatory disorders such as atopic dermatitis or osteoarthritis can improve as HAC develops.

Cats present with more vague and less well-defined clinical signs than dogs[4,5]. These may be similar to the range seen in dogs, but affected cats often present with cutaneous atrophy and skin fragility. Such cats must be handled with extreme care to prevent further damage to the skin. Many cats with HAC present as insulin-resistant diabetes mellitus.

DIFFERENTIAL DIAGNOSES
- Hypothyroidism
- Sertoli cell neoplasia and other sex hormone dermatoses
- Adrenal sex hormone dermatoses or alopecia of follicular arrest ('alopecia X')
- Follicular dysplasias
- Telogen effluvium and anagen defluxion
- Diabetes mellitus

DIAGNOSIS
Routine hematology, biochemistry, and urinalysis[6]
- Stress leucogram: neutrophilia, lymphopenia, eosinopenia, monocytosis (rare).
- Hypercholesterolemia.
- Mild to moderate hyperglycemia.
- Increased ALT and AP; the latter is very common in dogs (which have a steroid-induced isoenzyme) and usually out of proportion with the increase in ALT.
- Decreased total T4 due to cortisol inhibition.
- Urine specific gravity generally <1.015 (i.e. hyposthenuric).
- Presence of urinary white blood cells, blood, and protein due to urinary tract infections; these are common, but clinical signs can be masked by the anti-inflammatory action of cortisol.

Histopathologic examination of biopsy samples may be helpful, but in many instances the cutaneous changes are non-diagnostic[6], although the presence of calcinosis cutis is highly specific for HAC.

Imaging
- Radiography[6]:
  - 'Pot belly' and good contrast due to increased intra-abdominal fat.
  - Distended bladder (PU/PD).
  - Hepatomegaly.
  - Osteoporosis.
  - Dystrophic calcification of skin (calcinosis cutis), airways, blood vessels, kidneys, etc.
  - 50% of canine adrenal tumors calcified (no link to malignancy; normal aging change in cats).
  - Enlarged adrenals are otherwise difficult to see.
  - Thoracic metastasis of adrenal carcinoma.
- Ultrasonography can be very useful to detect and assess adrenal tumors[6] and will also detect bilateral hypertrophy in PDH[7].
- MRI and CT will detect pituitary tumors[6,8]; CT can also image the adrenal glands, but is less sensitive than MRI at detecting pituitary masses.

Urinary cortisol:creatinine ratio (UCCR)
UCCR measurement is cheap and highly sensitive but poorly specific for HAC[6]. A normal UCCR makes HAC very unlikely, but raised UCCRs are commonly seen in many other diseases associated with inflammation, systemic illness, and PU/PD. Stress can also result in a raised UCCR, so samples should be collected by the owner before visiting the veterinary clinic. Multiple UCCRs are more specific, but are more expensive.

ACTH stimulation test
Synthetic ACTH can be used to stimulate cortisol production from the adrenal cortex (**264**). It is more specific but less sensitive than a low-dose dexamethasone suppression test (LDDST) (i.e. there are fewer false positives [approximately 15%, due to stress or other illness], but more false negatives [approximately 15%; adrenal tumors in particular may fail to show elevated cortical post-ACTH]). ACTH stimulation tests are also used to monitor adrenal function during therapy[6].

Each laboratory has a normal range based on its protocol, so contact them if unsure. Most tests involve taking blood samples prior to and 30–90 minutes after 250 µg ACTH given intravenously or intramuscularly.

Serum 17-OH-progesterone levels are also elevated post-ACTH and these may be of diagnostic significance in equivocal cases[9].

Low-dose dexamethasone suppression test
An LDDST assesses the ability of the hypothalamic–pituitary–adrenal axis to respond to negative feedback, resulting in decreased ACTH release and adrenal cortisol production (**265**). These tests are more sensitive (5–10% false negatives) but less specific than ACTH stimulation tests (50% false positives)[6]. Dexamethasone is used as it does not cross-react with cortisol assays. The exact protocol varies with the laboratory, so it is advisable to check with the individual laboratory first. LDDSTs generally involve taking blood samples immediately before, four, and eight hours after giving 0.01–0.015 mg/kg dexamethasone intravenously.

In about 30% of dogs there is adequate suppression at four hours, but 'escape' at eight hours with cortisol concentrations rising again, which is diagnostic for PDH. In most cases of adrenal neoplasia, and some 25% of all spontaneous HAC cases (including PDH), there is no suppression whatsoever, and in other cases there may be suppression, but it does not fall below 50% of baseline.

High-dose dexamethasone suppression test (HDDST)
This tests the resistance of the pituitary–adrenal axis to high doses of dexamethasone, since in dogs with PDH it has been documented that the LDDST can be overridden. A basal blood sample is taken and dexamethasone injected (1 mg/kg i/v). Subsequent blood samples are taken after four and eight hours and submitted for cortisol assay. Any significant suppression (>50%) is diagnostic for PDH. Resistance to HDD is seen in about 15% cases of PDH and the majority of dogs with adrenal neoplasia[6]. However, given the relative frequencies of PDH and adrenal tumors, this results in only 50% specificity. HDDSTs are therefore now used less often[6,7].

264 ACTH stimulation tests. Typical results for various forms of HAC.

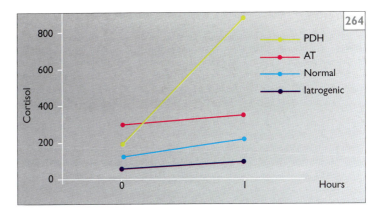

265 Low-dose dexamethasone suppression test. Typical results from cases of PDH and adrenal tumors following an LDDST.

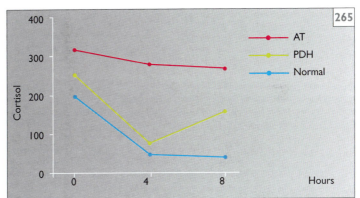

Endogenous ACTH assay

It is now possible to measure the circulating endogenous ACTH concentration to differentiate the etiology of spontaneous HAC. PDH cases have normal or high (>25 pg/ml) levels due to ACTH secretion from a functional pituitary tumor independent of negative feedback from elevated cortisol. Adrenal tumors have low ACTH levels (<5 pg/ml) due to negative feedback from ACTH-independent cortisol production[6,7]. ACTH is, however, very labile. Blood samples must be taken into chilled EDTA tubes and centrifuged in a chilled centrifuge (placing a mini-centrifuge in a refrigerator at 4°C for an hour is usually sufficient). The plasma should be immediately frozen and sent by overnight or same day courier in a freezer pack.

Diagnosis in cats

Confirmation of HAC in cats can be difficult. Screening tests are often non-specific (cats in particular lack steroid-induced ALP) and often simply reflect diabetes mellitus[4,5,10]. Adrenal function tests are possible in cats[4,5,10]. Results from UCCRs are similar to those in dogs. ACTH stimulation tests are similar to those in dogs (although giving 125 µg synthetic ACTH i/v and collecting the second blood sample after 90 minutes is also done), but the results are less specific and less sensitive[10,11]. LDDSTs have been performed, giving 0.1 mg/kg dexamthasone intravenously, as up to 20% of normal cats fail to suppress with 0.01 mg/kg. At the higher dose the results appear to be very sensitive but less specific. Plasma ACTH levels appear to be elevated in PDH and low with adrenal tumors.

MANAGEMENT
Trilostane
Trilostane is highly effective in canine HAC[12] and is the licensed treatment in the UK. Starting doses of 2–12 mg/kg p/o once daily are administered for 7–10 days. Cortisol levels following an ACTH stimulation test 4–6 hours post-injection should be <150 nmol/l (<5.4 µg/dl). The dose of trilostane should be adjusted as necessary; maintenance doses are usually in the range 3–4 mg/kg. The half-life of trilostane in some dogs is very short and these will require twice daily dosing[13,14]. These dogs typically have appropriate cortisol levels post-ACTH, but clinical signs such as PU/PD fail to resolve. Trilostane is a steroid synthesis inhibitor; therefore, while it controls the clinical signs associated with excess cortisol production, the underlying disease is not affected. Dogs therefore generally require lifelong treatment once or twice daily with regular ACTH stimulation tests. The latter group will need two tests to cover both dosing intervals. Trilostane is usually well tolerated, although there have been idiosyncratic cases of adrenal necrosis and sudden death following treatment[15]. Survival times of dogs treated with trilostane and mitotane do not differ significantly [16].

Mitotane (o,p'-DDD)
Once the treatment of choice, mitotane is used less now that trilostane is available. An induction dose (25–50 mg/kg q24h) is usually given with food until effect (PU/PD: water intake <60 ml/kg/day; polyphagia resolves; or if signs of hypoadrenocorticism occur) and an ACTH test performed to assess the adrenal reserve. Both basal and post-ACTH cortisol concentrations should be in the normal resting range. About 15% of dogs with PDH will still have elevated post-ACTH cortisol concentrations, and the induction course should be continued until the ACTH test is suppressed adequately. About 30% of dogs will have subnormal pre- and post-ACTH cortisol concentrations, and in these cases mitotane is withheld until normal cortisol concentrations recover. At this point, maintenance doses of mitotane (25–50 mg/kg/week) are given in 2–3 divided doses.

The prognosis for dogs treated with mitotane is fair, but an appreciable number of dogs prove very hard to stabilize, with frequent relapses and/or hypoadrenocortical (addisonian) crises. An alternative protocol is to continue the induction course at doses of 50–75 mg/kg until there is no adrenal reserve left, and then manage the dogs for hypoadrenocorticism[17]. This protocol is uncommon now, as there are frequent crises during induction and many dogs eventually relapse.

Very high-dose mitotane therapy (50–75 mg/kg/day) for up to 11 weeks (with regular ACTH tests to assess response) may be necessary to reduce serum cortisol to normal levels in cases of adrenal tumors. These dogs may also need higher doses to maintain remission.

Other treatment options
Adrenal neoplasia may be managed by surgical resection[18,19]. Surgery is difficult, has a significant complication rate, including perioperative death, and hypoadrenocortical crises are common. Histopathologic features, tumor size, and age do not appear to affect the outcome. Medical therapy with trilostane or mitotane can effectively control clinical signs in inoperable or partially resected adrenal tumors, although metastatic disease can still occur.

Microsurgical trans-sphenoidal hypophysectomy is a safe and effective treatment for canine and feline HAC[20], but it is a very diffcult technique requiring a high standard of surgical and technical expertise. Residual cells appear to maintain normal adrenal cortex function postoperatively.

Ketoconazole inhibits adrenal steroid synthesis and has been used at 5–10 mg/kg p/o once daily to manage HAC. Its activity, however, is less specific and efficacious than trilostane, and it is not widely used.

Early reports suggested that selegiline (l-deprenyl) (2 mg/kg p/o q24h) could be useful in the treatment of PDH[21], but later clinical trials demonstrated poor efficacy[22] and it is rarely used.

Recently, radiation therapy was found to be effective in cats with PDH and concurrent neurologic signs[23]. Irradiation of pituitary adenomas in dogs was also successful in controlling neurologic signs, but resolution of clinical HAC required further medical therapy[24]. Radiotherapy appeared to be well tolerated in both species.

Treatment in cats

Management of HAC in cats can be difficult, especially with insulin-resistant diabetes mellitus and skin fragility. Mitotane is of limited efficacy and often poorly tolerated. Ketoconazole and selegiline are also of limited efficacy, but metyrapone (65 mg/kg p/o q12h) may be more effective[5,10]. Early reports suggest that trilostane is well tolerated and of moderate efficacy[25-27], although concurrent insulin therapy is often required. Bilateral adrenalectomy has been the treatment of choice for feline PDH[4,5,10]. The prognosis appears to be better if cats are stabilized on medical therapy first and postoperative glucocortiocoids and mineralocorticoids are administered[28,29].

Hypoadrenocortical (addisonian) crisis

Most adverse effects from therapy are associated with falls in serum cortisol such that an addisonian crisis develops, with signs such as lethargy, weakness, inappetence, vomiting, diarrhea, bradycardia, and collapse[30]. Owners should be aware of these signs and instructed to withdraw therapy temporarily and administer prednisolone (0.2–0.25 mg/kg p/o) as necessary. Severe cases that present with circulatory collapse will need intravenous fluid support. Prednisolone treatment should cease for a minimum of 25 hours before an ACTH stimulation test, as it will interfere with the cortisol assay.

Calcinosis cutis

Exacerbation of or the appearance of calcinosis cutis post medical or surgical treatment is reasonably common. This usually resolves over the course of therapy. Severe cases of calcinosis cutis may not fully resolve even with good control of HAC. Benign neglect is appropriate if the lesions are quiescent and with no ulceration or secondary infection. Symptomatic lesions could be surgically removed, although this may involve extensive areas and necessitate plastic surgery to close the wound. Daily topical application of dimethyl sulfoxide (DMSO) has been effective, but treated animals should be closely monitored for signs of hypercalcemia.

KEY POINTS

- History and clinical signs are highly suggestive.
- Diagnosis often requires multiple tests.
- Therapy can be expensive and difficult.
- Iatrogenic hypoadrenocorticism is common.

Hyperandrogenism

ETIOLOGY AND PATHOGENESIS

Most cases of hyperandrogenism result from excessive androgen stimulation caused by increased production by testicular neoplasms[1,2], particularly interstitial cell tumors (see Sertoli cell and other testicular neoplasia, p. 246), or an imbalance associated with altered peripheral sex steroid metabolism, and/or alterations in the number or activity of peripheral receptors. Hyperandrogenism can, therefore, occur in males with normal testes and, rarely, in neutered males or females as a consequence of adrenal androgen synthesis[3]. This has been noted with adrenal tumors[4].

The androgen dependent tissues are the tail gland and the prostate gland in the male, and perianal gland tissue in both males and females. Under androgen influence these tissues exhibit hyperplasia and, occasionally, adenomatous change[1]. Androgens also stimulate epidermal hyperproliferation, enhance sebum secretion, and retard the initiation of anagen[2].

Neutered females and entire males are predisposed to perianal gland neoplasia compared with entire females or neutered males. Cocker Spaniels of both sexes are predisposed to perianal gland neoplasia and male English Bulldogs, Samoyeds, and Beagles are predisposed to perianal gland adenomas[1,2].

CLINICAL FEATURES

Hyperandrogenism is most commonly seen in elderly, entire male dogs. There is hyperplasia of the tail gland (**266**), perianal gland hyperplasia, and prostatomegaly. There is often macular hyperpigmentation of affected perianal and perigenital skin[1,2]. Benign perianal adenomas frequently appear as single to multiple, well-defined, soft, mobile nodules in the perianal skin (**267**). Testicular neoplasia may be palpable as a discreet mass or manifest as a difference in the size, shape, and/or texture of the testes. Ultrasonography is highly sensitive for detecting small, non-palpable testicular tumors. Other cutaneous manifestations include greasy seborrhea, seborrheic dermatitis (particularly of the tail gland), otitis, alopecia, and hypertrichosis (caused by abnormal retention of hairs)[1] (**268**). Aggression and hypersexuality are uncommon. Female dogs may exhibit masculine behavior such as mounting[2].

DIFFERENTIAL DIAGNOSES

- Perianal gland adenocarcinoma
- Lipoma
- Other cutaneous neoplasia
- Other endocrinopathies

DIAGNOSIS

The triad of tail gland hyperplasia, perianal gland hyperplasia, and prostatomegaly in an elderly male dog is diagnostic. Tape-strip or impression smear cytology will identify secondary bacterial or *Malassezia* infections. Serum testosterone concentrations may be elevated. Fine needle aspirate cytology is usually sufficient to identify a benign, epithelial cell tumor consistent with a perianal adenoma. However, a small number of these tumors can be malignant, so histopathology should be performed to confirm their benign nature and assess the surgical margins. Radiography, ultrasonography, and adrenal function tests should be considered if adrenal gland neoplasia or hyperplasia is suspected.

MANAGEMENT

The adenomatous changes and hyperplasia are androgen dependent and castration is the treatment of choice. Surgical excision is effective for perianal adenomas, although dogs should also be castrated to prevent recurrence and development of new tumors. Secondary infections should be managed with the appropriate topical and/or systemic antimicrobials. Adrenal disease should be managed as for hyperadrenocorticism.

KEY POINT

- Common, especially in elderly entire males.

266, 267
Hyperandrogenism in an adult male Staffordshire Bull Terrier. There is a nodular alopecic swelling of the tail gland (**266**); hyperplasia of the perianal tissues (**267**).

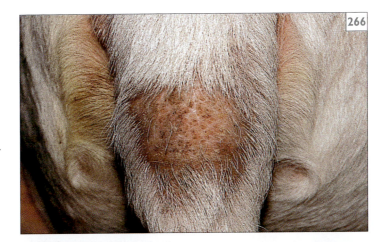

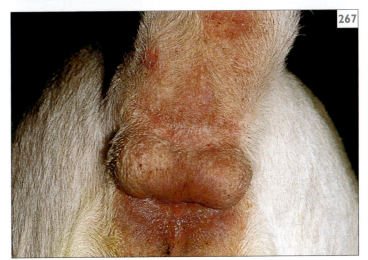

268 Hypertrichosis, greasy coat, and scaling in a Bouvier with hyperandrogenism.

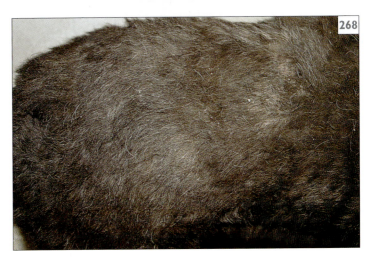

Sertoli cell and other testicular neoplasia

ETIOLOGY AND PATHOGENESIS

Sertoli cell neoplasms, seminomas, and interstitial cell tumors are potentially malignant neoplasms of the testicle arising, respectively, from the sustentacular, germinal, and Leydig cells. The etiology of testicular neoplasia is unknown. Boxers and, perhaps, Cairn Terriers, Border Collies, Shetland Sheepdogs, and Pekingese are predisposed to testicular neoplasia and tend to be affected at an earlier age (mean 7.2 years) than other breeds (mean 9–10 years)[1,2].

Interstitial cell tumors are the most common testicular tumors in dogs[1,2]. They are usually very small, often not palpable, and are confined to scrotal testes. Interstitial cell tumors are often associated with testosterone production, but they rarely display malignant behavior. Sertoli cell tumors are more common and appear earlier in retained abdominal or inguinal testes than in scrotal testes[1,2]. Functional estrogen-secreting tumors occur in about 30% of cases and are more common in retained testes. Malignancy and metastasis occur in about 10% of Sertoli cell tumors and 5% of seminomas[1,2].

CLINICAL FEATURES

Scrotal tumors are usually associated with enlargement and/or distortion of the affected testis, although this may be difficult to appreciate in early cases or with small tumors. The contralateral testis is often atrophied. Non-scrotal tumors can form masses in the inguinal area or abdomen. Rare interstitial and Sertoli cell tumors have been seen in extratesticular tissues[3]. Most seminomas are scrotal in location, usually palpable, and very rarely associated with clinical signs other than testicular enlargement, although they can occasionally metastasize[1]. Estradiol levels are frequently low, but this is of little clinical significance[4]. Rare cases are associated with hyperestrogenemia and alopecia[5].

Functional interstitial cell tumors can result in hyperandrogenism or, rarely, feminization[1,2]. Clinical signs of hyperandrogenism include prostatomegaly, perianal and tail gland hyperplasia, perineal hyperpigmentation, and perineal hernia (see Hyperandrogenism, p. 244). Other less common problems include a greasy coat (**269, 270**) and seborrheic otitis externa. Symmetrical alopecia is uncommon.

Functional Sertoli cell tumors frequently result in feminization and symmetrical alopecia[1,2], which may be more related to decreased testosterone/estradiol ratios than to the absolute level of estradiol[6]. Clinical signs include gynecomastia, pendulous prepuce, squatting to urinate instead of cocking a leg, and attractiveness to male dogs. Linear preputial erythema (**271**), if present, is highly suggestive of a Sertoli cell tumor. Alopecia is symmetrical, often diffuse, and may initially affect the perineum, neck (**272**), and hindlimbs (**273**). Affected skin can develop macular hyperpigmentation. Hyperestrogenemia can occasionally induce profound bone marrow suppression, which may be life threatening[7].

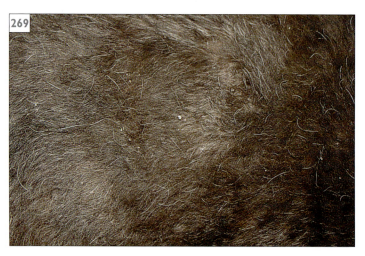

269 Poor quality, seborrheic coat in a Bouvier with hyperandrogenism. Same dog as in figure **268**.

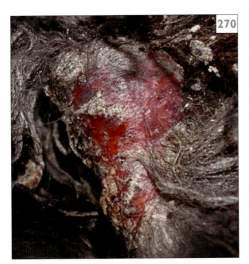

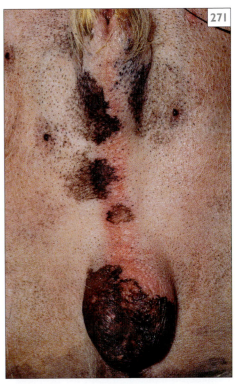

270 Inflamed caudal gland with seborrheic dermatitis in a dog with hyperandrogenism.

271–273 Linear preputial erythema (**271**) and alopecia (**272, 273**) in a Bearded Collie with an intra-abdominal Sertoli cell tumor.

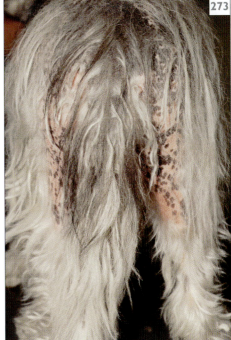

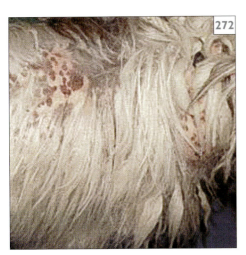

DIFFERENTIAL DIAGNOSES

- Hypothyroidism
- Hyperadrenocorticism
- Adrenal sex hormone production (alopecia X)
- Follicular dysplasia
- Cyclical flank alopecia
- Sebaceous adenitis

DIAGNOSIS

Physical examination will often reveal a scrotal or inguinal enlargement or suggest cryptorchidism. Bilaterally cryptorchid dogs may be presented as neutered. Routine hematology and biochemistry, thyroid assays, and dynamic adrenal function tests will help eliminate differential diagnoses and identify bone marrow suppression. Abdominal radiography and ultrasonography can detect internal tumors[8]. Testicular ultrasonography can be used to detect small, non-palpable tumors[8]. Cytology can reliably distinguish different testicular tumors and the degree of malignancy[9]. Sex hormone levels are unreliable due to episodic secretion and wide variation in normal levels[1,2].

MANAGEMENT

Castration is indicated if testicular neoplasia is suspected. Alopecia, feminization, and hyperandrogenism usually resolve within 2–6 weeks unless functional metastases and/or extratesticular tumors are present[1,2].

KEY POINTS

- Always examine/palpate the scrotum in male dogs.
- If the clinical signs fit, look for retained testes in apparently neutered dogs.
- The prognosis is good unless metastasis occurs.

Pituitary dwarfism

DEFINITION

Pituitary dwarfism is an hereditary hypopituitarism resulting in a failure of growth plus a variable coat and thyroidal, adrenocortical, and gonadal abnormalities.

ETIOLOGY AND PATHOGENESIS

The presence of a cyst (Rathke's cleft cyst) in the pituitary gland, resulting in varying degrees of anterior pituitary insufficiency, is responsible for the majority of cases. However, the condition has been described in dogs with either hypoplastic or normal anterior pituitary glands[1,2]. The condition is thought to be inherited as a simple autosomal recessive condition[3,4].

CLINICAL FEATURES

Pituitary dwarfism is seen primarily in German Shepherd Dogs and Carnelian (Karelian) Bear Dogs[3,5]. Affected dogs often appear normal during the first 2–3 months of life. After this time, a failure to grow properly in stature and retention of puppy coat become apparent (**274**). Partial loss of the puppy coat then occurs, resulting in a bilateral symmetrical alopecia over the neck, caudolateral aspects of the thighs, and, occasionally, the trunk. Secondary bacterial and/or yeast infections are common. Growth of primary hair is generally limited to the face and distal extremities. The skin becomes hyperpigmented, hypotonic, and scaly, and comedones may develop. Gonadal status may be altered with testicular atrophy occurring in males and anestrus in females. Affected animals may also show evidence of personality changes such as aggressiveness and fear biting[1]. Clinical signs of hypothyroidism and adrenocortical insufficiency will be noted if there is a lack of TSH or ACTH. The condition is generally compatible with life, but most animals only live to 3–8 years of age[6].

DIFFERENTIAL DIAGNOSES

- Congenital hypothyroidism
- Malnutrition
- Skeletal dysplasias
- Gonadal dysgenesis
- Severe metabolic diseases

DIAGNOSIS

History and clinical findings are usually diagnostic of an endocrinopathy and highly suggestive of pituitary dwarfism. Affected dogs usually have subnormal insulin-like growth factor 1 (IGF1) levels. They will also fail to have an increase in plasma growth hormone levels (normal levels 1–2 ng/ml) after the injection of xylazine (0.1–0.3 mg/kg i/v) or clonidine (0.01–0.03 mg/kg i/v)[3]. Severe prolonged hypoglycemia occurs after injection of regular insulin (0.025 IU/kg i/v)[3,4]. Histopathologic examination of biopsy material that reveals evidence of a decreased amount and size of elastin fibers is highly suggestive. Appropriate evaluations of thyroidal, adrenal, and gonadal status will allow a definitive diagnosis.

MANAGEMENT

Bovine somatotropin (10 IU s/c q48h for 30 days) with retreatment necessary every three months to three years[3–7]. Repeated injections of bovine somatotropin have the potential to result in hypersensitivity reactions or diabetes. Improvement in the skin and hair will generally be noted within 6–8 weeks. An increase in stature is generally not achieved, as the growth plates close rapidly[1]. Progestin therapy, which stimulates the mammary glands to produce growth hormone, has been used to induce hair regrowth and increase body weight and size. Either medroxyprogesterone acetate (2.5–5 mg/kg s/c) or proligestone (10 mg/kg s/c) can be administered every 3–6 weeks[8]. Progestin therapy may induce diabetes mellitus, acromegaly, and, in intact bitches, cystic endometrial hyperplasia and pyometra. Appropriate therapy for adrenocortical insufficiency and/or hypothyroidism, as well as secondary bacterial or yeast infections, should be instituted if they are present.

KEY POINT

- A well-recognized disease, but very uncommon.

274 Pituitary dwarf.

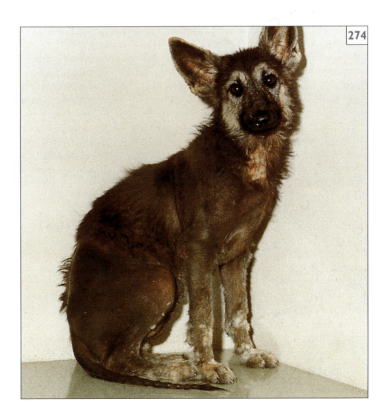

Alopecia X (adrenal sex hormone imbalance, follicular dysfunction of plush-coated breeds, adrenal hyperplasia-like syndrome, growth hormone/castration responsive dermatoses, adult-onset hyposomatotropism, pseudo-Cushing's disease, alopecia of follicular arrest)

DEFINITION
An uncommon skin condition with characteristic areas of alopecia and hyperpigmentation and distinct breed predisposition.

ETIOLOGY AND PATHOGENESIS
Abnormal growth hormone response tests coupled with response to treatment with growth hormone in some animals led to the theory of this condition being hyposomatotropism[1]. However, this theory does not explain why some animals with the condition do not respond to growth hormone (or relapse while on growth hormone therapy) and have normal growth hormone response tests[1]. It has been proposed that acquired or congenital deficiency in 11β-hydroxylase, 21-hydroxylase, or 3β-hydroxysteroid dehydrogenase results in accumulation of progesterone, 17-hydroxypregnenolone, or dehydroepiandrosterone, respectively[2,3]. Binding of these hormones to certain susceptible hair follicles was speculated to result in alopecia[2,3]. However, a recent study has shown that there is no consistent abnormality of sex hormone levels or their intermediates in dogs suspected of having alopecia X[4]. This has led to the theory that the condition may be due to abnormalities in hormone receptors of the hair follicle[4].

CLINICAL FEATURES
Pomeranians, Chow Chows, Siberian Huskies, Keeshonds, Samoyeds, Alaskan Malamutes, and Miniature Poodles are predisposed[2-5]. Most animals are affected at between one and two years of age, although older animals may also be presented. Either sex may be affected and the dermatosis may occur before or after neutering. The clinical signs are confined to slowly developing symmetrical alopecia of the trunk, caudal thighs, and cervical regions (**275, 276**). Animals are not systemically affected. Alopecia may eventually affect the entire trunk, sparing the head and limbs[2-5]. Primary hairs are lost at

first, but with time the secondary hairs also disappear. Hair may fail to regrow after clipping and, paradoxically, some affected cases exhibit local regrowth of hair after biopsy or local trauma[2-5]. Areas of alopecia may become hyperpigmented and, occasionally, mild secondary seborrhea and superficial pyoderma are present.

DIFFERENTIAL DIAGNOSES
- Hypothyroidism
- Hyperadrenocorticism
- Sex hormone endocrinopathies
- Follicular dysplasia
- Cyclic flank alopecia
- Telogen or anagen defluxion

DIAGNOSTIC TESTS
Diagnosis of alopecia X is based on history and physical examination findings and ruling out other endocrinopathies and follicular dysplasias. A full blood and biochemical screen and appropriate endocrine testing should be performed to rule out hypothyroidism, hyperadrenocorticism, and sex hormone endocrinopathies. Histopathologic examination of biopsy material will allow ruling out of follicular dysplasia and defluxion, but it is unlikely to differentiate between the endocrinopathies. Some features (e.g. haired telogen follicles with prominent tricholemnal keratinization, flame follicles [hairless follicles with exaggerated, fused tricholemnal keratinization], and follicular dysplasia) are indicative of the condition, but these are not specific and should be interpreted in the light of other findings. Measuring sex hormones before and after administration of ACTH or cosyntropin (synthetic ACTH) has been advocated[2,3]. However, as there is no consistent abnormality in these hormones or their intermediates, this testing is of limited value.

MANAGEMENT
As a specific etiology for this condition has not been determined, there is no specific therapy. Various treatment modalities have been advocated, but none are effective in all cases:
- As the condition is purely cosmetic and the health of affected animals is not impaired, foregoing treatment is a reasonable option.
- Entire animals should be neutered. Approximately 75% will regrow hair after neutering, but this may be temporary[5].

275 Alopecia and hyperpigmentation about the neck, trunk, and tail of a Pomeranian with alopecia X.

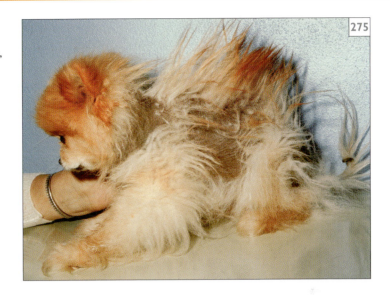

276 Alopecia and hyperpigmentation over the trunk of a Chow Chow with alopecia X.

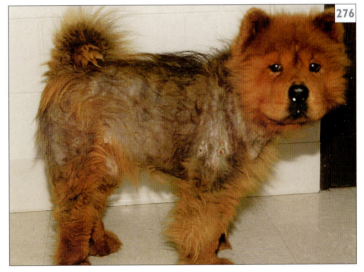

- Melatonin (3–12 mg/kg p/o q12h) has resulted in hair regrowth in approximately 30% of cases within 3–4 months[5]. Once hair has regrown it may be discontinued, but restarted if the coat starts to thin again.
- Treatment with oral trilostane was found to result in hair regrowth within 4–8 weeks in 85% of cases in one study[6]. Dogs <2.5 kg were administered 20 mg p/o with food q24h; dogs between 2.5 and 5 kg were

administered 30 mg p/o with food q24h; and dogs between 5 and 10 kg were administered 60 mg p/o with food q24h. Two of the 14 cases did not respond to initial treatment after 4–6 months, so the dose of trilostane was doubled, resulting in hair growth. Once hair regrowth was obtained, the frequency of trilostane administration could be reduced to 2–3 times a week for some cases. As trilostane is a competitive inhibitor of the enzyme necessary for the formation of cortisol, aggressive therapy may result in adrenal insufficiency. Owners should be instructed to stop treatment if depression, inappetence, vomiting, or diarrhea occur and present the animal for examination. Pre- and post-ACTH cortisol concentrations should be obtained to monitor the animal. Cortisol levels return rapidly once trilostane administration is stopped, and the drug can be reinstituted at a lower dose in 5–7 days. Trilostane is contraindicated in pregnant and lactating dogs and in dogs with hepatic disease or renal insufficiency.

- Therapy with mitotane (o,p'-DDD) may also be tried[3,5]. It is administered at induction doses of 15–25 mg/kg p/o daily for 2–5 days, with ACTH testing after seven days. Cortisol concentrations should be in the range 138–193 nmol/l (5–7 µg/dl). Initial treatment may be followed by a maintenance dosage of 15–25 mg/kg at bi-weekly intervals[3,5]. Favorable results should be seen within three months. Dogs should be monitored carefully for evidence of hypocortisolemia.
- Growth hormone (bovine, porcine, or synthetic somatotropin) may be tried (0.1 IU/kg s/c or i/m 3 times a week for 6 weeks) (**Note:** 1 IU is approximately 1.8 mg bovine somatotropin)[3]. Regrowth of hair is evident in 4–6 weeks. A full coat is generally maintained for 2–3 years, after which retreatment may be necessary. The treatment is very expensive and diabetes mellitus is a possible complication of growth hormone therapy. Because of this, weekly blood glucose determination should be made during therapy. If diabetes mellitus does develop, it will generally resolve when growth hormone therapy is discontinued.

- Methyltestosterone (1 mg/kg p/o to a maximum dose of 30 mg/dog) every other day for a period of three months (or for a shorter duration if a clinical response is noted) may result in hair regrowth in some intact or neutered dogs[3]. Liver enzymes should be monitored every 1–3 months in animals treated with methyltestosterone.

KEY POINTS
- Theories on etiology, classification, and management of disease in this area are far from satisfactory.
- The prognosis for hair regrowth is guarded.

Otitis externa

General approach

- Always attempt to make a definitive diagnosis – do not rely on polypharmacy
- Remember that otitis commonly results from underlying disease

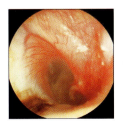
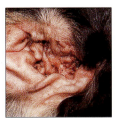
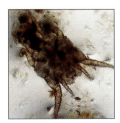
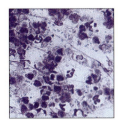

Otitis externa

DEFINITION

Otitis externa results from inflammation of the epithelial lining of the external auditory canal. The inflammation may arise within the external ear canal (e.g. following grass seed penetration) or result from conditions affecting the pinnae or middle ear.

ETIOLOGY AND PATHOGENESIS

Otitis externa may result from many causes and it has proven useful to classify these as primary, predisposing, and perpetuating[1]. Bacterial and *Malassezia* infections are important perpetuating factors, but they may also be regarded as separate, secondary factors.

Primary factors

Primary factors directly induce inflammation within the external ear canal. These include:
- Hypersensitivities, including atopic dermatitis and cutaneous adverse food reactions, which are the most common triggers for recurrent otitis in dogs.
- Ectoparasites, especially *Otodectes*.
- Foreign bodies.
- Disorders of keratinization.
- Autoimmune conditions.
- Contact reactions to ear cleaners and medications.
- Hypothyroidism, hyperadrenocorticism, and sex hormone dermatosis, which can give rise to immunologic and cutaneous changes.
- Dermatophytosis (a rare cause).

Predisposing factors

Predisposing factors alter the environment within the external ear canal, which may result in quantitative and qualitative changes in otic microflora. These make an individual more prone to develop otitis, and include:
- Conformation.
- Otic neoplasia or nasal–pharyngeal polyp formation, which obstructs the ear canal. Rarely, tumors adjacent to ears may compress or invade the ear canals and middle ears. (**Note:** Tumors and polyps can also be regarded as primary causes of otitis.)
- Errors in otic pharmacy or errors in the management of ear disease.
- Environmental temperature and humidity, lifestyle (particularly swimming).

Perpetuating factors

Perpetuating factors arise within the external ear canal as a consequence of primary or predisposing conditions. They exacerbate the otitis and prevent resolution and include:
- Changes in microflora leading to overgrowth and infection. Virtually all staphylococcal and *Malassezia* infections are secondary, but one author (TJN) occasionally sees apparently primary *Pseudomonas* infections in dogs akin to swimmer's ear in humans.
- Otitis media.
- Progressive chronic pathologic changes in the otic epithelium and underlying cartilage.

CLINICAL FEATURES

Clinical features will vary from individual to individual because of variation in primary cause, predisposing conditions, perpetuating factors, and individual expression[1,2]. In particular, the clinician should bear in mind a few key points:
- Acute, unilateral otitis externa is common in the dog and typically reflects a foreign body penetration. Acute, unilateral otitis externa is unusual in the cat.
- Chronic unilateral otitis externa in the cat is often associated with neoplasia or polyp formation, whereas bilateral otitis externa in the cat is considered otodectic mange until proven otherwise.
- Bilateral otitis externa in the dog, particularly if recurrent, is highly suggestive of hypersensitivity (e.g. atopic dermatitis, cutaneous adverse food reaction, or topical neomycin sensitivity). Note that atopic dermatitis and adverse food reactions can present with unilateral otitis, although mild clinical signs are usually also present in the unaffected ear, and that clinical otitis may affect both ears sequentially.
- Chronic otitis externa results in a quantitative (more bacteria) and qualitative (initially more gram-positive and then more gram-negative bacteria) shift in microbial flora[3].
- Erythematous ulceration of the external ear canal suggests gram-negative infection or an immune-mediated disease (rare in the absence of clinical signs elsewhere).
- Pustules are rare on the concave aspect of the pinna and are often associated with pemphigus foliaceus rather than superficial pyoderma.

- An abundant slimy, ropy, often dark exudate from the ear is a good indication that the tympanic membrane is ruptured. This type of exudate results from irritation of the goblet cells in the tympanic bulla, which are stimulated to produce more mucus.
- Otitis media can cause depression, pain, head tilt, and difficulty in eating, but most cases are clinically indistinguishable from otitis externa alone.
- A good guide to the severity and/or chronicity of the problem is the degree of pain, firmness, and mobility of the ear canal on palpation. Very firm, immobile ear canals are often irreversibly fibrosed or mineralized.
- Sedation of the animal and cleaning of the ear are often necessary to perform a thorough otoscopic evaluation in severe cases. The normal tympanum should be translucent with radiating stria (**277**).

Foreign bodies

Foreign bodies, particularly grass seeds, are usually easily seen on otoscopic examination (**278**), although in some cases the ear canal needs to be cleaned before they can be visualized.

277, 278 Otitis externa. Normal view of the tympanum (**277**) and of a foreign body (grass seed) adjacent to the tympanum (**278**).

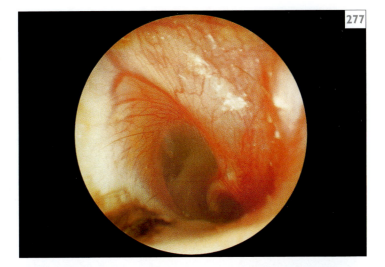

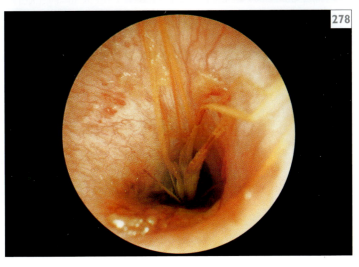

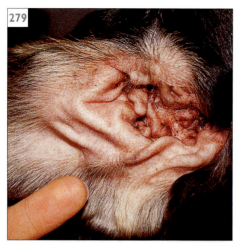

Otodectes cynotis

Otodectes cynotis infestation has a characteristic appearance and is associated with large amounts of dry, dark brown, waxy debris with variable amounts of inflammation (**279**). Careful otoscopic examination may allow for visualization of the mites as they move within the canal (**280**). Mites may also be seen on microscopic examination of scrapes from the external ear canal (**281**). Some cats respond to acaricidal treatment, even though no mites can be found. It is possible that they develop a hypersensitivity reaction to the mites akin to the situation with *Sarcoptes* in dogs. Otodemodicosis (due to *Demodex canis*) is a rare cause of chronic otitis externa in dogs and cats.

Bacterial infection

Infection with *Staphylococcus* spp., *Streptococcus* spp., and *Proteus* spp. is often, although not exclusively, associated with a light yellow exudate. The discharge becomes progressively darker if there is concomitant wax production.

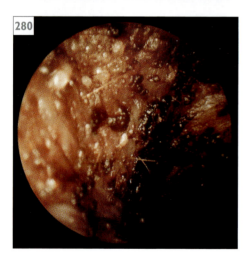

Pseudomonas spp.

Pseudomonas spp. are often found in ears that are very painful, inflamed, eroded, or ulcerated and have copious amounts of bright yellow to green, foul smelling exudate (**282, 283**). This organism is more likely to be present if the case is chronic, although acute suppurative otitis due to *Pseudomonas* spp. is not uncommon.

Yeast infection

Infection, particularly by *Malassezia* spp., may result in a chocolate-brown waxy discharge. However, in some cases a more liquid discharge may be noted. In cats, *Malassezia* spp. have been associated with chronic pruritic otitis externa characterized by minimal discharge. The status of *M. pachydermatis* as an otic pathogen in cats is uncertain[4].

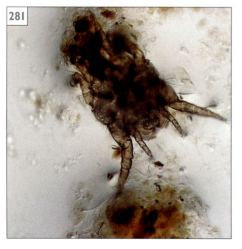

279–281 Otitis externa. Otic discharge secondary to *Otodectes cynotis* infection (**279**); the mites seen on otoscopic (**280**) and microscopic (**281**) examination.

282, 283 Otitis externa. The typical brown discharge that is often associated with *Malassezia pachydermatis* infection (**282**); extensive ulceration associated with *Pseudomonas aeruginosa* infection (**283**).

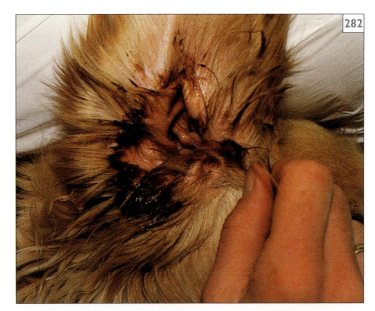

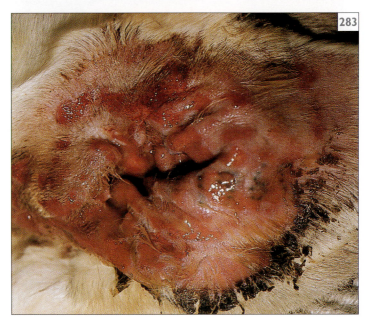

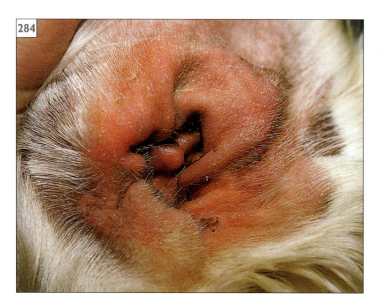

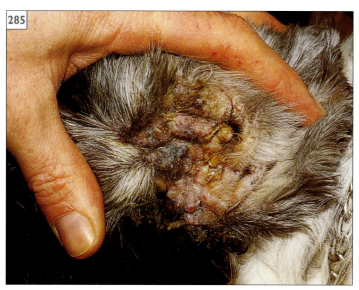

284, 285 Chronic otitis externa associated with atopic dermatitis (**284**); a defect in keratinization (**285**).

Hypersensitivities

Hypersensitivities (see Canine atopic dermatitis, p. 20, and Cutaneous adverse food reaction, p. 31) are some of the most common causes of chronic otitis externa, particularly in dogs (**284**). Early cases may exhibit erythema and lichenification of the concave aspect of the pinna and the vertical portion of the external ear canal. In these early cases the horizontal ear canal may appear quite normal. Although most cases will be associated with pruritus and clinical signs elsewhere (e.g. face, feet, and ventrum), a few dogs will present with otitis externa alone. Eosinophilic granuloma syndrome lesions (see p. 102) may be seen in the ear canals of cats with or without lesions elsewhere.

Defects in keratinization

These are often associated with chronic otitis externa (**285**). Some breeds (notably Cocker Spaniels) are prone to both otitis externa and idiopathic defects in keratinization. This is often accompanied by conformational problems such as narrow, hirsute ear canals[5]. Most affected animals have generalized clinical signs.

Autoimmune diseases

These may be associated with pustules and crusts on the pinnae and otic epithelium. However, a recent case report described two dogs with immune-mediated ear canal ulceration that resembled *Pseudomonas* otitis externa[6]. By far the most common of these diseases is pemphigus foliaceus, and the lesions may on rare occasions be confined to the pinnae and ear canal. More commonly there is extensive pustule and crust formation. The diseases that cause deeper lesions (e.g. pemphigus vulgaris and bullous pemphigoid) may cause ulceration in the ear canal, but will be associated with lesions elsewhere and systemic disease.

Chronic pathologic changes

Whatever the cause of the otitis externa, the chronic changes to the external ear canal are associated with hyperplasia of the apocrine glands[7], thickening of the otic epithelium, a reduction in the effective diameter of the ear canal, decreased epidermal cell migration, and an increase in the humidity within the canal lumen[5,7]. Maceration of surface debris occurs and there is potential for further microbial multiplication and continued inflammation. In severe, long-standing cases of otitis externa, chronic fibrosis and, later, ossification of the external ear canal and associated cartilage may occur. Other changes include tympanic membrane hyperplasia, diverticula, and rupture, as well as otitis media with mucosa proliferation and increased secretion, inspissated debris, cholesteatoma, mineralization, and osteomyelitis.

DIFFERENTIAL DIAGNOSES

The differential diagnoses for otitis externa are formulated on the basis of history, clinical examination, and the observation of any association, or otherwise, with systemic or generalized disease. Broadly, all primary and most predisposing conditions should be considered. The history and clinical signs must therefore be evaluated carefully.

DIAGNOSIS

Appropriate clinical, diagnostic, and laboratory procedures should be performed to rule in or out the various primary, predisposing, and perpetuating factors.

Cytologic evaluation of otic exudates or debris should be the initial diagnostic procedure. Smears should be stained with either Gram's stain or a modified Wright's stain (e.g. Diff-Quik) and examined for numbers and morphology of leukocytes (**286**), squames and/or acanthocytes,

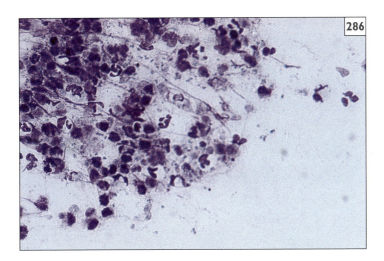

286 Otitis externa. Otic cytology may reveal many leukocytes.

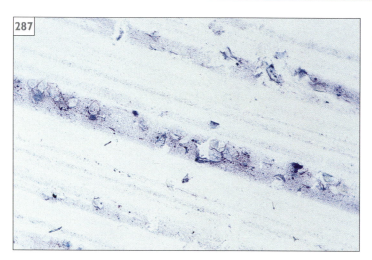

287 Otitis externa. Otic cytology may reveal masses of bacteria.

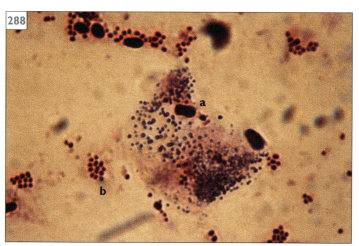

288 Modified Wright's (Diff-Quik) stain showing peanut-shaped yeast (a) and packets of cocci (b).

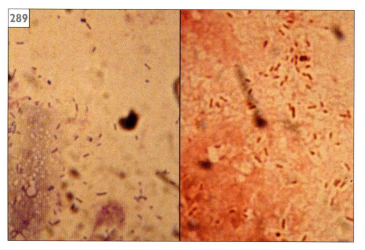

289 *Pseudomonas* spp. organisms appearing as blue-purple rods with modified Wright's (Diff-Quik) stain (far left) and gram-negative rods with Gram's stain (near left).

neoplastic cells, yeast, and bacteria (**287**). The presence of cocci is indicative of *Staphylococcus* spp. (**288**) or *Streptococcus* spp., while the presence of gram-negative rods may indicate either *Pseudomonas* spp. or *Proteus* spp. Peanut-shaped yeast are characteristic of *Malassezia* spp. (**288**), which are the most commonly found yeast in the ear. Most cocci and *Malassezia* spp. infections are associated with overgrowth in the absence of neutrophils. Most rod and severe cocci infections are associated with large numbers of degenerate neutrophils with intracellular bacteria. Neutrophils can also be seen in contact reactions, and the presence of both red blood cells and neutrophils is common with ulceration of the ear canal. In addition to stained smears, debris from the ear canal can be mixed with mineral oil and examined for ectoparasites and their eggs or larvae.

Samples of ear exudate should be submitted for culture and sensitivity when the presence of gram-negative rods (**289**) is noted on cytology. This is because of the high likelihood of *Pseudomonas* spp., which can become resistant to a majority of antibacterial agents. Samples for culture and sensitivity should also be submitted when there has not been significant response to initial treatment.

To diagnose a tumor or to differentiate neoplasia from proliferative tissue in the ear canal, a small pinch biopsy may be obtained with an endoscopic forceps passed through the otoscope cone.

The integrity of the tympanic membrane can be assessed by probing gently with a soft tube under direct visualization. Debris can often mimic a tympanic membrane; a feeding tube or catheter, will, however, pass through into the middle ear without resistance. Even if the tympanic membrane is not visible, being able to pass a tube beyond the depth it should be at indicates it is ruptured.

Radiographic changes are reasonably specific but poorly sensitive at detecting otitis media. The changes, furthermore, can be very subtle. Evaluation should be by taking a series of left and right lateral obliques, dorsoventral skull, and if necessary, open mouth rostrocaudal views under general anesthesia. Look for occlusion and bony change in the ear canals, soft-tissue opacity of the middle ear cavity, and lysis or proliferation of the bulla wall. Osseous changes should prompt a consideration of surgery, as the prognosis with medical treatment alone is guarded. CT and MRI detect ear canal pathology and occlusion and otitis media very accurately, but are expensive and availability may be limited. Ultrasound can also be used to detect fluid and soft tissue within the tympanic bullae, but the technique requires practice and is in its infancy.

MANAGEMENT
Any predisposing conditions should receive appropriate treatment for the specific disease or factor.

In-hospital ear cleaning
To ensure that the ear canals are free of exudate and debris prior to topical treatment, it is recommended that the clinician, or an experienced technician, perform the initial cleaning. Ears with minimal secretions and patent canals may be cleaned without sedation. However, sedation is generally appropriate for the initial cleaning, as it allows for a more thorough cleaning and better visualization of the ear canal and tympanic membrane. A combination of ketamine (1.36–2.2 mg/kg), diazepam (0.45 mg/kg), and acepromazine (0.23 mg/kg) mixed together and given intravenously has been used satisfactorily for both examination and cleaning of the ears. The higher dose of ketamine (2.2 mg/kg) is preferred, and it provides ample restraint for about 20 minutes. Alternatively, a combination of medetomidine (10 mg/kg) and butorphanol (0.1 mg/kg) intravenously can be given, with further incremental half doses given as necessary. General anesthesia using a cuffed ET tube is recommended if the ears are severely involved and painful or if a video otoscope is to be used. If the ears are hyperplastic and stenotic, 2–3 weeks of topical and/or systemic glucocorticoids (prednisone or prednisolone 1–2 mg p/o q24h or methylprednisolone 0.25 mg/kg p/o q12h) may decrease the swelling and allow access for evaluation and flushing.

The status of the tympanic membrane should be established before cleaning. If it cannot be visualized due to exudate or debris, or if it is known to be ruptured, saline can be used to rinse the ear. If an animal swallows, gags, or coughs when fluid is placed in the ear, it is a good indication that the tympanic membrane is ruptured. If saline is not able to rinse away the exudate or debris, then a solution containing propylene glycol, malic acid, benzoic acid, and salicylic acid can be used[2,8].

One author (TJN) has also safely used Epi-Otic® (Virbac). These solutions have been used for cleaning ears with ruptured tympanic membranes without any apparent signs of ototoxicity. However, the middle ear is always flushed afterwards with saline. (**Note:** It must be appreciated that there is no completely safe solution for cleaning the middle ear. Even water may cause a loss of cochlear and/or vestibular function[8,9].)

If the tympanic membrane is intact, the ear canal is filled with appropriate cleaning solution and the ear canal is then massaged for 1–2 minutes to loosen and dissolve the debris. The excess solution and debris that has floated to the surface are wiped away with a cotton ball. The process is repeated until the solution comes out clear of exudates or debris. Dry, waxy, and adherent debris can be removed by filling the ear canal with a ceruminolytic solution for 15–20 minutes to soften the debris, which can then be either massaged free or flushed out of the ear canal using a bulb syringe. The latter is much more effective; however, care must be taken not to seal the nozzle in the canal, but to leave an exit channel for the flushing solution and debris to avoid damage to the middle ear.

Flushing and aspirating using a urinary catheter or feeding tube of appropriate diameter, inserted under direct visualization through an operating head otoscope, is a very effective way of removing any remaining water and debris and of verifying complete cleaning. A three-way tap is used to connect a syringe, fluid supply, and urinary catheter, tomcat catheter, or feeding tube of appropriate length and diameter. The catheter tip is placed adjacent to the tympanic membrane or into the middle ear under visualization through an operating otoscope. It is important to angle the tip ventrally to avoid the sensitive structures in the dorsal part of the middle ear cavity. The syringe and three-way tap are used to flush and aspirate the ear canal, and middle ear if necessary, until free of debris or exudates. Finally, an astringent can be used to dry the ear canal. Retrograde flushing using this technique is very effective at removing deep material and is the only effective way to clean the middle ear.

Ear cleaning can be greatly facilitated with the use of instruments that can both flush and aspirate (e.g. Earigator® [MedRx] and systems by Karl Storz) through a catheter advanced through the working channel of a video otoscope. General anesthesia is required when flushing and aspirating techniques are performed.

Ear curettes or loops are very helpful in removing stubbornly adherent material, but they should be used with care and under general anesthesia to avoid damaging the ear canal or tympanic membrane. The loop is introduced into the ear through an operating otoscope and gently hooked over the obstruction. Drawing the edge outwards along the epidermal surface removes the obstruction. Alligator forceps are also useful, especially for keratin plugs, hair, and foreign bodies, but it may be difficult to open their jaws sufficiently in narrow ear canals.

The normal ear drum should have a taut, translucent, gray white pars tensa that is angled dorsolateral to ventromedial. There should be a slightly bulging, pink pars flaccida dorsally. The attachment of the malleus appears as a white C-shaped structure facing rostrally at the cranial border. Bubbles usually appear during ear flushing if the tympanic membrane is ruptured. A bulging, opaque, discolored, or inflamed membrane is an indication for a myringotomy. This is best performed using a stylette, curette, or firm ENT swab through a video or operating otoscope to puncture the caudoventral membrane. Samples can be taken for cytology and culture using an ENT swab or by instilling and aspirating a small volume of sterile saline. The tympanic bulla can be flushed as previously described, making sure to angle the catheter ventrally to avoid damage to the sensitive structures located dorsally.

It should be noted that in many cases of *Pseudomonas* infection or cases where there is extensive mucus secretion in the middle ear, the results of in-hospital cleaning will be very transient as the ear will again be filled with secretions in 12–24 hours. In these cases, at-home cleaning and/or flushing becomes of paramount importance. In-hospital cleaning is always beneficial, but it is not always necessary.

At-home ear cleaning

Periodic cleaning by the patient's owner is often necessary to remove secretions associated with continued inflammation or infection. The interval for this cleaning will vary from twice daily to weekly or longer, depending on the rate of accumulation of exudate or wax in the ear.

For removal of a waxy debris, products containing a ceruminolytic (organic oils and solvents such as propylene glycol, lanolin, glycerine, squaline, butylated hydroxytoluene, cocamidopropyl betaine, and mineral oils) can be used. Two *in vitro* studies recently found that there was wide variation in the ceruminolytic activity of a number of ear cleaners[10,11]. Surfactants help expedite the cleaning process by emulsifying debris, breaking it up, and keeping it in solution. Some detergents, however, can be irritating, particularly to the middle ear mucosa, and are contraindicated if the tympanic membrane is ruptured. Useful surfactants include dioctyl sodium sulfosuccinate (DSS or docusate), calcium sulfosuccinate, and other detergents. Urea and carbamide peroxide release oxygen *in situ*. This helps disperse debris and aerates the canals. Some animals may find the foaming sensation and sound unsettling. Astringents dry the ear canal surface, preventing maceration. They are often combined with ceruminolytics and surfactants in cleaning/drying products, but they can also be used separately after ear cleaning or prophylactically after bathing or swimming in dogs with underlying dermatosis that makes them prone to otitis. Commonly employed astringents include isopropyl alcohol, boric acid, benzoic acid, salicylaicte acid, aluminum acetate, and silicon dioxide. Sulfur is astringent, antimicrobial, keratolytic, and keratoplastic. Salicylic acid is keratoplastic at low concentration and keratolytic at higher concentrations (above 2%). These qualities may be of use in seborrheic and proliferative ears.

Various antimicrobial compounds are frequently incorporated in ear cleaners to retard microbial proliferation. A recent *in vitro* study found that there was wide variation in antimicrobial activity between ear cleaners, and that efficacy appeared to be associated with isopropyl alcholol, parachlorometaxylenol (PCMX), and a low pH[12]. Other studies have shown that PCMX[13,14,15] and acidified sodium chlorite[16] are effective against *S. intermedius*, *P. aeruginosa*, *Proteus* spp., and *M. pachydermatis in vitro* and *in vivo*. A 2% acetic acid/2% boric acid combination helped resolve *Malassezia* otitis in one study, but relapses were common[17]. Other *in vitro* studies reported that a triz-EDTA ear cleanser was effective against *Pseudomonas*, although the inclusion of benzyl alcohol increased the efficacy against *Pseudomonas*

and extended the spectrum to include *Proteus* and β-hemolytic streptococci[18].

Chlorhexidine 0.15%/tris-ethylenediamine tetra-acetic acid (triz-EDTA) is also active against *Pseudomonas* and *M. pachydermatis*, but less so against *S. intermedius*[12]. Recent studies have shown that the inclusion of monosaccharides significantly reduces adherence of *Malassezia*, staphylococci, and *Pseudomonas* to canine keratinocytes[19–21].

At-home cleaning is especially important if *Pseudomonas* spp. are present. This is because ulceration of the canal results in an increased rate of exudate formation and may necessitate cleaning once or twice daily. Flushing the ear with a bulb syringe containing cleaning agents is often very beneficial for obtaining a thoroughly clean ear. One of the following would be beneficial if *Pseudomonas* spp. are present:

- A low pH solution (2.0–2.5%) for flushing ears can be made by diluting distilled malt vinegar (which contains very few impurities: acetic acid content usually 5–8%) with distilled water or saline. This can be diluted further if it proves irritating. The low pH of this solution is especially detrimental to *Pseudomonas* spp. If the ear canal is severely ulcerated, this solution may be very painful to the animal and inappropriate to use.
- A solution containing phytosphingosine.
- A solution releasing chlorine dioxide, which is a very good cleaning solution and will kill *Pseudomonas* spp.
- A solution containing PCMX and monosaccharides, which is a very good cleaning solution and also inhibits *Pseudomonas* spp. from adhering to the epithelial surface.
- A solution containing acetic acid and aloe, which also lowers the pH but is less irritating than the vinegar and water solution.
- A solution containing triz-EDTA, which promotes increased permeability to extracellular solutes and increased sensitization to antibiotics. This solution is generally non-irritating and is routinely used just before instilling antibacterial drops.
- Triz-EDTA/0.15% chlorhexidine solution.

Topical treatment
Topical antibacterial treatment

If doublets or packets of gram-positive cocci are present (most likely to be *Staphylococcus* spp.), topical preparations containing one of the following would be appropriate: neomycin, gentamicin, polymixin B, or fusidic acid.

If chains of gram-positive cocci are present (most likely to be *Streptococcus* spp.), a topical preparation containing one of the penicillins would be appropriate. Alternatively, antibacterial choice can be based on culture and sensitivity.

If gram-negative rods are present (most likely to be *Pseudomonas* spp.), preparations containing one of the following would be appropriate pending the results of culture and sensitivity:

- Gentamicin.
- Polymyxin B. (**Note:** There is evidence that polymyxin B and miconazole have synergistic activity against staphylococci and *Pseudomonas*.)
- Amikacin sulfate (50 mg/ml): undiluted, 0.15–0.3 ml instilled q12h.
- Enrofloxacin (22.7 mg/ml): undiluted, 0.15–0.3 ml instilled q12h.
- Tobramycin injectable (40 mg/ml): diluted with saline to 8 mg/ml and 0.15–0.3 ml instilled q12h.
- Ciprofloxacin (0.2%): instill 0.15–0.3 ml q12h.
- 1% silver sulfadiazine ointment diluted in saline or triz-EDTA to achieve a 0.05–0.1% suspension: 0.15–0.3 ml instilled q12h.
- Clavulanate-potentiated ticarcillin: comes as a powder for injection. Reconstitute as directed and freeze in 1 ml tuberculin syringes. Daily thaw a syringe and instill 0.15–0.3 ml q12h.
- Ofloxacin (Ofloxacin otic 0.3%): instill 0.15–0.3 ml q12h.
- Marbofloxacin (Aurizon otic, Pfizer) (available in Europe, but not the United States).
- Ceftazidime: reconstitute the injectable solution as per manufacturer's directions and instill 0.15–0.3 ml q12h.
- One author (TJN) routinely dilutes several antibiotics in triz-EDTA to achieve solutions of approximately 0.6% enrofloxacin, 0.2% marbofloxacin, 2.8% ticarcillin, and 1.7% ceftazidime. This is used to fill the ear canal once (if using ear wicks) to twice daily.

Neomycin, some proprietary gentamicin preparations, ticarcillin, chloramphenicol, polymyxin B, and amikacin are potentially ototoxic and should be used with great care if the tympanic membrane is ruptured[8,9]. Antibacterials that would be appropriate for this situation include enrofloxacin, penicillin, aqueous gentamicin, and silver sulfadiazine.

Topical anti-yeast treatment

If yeasts are present, topical preparations containing one of the following would be appropriate: clotrimazole, miconazole, cuprimyxin, nystatin, or amphotericin B.

Topical anti-inflammatory treatment

Many otic preparations contain glucocorticoids, which will benefit most cases of otitis externa by reducing pruritus, swelling, exudation, and tissue hyperproliferation. Hyperplasia of tissues lining the ear canal is reduced by treatment with a solution containing fluocinolone acetonide in 60% dimethylsulfoxide. Long-term topical use of glucocorticoids in ears may result in systemic absorption, resulting in elevations of liver enzymes and suppression of the adrenal response to adrenocorticotropic hormone[22]. One author (TJN) uses 0.2% dexamethasone added to triz-EDTA/antibiotic solutions initially, and then switches to topical eye or ear products containing 1% prednisolone or hydrocortisone or 0.1% betamethasone as necessary for maintenance. Hydrocortisone aceponate 0.0584% can also be sprayed onto the pinna and opening of the ear canal (where some will run in) or 2–3 drops can be directly applied into the ear canal. (**Note:** This is off-label use.)

Ear wicks

Polyvinyl acetate ear wicks are an alternative to repeated topical treatments. These are inserted into the ear canal under general anesthesia, soaked with an antibiotic plus triz-EDTA, and left for 3–10 days, applying the antibiotic solution once daily. The wicks absorb discharge, draw the antibiotic solution into the ear canal, and act as a reservoir. The ears are cleaned and re-examined under general anesthesia, replacing the wicks as necessary. Steroid-soaked wicks can be effective in resolving stenosis of the ear and preventing cicatricial stenosis following sharp or laser surgery to remove polyps and other masses in the ear canal.

Anti-parasitic treatment

Ears with *O. cynotis* infestation should first be cleaned of excess wax. Topical treatments have generally been superseded by use of the following systemic acaricides:

- Ivermectin: 0.3 mg/kg s/c q10–14 days for three treatments to the affected animal as well as all contact animals[23] or 1% ivermectin diluted 1:9 with mineral oil or propylene glycol (2–4 drops in ear q24h for 3–4 weeks). (**Note:** Systemic ivermectin is contraindicated in Collies, Shetland Sheepdogs, and certain other herding breeds, and is not licensed for use in cats and dogs.)
- Selamectin: 6–12 mg/kg applied topically twice at one monthly intervals.
- Moxidectin (dogs): 0.2 mg/kg p/o or s/c 3 times at 10 day intervals.
- Fipronil: 0.1–0.15 ml in each ear q14 days for 3 treatments.

In addition, all contact animals (both dogs and cats) should be treated as asymptomatic carriers as they may be a source of reinfection. The use of systemic treatments also ensures that *O. cynotis* on other body areas will be killed.

Systemic anti-inflammatory treatment

Prednisolone (0.5–1.0 mg/kg p/o q12–24h) or methylprednisolone (0.4–0.8 mg/kg p/o q12–24h) may be administered for 10–14 days to reduce severe inflammation and swelling due to hypersensitivity states or the foreign body reaction that occurs due to rupture of cystic apocrine glands.

Systemic antibacterial agents are indicated when the tympanic membrane is ruptured and infection is present in the middle ear, or when there is poor response to topical treatment. Choice should be made according to culture and sensitivity results.

Some dogs with extensive hyperplasia of the ear canals may respond to a 4–8 week course of therapy with ciclosporin (cyclosporine) (5 mg/kg p/o q24h).

Indications for surgery

Surgery is indicated when a tumor or polyp is present in the ear canal or when the hyperplasia of the ear canal is so great that the resulting stenosis precludes appropriate cleaning and application of medications. A surgical text should be consulted for the exact procedures, as techniques will vary depending on the extent and location of the lesions. Generally, most end-stage ear disorders require a total ear canal ablation and lateral bulla osteotomy. Vertical canal ablation and lateral wall resection are only appropriate if lesions are limited to the vertical canal, although they can be considered prophylactically to improve access to the horizontal canal in dogs with conformational problems. Ventral bulla osteotomies are most commonly performed in cats to remove inflammatory polyps from the middle ear.

KEY POINTS

- Do impression smears of otic exudates to determine which bacteria or yeast are present.
- Because otitis is often secondary to other conditions, it often can just be controlled and not cured.
- Diagnose and treat any underlying disease.

Disorders of the nails

General approach
- Diagnosis is difficult
- Treatment is often very prolonged and good communication is important

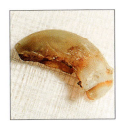
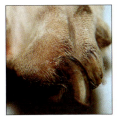
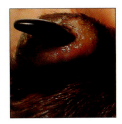

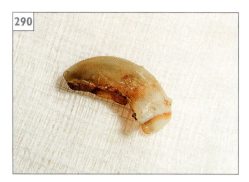

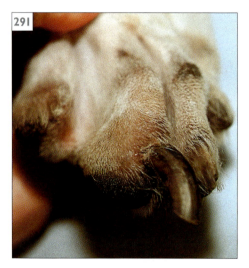

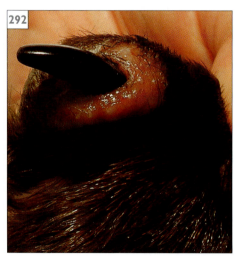

290–292 Shedding of nails (**290**) and paronychia (**291, 292**). Note the erythematous swelling around the base of a nail in **292**.

Disorders of the nails

DEFINITION

Claw abnormalities are defined by certain terms. The following is a partial list of these terms and includes those that are used more frequently in association with conditions of the dog and cat[1]:

- Macronychia: unusually large claws.
- Onychalgia: claw pain.
- Onychia (onchitis): inflammation somewhere in the claw unit.
- Onychoclasis: breaking of claws.
- Onychocryptosis (onyxis): ingrown claws.
- Onychodystrophy: abnormal claw formation.
- Onychogryphosis: hypertrophy and abnormal curvature of claws.
- Onychomadesis: sloughing of claws (**290**).
- Onychomalacia: softening of claws.
- Onychomycosis: fungal infection of claws.
- Onychorrhexis: longitudinal striations associated with brittleness and breaking of claws.
- Onychoschizia: splitting and/or lamination of claws, usually beginning distally.
- Onychopathy: disease abnormality of claws.
- Paronychia: inflammation/infection of claw folds (**291, 292**).

ETIOLOGY AND PATHOGENESIS

Onycopathy may occur due to trauma, bacterial infection, neoplasia, dermatophytosis, pemphigus foliaceus, lupus erythematosus, other autoimmune diseases, deep mycotic infections, leishmaniasis, severe generalized systemic disease, severe nutritional deficiencies, and idiopathic changes[1-4].

CLINICAL FEATURES
Trauma

Trauma is the most common cause of damage to the claws of dogs and cats. This often occurs when a long claw is caught in a carpet or rug, resulting in avulsion of the claw plate. Damage can also occur with bite wounds or when a foot is run over by a motor vehicle or is stepped on. It may also occur in hunting dogs and racing Greyhounds due to the severe strain that is placed on the claws while the dogs are working. Onychalgia, onychoclasis, onychomadesis, and, occasionally, onychorrhexis are noted. Secondary bacterial infection with exudate formation is a frequent finding associated with trauma[1].

Bacterial infection

This is generally thought to be secondary to other conditions such as trauma, and it has been reported in association with systemic diseases such as hypothyroidism, hyperadrenocorticism, and atopic dermatitis[1]. However, it can occasionally occur as primary disease[4].

Idopathic onychoclasis and onychomadesis

Onychoclasis and onychomadesis may occur with or without onychorrhexis. The etiology is unknown, but many of the animals respond to biotin therapy[5]. Small pieces of the claw break off or the claws may slough, with or without longitudinal cracking. Generally, many but not all nails are affected. In the absence of infection, there is usually no inflammation associated with these conditions.

Onychomycosis

Onychomycosis is a rare condition and is usually due to infection with *Trichophyton mentagrophytes*[1,2]. Onychodystrophy is the predominant clinical finding, with the nails appearing friable and misshapen. Generally, only one or two nails are affected, but many or all can suffer from the disease. *Malassezia* infection can also result in paronychia, especially in animals with atopic dermatitis[1]. This is characterized by tightly adherent brown debris extending out from the claw fold onto the nail. It does not extend to the full length of the nail.

Autoimmune/immune-mediated diseases

Pemphigus vulgaris, pemphigus foliaceus, bullous pemphigoid, systemic lupus erythematosus, a lupus-like syndrome, cold agglutinin disease, drug eruption, and vasculitis have all been associated with onychomadesis and onychodystrophy[2]. Often, most claws on many of the feet are affected[2]. Macronychia and onychomalacia were the only clinical signs in one dog with pemphigus foliaceus[5].

Lupoid onychodystrophy
(lupoid onychitis, symmetrical lupoid onychodystrophy)

Onychomadesis with exudate under the claw plate of one or a few claws is the most common clinical presentation. In some cases, involvement will initially occur in only 1–3 nails, but slowly over a 4–8 month period many, if not all, of the claws will become involved[6]. After sloughing, dry, brittle, misshapen nail plates regrow. If untreated, re-sloughing may occur. Pain is pronounced at the time of nail plate sloughing. Secondary infection is common.

Neoplastic diseases

Squamous cell carcinoma, melanoma, mast cell tumor, keratoacanthoma, inverted papilloma, lymphosarcoma, eccrine adenocarcinoma, neurofibrosarcoma, hemangiopericytoma, fibrosarcoma, and osteosarcoma have all been reported to occur in the digit, claw, and/or the claw fold[2]. Animals are presented for swelling of the claw or digit and variable degrees of paronychia, erosion, and ulceration. Squamous cell carcinoma arising from germinal claw epithelium is the most common digital tumor of the dog[2]. It develops more frequently in black Standard Poodles and black Labrador Retrievers, and multiple digits may be involved over a course of 2–6 years[2,4].

DIFFERENTIAL DIAGNOSES

See the conditions listed under 'Etiology and pathogenesis'.

DIAGNOSIS

Bacterial culture and sensitivity of any exudates, after appropriate cleaning, should be carried out. Fungal culture of dystrophic claws should also be performed. Biopsy is difficult since the nail bed is essential for a definitive diagnosis. This is achieved by amputating P3 and its associated claw, or a proximal transection of the claw, but there is often considerable owner resistance to this procedure. Careful evaluation of the history and clinical signs and appropriate diagnostic tests to rule in or out systemic diseases in the differential diagnosis would also be indicated.

MANAGEMENT
Trauma

Any loose fragments of the claw plate should be removed. If large amounts of the claw plate are missing, the area can be dressed with silver sulfadiazine and bandaged for 2–3 days. Systemic antibiotics (if possible based on culture and sensitivity) are appropriate for 4–6 weeks, as secondary infection is common with trauma[1,2].

Bacterial infection

The animal should be anesthetized and all loose claw plates removed. Treatment as described for trauma should then be carried out.

Onychoclasis and onychomadesis

The claws should be kept trimmed short. Owners should use a nail file or an electric disk sanding tool designed for use on nails, as they do not split or crack the nails. Biotin (0.05 mg/kg p/o q24h) is beneficial in many cases[2,4]. Gelatin (10 grains p/o q12h) has also been reported to be beneficial[1].

Onychomycosis

Onychomycosis should be treated with micronized griseofulvin (50–75 mg/kg p/o q12h with a high-fat meal) if the cause is a dermatophyte infection, or with itraconazole (5–10 mg/kg p/o q24h with food) or ketoconazole (5–10 mg/kg p/o q12h with food) if the cause is a dermatophyte or yeast infection. Treatment should be continued until the nails are normal in appearance and cultures for dermatophytes or smears for yeast are negative. Some nail infections can be difficult to clear and may require treatment with other anti-fungal drugs (see Dermatophytosis, page 278).

Autoimmune/immune-mediated diseases

These and other systemic diseases are treated as appropriate for the specific disease.

Lupoid onychodystrophy

Lupoid onychodystrophy can be treated with tetracycline and niacinamide therapy (250 mg tetracycline and 250 mg niacinamide for dogs <15 kg, and 500 mg each for dogs >15 kg p/o q8h; doxycycline [10 mg/kg p/o q24h] can be used instead of tetracycline). Systemic glucocorticoids at anti-inflammatory (0.5–0.7 mg/kg p/o q12h) or moderate (1.0–1.2 mg/kg p/o q12h) immunosuppressive doses have also been used successfully to treat some cases[6]. Also omega-6 fatty acids or mixtures of omega-6 and omega-3 fatty acids have been helpful in the long-term management of lupoid onychodystrophy[6]. Topical glucocorticoids, topical tacrolimus, and systemic ciclosporin (cyclosporine) have also been used. Some dogs appear recalcitrant to therapy and require treatment as for immune-mediated diseases (see Pemphigus foliaceus, p. 155). Radical, total P3 amputation may be considered in dogs that do not respond to medical therapy.

Neoplasitic diseases

Surgical removal of the affected digit or digits is the treatment of choice. The lung fields should be radiographed prior to surgery to demonstrate the presence, or otherwise, of metastases. The prescapular lymph node should be excised and submitted for histopathologic examination.

KEY POINT
• Nail disorders are frustrating for owners and clinicians.

Dermatoses characterized by patchy alopecia

General approach

- The differential diagnosis is dominated by demodicosis, dermaphytosis, follicular dysplasias, and immune-mediated diseases – scrape, pluck, culture, and biopsy
- Screening blood tests and endocrine tests are much less helpful than with symmetrical alopecia – use as a last resort
- Dermatophytosis may be zoonotic

Common conditions

- Canine demodicosis
- Dermatophytosis
- Follicular dysplasias
- Cyclical flank alopecia
- Acquired pattern alopecia (pattern baldness)
- Telogen effluvium

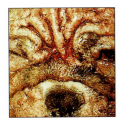
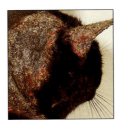
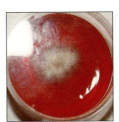
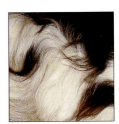

Canine demodicosis
(red mange, demodectic mange, demodicosis, demodectic acariosis, follicular mange)

ETIOLOGY AND PATHOGENESIS

Demodicosis results from proliferation of *Demodex* mites. Most cases are associated with the long-bodied mite *Demodex canis*, which is found in the hair follicles and the sebaceous and apocrine glands. There also appear to be two other species: a short-bodied mite living on the skin surface and follicular openings[1]; and an extra-long bodied form (*D. injai*) associated with pilosebaceous units[2].

Transmission from animal to animal is thought to be restricted to mother and offspring during the immediate post-natal period. The life cycle requires 20–35 days and consists of five stages: spindle-shaped eggs; small larvae with six short legs; six-legged protonymphs; nymphs with eight short legs; and adults with an obvious head, thorax, and four pairs of jointed legs (**293**). Adult mites survive for only a short period of time off the host[3].

Demodex appear to be commensal in most healthy dogs. Demodicosis is, therefore, associated with intrinsic host factors that permit proliferation rather than simple acquisition of parasites. A serum factor that suppresses lymphocyte activity has been found with heavy infestations complicated by bacterial pyoderma[4,5]. Demodicosis is also more common in purebred dogs. Studies suggest an autosomal recessive inheritance[6] and elimination of affected dogs, parents, and siblings from a breeding program reduces the incidence of clinical disease[3].

CLINICAL FEATURES
Localized demodicosis

Localized demodicosis is more common in younger dogs. Lesions consist of up to five areas of multifocal, asymmetrical, and well-circumscribed scaling, thinning of the hair, alopecia, and/or erythema (**294**). The skin can have a blue-gray color, comedones, follicular casts, and a musty smell. Commonly affected sites are the face, head, neck, forelimbs, and trunk. Demodicosis is a rare cause of otitis externa. Secondary bacterial or *Malassezia* infection is uncommon, but can cause papules, pustules, scaling, crusts, seborrhea, pruritus, and pain. Approximately 90% of cases self-cure, while 10% progress to generalized disease[6].

Generalized demodicosis

There is some overlap with localized disease, but generalized demodicosis is associated with more than 12 lesions, an entire body region, or one or more feet (pododemodicosis). The clinical signs include multifocal to generalized alopecia with scaling, hyperpigmentation, comedones, and follicular casts (**295**). Secondary bacterial infection, with papules, pustules, furunculosis, draining sinus tracts, crusts, pruritus, and pain is common (**296**). Severe secondary infections can be associated with enlarged lymph nodes, pyrexia, depression, septicemia, and death. Pododemodicosis is characterized by swelling of the feet, interdigital furunculosis ('cysts'), draining sinus tracts, pain, and lameness (**297**).

Some dogs, especially West Highland White Terriers, present with a pruritic form of demodicosis affecting the face, ears, feet, ventral body, and trunk, which could be confused with

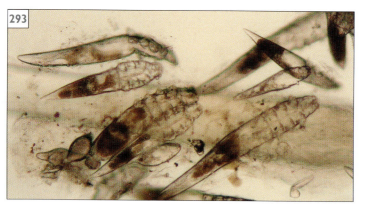

293 *Demodex canis* adults, eggs, and larvae.

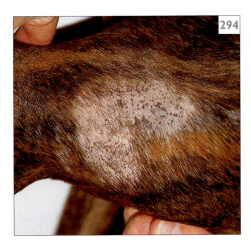

294 Localized demodicosis on the forelimb of a Boxer.

295 Generalized alopecia and hyper-pigmentation in a Dachshund.

296 Generalized demodicosis. Multiple erosions and furunculosis on the face of a six-month-old English Bulldog.

297 Severe pododemodicosis and pyoderma.

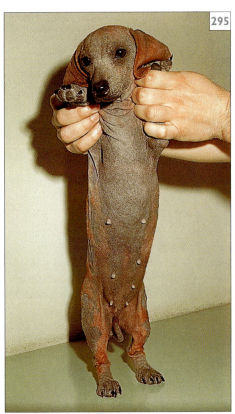

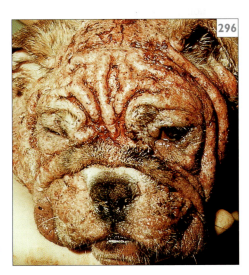

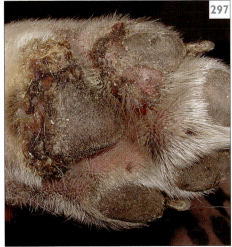

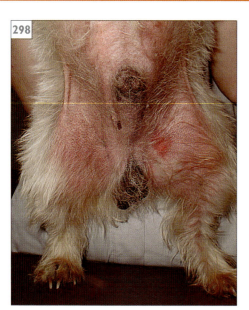

298 Pruritic demodicosis in a West Highland White Terrier. This can be very similar to atopic dermatitis, but note the follicular papules, erythema, and casts compared with the more diffuse erythema seen in atopic dermatitis.

atopic dermatitis. However, the clinical lesions usually outweigh the pruritus. Furthermore, the erythema is follicular rather than diffuse and associated with comedones and follicular casts (**298**).

Juvenile- and adult-onset disease
Juvenile-onset disease can occur at any age from 1–10 months, but is most common from 3–6 months. It has been associated with endocrine, immunologic, and cutaneous changes during adolescence and usually resolves with sexual maturity. Generalized disease, however, is less likely to resolve spontaneously. True adult-onset disease can be secondary to immunosuppressive conditions including[7]:
- Hyperadrenocorticism.
- Hypothyroidism. (**Note:** Euthyroid sick syndrome is a common finding in severe demodicosis.)
- Diabetes mellitus.
- Systemic neoplasia.
- Immunosuppressive therapy.
- Other debilitating conditions including systemic illness, lactation, poor nutrition, and stress.

DIFFERENTIAL DIAGNOSES
Multifocal inflammatory alopecia
- Dermatophytosis
- Follicular dysplasia
- Color-dilution alopecia
- Sebaceous adenitis
- Alopecia areata
- Superficial bacterial folliculitis (**Note:** Often a secondary problem in demodicosis.)
- Pemphigus foliaceus
- Post-injection/vaccine alopecia
- Drug eruption
- Dermatomyositis
- Leishmaniasis
- Epitheliotropic lymphoma
- Zinc responsive dermatitis

Furunculosis and draining sinus tracts
- Deep bacterial furunculosis (**Note:** Often a secondary problem in demodicosis.)
- Subcutaneous fungal infection
- Juvenile cellulitis and lymphadenitis (juvenile pyoderma/puppy strangles)
- Mycobacteria and filamentous bacteria (e.g. *Nocardia*, *Actinomyces*)

Pruritus
- Atopic dermatitis
- Cutaneous adverse food reactions
- Superficial bacterial folliculitis (**Note:** Often a secondary problem in demodicosis.)
- *Malassezia* dermatitis (**Note:** May be a secondary problem in demodicosis.)
- *Sarcoptes*, *Cheyletiella*, *Otodectes*, *Neotrombicula*, lice, and fleas
- Epitheliotrophic lymphoma

DIAGNOSIS
Adhesive-tape strips are minimally invasive, but not very sensitive[8]. Squeezing the skin can force mites onto the surface prior to collection. Hair plucks are more sensitive and can be useful for fractious animals and sites that are difficult to scrape. Skin scrapes are the most sensitive technique[8]; the skin is squeezed to push the mites further up the hair follicle and scraped until there is clear capillary ooze from the dermis. It can be difficult to scrape heavily scarred, ulcerating, and draining lesions, but squeezing can force purulent material and mites onto the surface where they can be collected on a microscope slide[9]. Skin biopsies may be necessary in dogs with severely scarred and/or thickened skin (e.g. Shar Peis).

In clinical demodicosis there are usually large numbers of mites. Because they are commensals, however, one or two adults are occasionally found in other dermatoses. Clinical judgment is important, but, if necessary, the demodicosis can be treated, the skin scrapes repeated, and any clinical improvement evaluated.

MANAGEMENT
Localized demodicosis
Simple monitoring is appropriate for localized demodicosis without secondary infection in young dogs that is expected to resolve spontaneously. Rotenone ointment and shampoo are licensed for localized demodicosis in the US and may be helpful. Re-examinations should be scheduled at 2–3 week intervals to assess whether the case is becoming generalized.

Generalized demodicosis: licensed drugs
Amitraz
Amitraz is applied in the US as a 250 ppm (0.025%) dip every 14 days and in Europe as a 500 ppm (0.05%) dip once weekly. In each case the dip is allowed to dry on the animal (wetting reduces efficacy). Long-haired animals should be clipped and bathed with benzoyl peroxide or other keratolytic shampoo to enhance contact. Reported efficacy ranges from 0–90%[10]. Off-license uses include applying 1000–1250 ppm solutions once or twice weekly to alternate halves of the body and using 0.15%–0.5% solutions in mineral oil daily for pododemodicosis and otitis externa[10,11]. Amitraz-impregnated collars are not effective.

Adverse effects include vomiting, sedation, hypothermia, hypotension, bradycardia, pruritus, exfoliative erythroderma, hyperglycemia, and death, especially in Chihuahuas. Some of the effects can be reversed with atipamezol or yohimbine. Amitraz is not pleasant to use and compliance can be poor. It should be applied in a well-ventilated area and the owners should wear impervious aprons and gloves. Potential adverse effects in humans include sedation, migraines, hyperglycemia, dyspnea, and contact reactions. Amitraz is a monoamine oxidase inhibitor (MAOI) and it can have potential adverse effects in individuals taking other MAOIs (e.g. some antihistamines, antidepressants, and antihypertensives).

10% imidacloprid/2.5% moxidectin spot-on
Preliminary studies indicate that once monthly application resulted in cure rates of 86–98%, although mites were still present in 14/18 dogs in one report. The majority of dogs will not have an adequate clinical response to once monthly dosing and further studies to determine the optimum dosing regime are under way. Repeated bathing and wetting are likely to reduce efficacy.

Adverse effects are uncommon, but can include seborrhea, erythema, and vomiting. Ingestion can result in ataxia, tremors, dilated pupils and poor papillary light reflex, nystagmus, dyspnea, salivation, and vomiting, especially in Collies, Old English Sheepdogs, and related breeds.

Generalized demodicosis: non-licensed drugs
Milbemycins
The response to milbemycin oxime (0.5–2 mg/kg p/o q24h) is reported to be 60–90%[10,12]. 0.5–0.75 mg/kg is usually given initially and the high doses reserved for recalcitrant cases. Adverse effects are rare, even in Collie-type breeds, and are generally limited to mild, transient ataxia and tremors, inappetence, and vomiting. These can be managed by reducing the dose and administering with food. Milbemycin is, however, expensive.

The success rate with moxidectin (200–400 µg/kg p/o q24h) is similar. It is less expensive, but side-effects including inappetence, vomiting, lethargy, ataxia, and tremors are more frequent[10].

Avermectins
Ivermectin (0.4–0.6 mg/kg p/o q24h) is successful in up to 85% of cases (higher doses are more effective)[10,13]. It is cheap and easily administered, but adverse effects are common in Collies and related breeds. Doses of 0.2 mg/kg can result in ataxia, tremors, depression, coma, and death. Test doses of 0.05–0.1 mg/kg, which induce ataxia but not coma in susceptible dogs, can be given. If this is tolerated, the dose can be increased incrementally. Alternatively, at-risk dogs can now be tested for the susceptible *mdr* (*abcb*) gene. There are, however, reports of neurologic side-effects including ataxia and blindness following long-term use in non-susceptible breeds. Pour-on solutions are not effective[14].

There is one report of successfully using doramectin (600 µg/kg s/c once weekly)[10]. No adverse effects were seen, but it is likely that they will be similar to those of ivermectin.

Other treatment considerations

Pyoderma should be treated with a bactericidal antibiotic for at least three weeks (superficial folliculitis) or for 4–6 weeks (furunculosis) (see p. 166). Topical antibacterials may also be beneficial, and will help remove surface scale and crust. Secondary *Malassezia* dermatitis can be managed with an antifungal shampoo, or systemically with itraconazole or ketoconazole (not licensed for dogs) (see p. 57).

Managing an underlying condition can result in remission of adult-onset demodicosis. A poor response to treatment, in contrast, is often associated with failure to control underlying conditions. Glucocorticoids should be avoided wherever possible; antihistamines or NSAIDs can be used to manage pruritus or pain if necessary. Relapses can be associated with estrus and affected bitches should be neutered. Affected dogs and their relatives should not be bred from.

Monitoring treatment

Skin scrapes and/or hair plucks should be repeated every 4–6 weeks and reveal an increasing ratio of dead and adult mites to live and immature mites. If not, the treatment should be re-evaluated and an underlying cause looked for. Treatment is continued until there have been 2–3 negative skin scrapes at 7–14 day intervals, and then for a further month. Apparently cured cases may relapse up to 12 months after treatment and will require further courses. Some cases with clinical but not parasitological cure may need maintenance treatment with the lowest frequency that controls clinical signs.

KEY POINTS

- Possibly the most serious non-neoplastic dermatologic disease. Client education and good communication are essential.
- Monitor carefully and repeat skin scrapings.

Feline demodicosis

ETIOLOGY AND PATHOGENESIS

Feline demodicosis is a rare disease caused by proliferation of the long-bodied *D. cati* and/or the short-bodied *D. gatoi*[1]. *D. cati* lives in pilosebaceous units and probably has a similar life cycle to *D. canis*. *D. gatoi* is found in the superficial epidermis and is potentially contagious[2]. It is unclear why the mites cause disease in some cats but not in others. There is no apparent age, sex, or breed predisposition, but juvenile disease (under three years) is usually idiopathic and has a better prognosis than adult disease (over five years), where underlying conditions are common[3–5]. These include hyperadrenocorticism, diabetes mellitus, hyperlipidemia, FIV and FeLV, multicentric squamous cell carcinoma in situ (Bowen's disease), and immunosuppressive drug therapy.

CLINICAL FEATURES

Demodicosis in cats can be localized, generalized, or otic. There may be variable, focal to multifocal or generalized alopecia and scaling, with occasional erythema, papules, erosions, crusting, comedones, and hyperpigmentation, especially of the eyelids, periocular area, chin, head, and neck (**299**). Infestation of the chin may result in the lesions of feline acne. The otic form may be associated with ears of normal appearance, where the mites are an incidental finding, or the ears may have a dark-brown ceruminous exudate[6]. *Demodex* have also been associated with facial or focal to generalized greasy seborrhea, especially in Persian cats. Pruritus is variable, but typically absent with *D. cati*. *D. gatoi*, in contrast, may cause moderate to severe pruritus of the head and neck or ventral body.

DIFFERENTIAL DIAGNOSES

- Dermatophytosis
- Bacterial folliculitis–furunculosis
- Psychogenic alopecia
- Atopic dermatitis
- Cutaneous adverse food reaction
- Contact dermatitis
- Flea bite hypersensitivity
- Infestation with *Cheyletiella*, *Notoedres*, *Sarcoptes*, and lice species

299 Focal alopecia and erythema due to feline demodicosis.

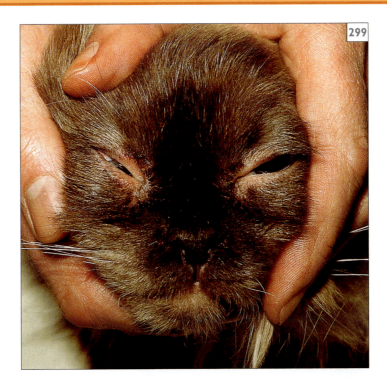

DIAGNOSIS
(See Canine demodicosis, p. 272)

MANAGEMENT
Because the mites are often superficial, many cases respond to 2% lime sulfur dips weekly for 4–6 weeks. If this should fail, 0.0125–0.025% (125–250 ppm) amitraz may be used as a weekly dip and continued for 3–4 weeks beyond the presence of negative skin scrapings[7]. Amitraz is not approved for use in cats and the strength is half that recommended by the manufacturer for dogs. Adverse effects at this strength include mild sedation, pytalism, anorexia, depression, and diarrhea.

Doramectin (600 µg/kg s/c once weekly) was successful and well tolerated in three cats[8]. There are also anecdotal reports of treatment with ivermectin (0.2–0.4 mg/kg p/o q24h), moxidectin (600 µg/kg p/o q24h), and milbemycin oxime (1–2 mg/kg p/o q24h. None of these drugs are licensed for feline demodicosis.

KEY POINTS
- Examination of skin scrapes is just as important in feline dermatology as it is in canine dermatology.
- Underlying conditions often mean a poor prognosis in adult-onset, generalized disease.

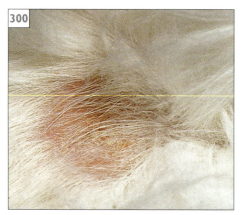

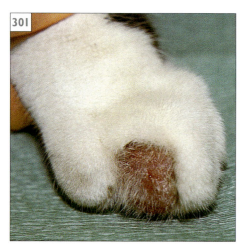

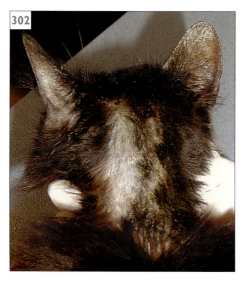

Dermatophytosis

ETIOLOGY AND PATHOGENESIS

Dermatophytosis is an infection of the skin, hair, or nails with fungi of the *Microsporum*, *Trichophyton*, or *Epidermophyton* genus. The most common cause in cats is *M. canis*; in dogs the most common causes are *M. canis* and *M. gypseum*. Other less frequent species include *T. mentagrophytes*, *M. persicolor*, *T. erinacei*, *M. verrucosum*, *M. equinum*, and *T. equinum*[1-4].

Isolation rates from healthy cats vary and probably reflect differences in environment and management. Dermatophytes are most likely to be isolated from colonies of cats, but they are rarely found in those that have never been exposed to infection. It is possible that culture-positive cats are transiently contaminated rather than true carriers[5-8].

Infection is by contact with infected animals or contaminated environments and the incubation period varies from 1–3 weeks. Dermatophytes infect growing hairs and living skin. Factors that influence the outcome of infection include a young age or the elderly, immunosuppression, high temperature and humidity, and skin trauma. *M. canis* is more common in Persian cats and Yorkshire Terriers (possibly due to ineffective grooming and/or impaired cell-mediated immunity) and Jack Russell Terriers are predisposed to *T. mentagrophytes* and *T. erinacei* (possibly because of their behavior)[2-4]. Most cats inoculated with spores do not develop dermatophytosis, as their grooming behavior efficiently removes the spores[9].

M. canis tends to induce a mild, self-limiting infection and a low-grade immune response. Antibodies are not protective and recovery is associated with cell-mediated immunity, which is nevertheless short-lived and induces relative and not absolute resistance[9,10]. Lesions typically resolve in 2–3 months, although animals may remain infective for several weeks longer. Infective fungal spores are readily shed into the environment and can remain viable for 18 months[11]. Control of contamination is of great importance in the management of dermatophytosis.

300–302 Dermatophytosis. *Microsporum canis* dermatophytosis usually results in focal alopecia (**300, 301**). Localized dermatophytosis with minimal inflammation and scaling in a cat (**302**).

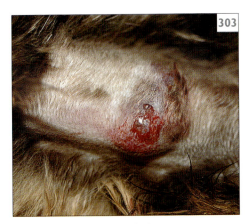

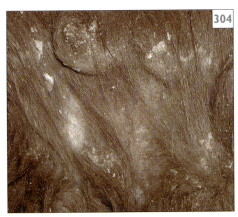

303 Ulcerated nodule with draining sinus tracts in a Maine Coon with dermatophyte mycetoma.

304 Generalized greasy scaling and poor hair coat in a Persian cat with dermatophytosis.

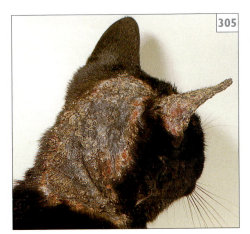

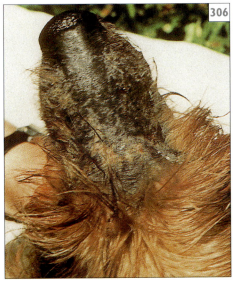

305, 306 Dermatophytosis. *Trychophyton mentagrophytes* infection usually results in well-demarcated inflammatory lesions in both cats (**305**) and dogs (**306**).

CLINICAL FEATURES

Classic signs include multifocal alopecia and scaling, typically on the face, head, and feet (**300, 301, 302**). Other clinical signs include folliculitis and furunculosis, feline acne, onychomycosis, granulomas, and kerions. Pruritus and inflammation are usually minimal, but occasionally pruritic, pustular, or crusting forms may mimic allergies, parasites, miliary dermatitis, pyoderma, or pemphigus foliaceus[9]. Dermatophyte mycetomas or pseudomycetomas are subcutaneous nodular and ulcerating forms with draining sinus tracts seen in Persian cats and, occasionally, in other long-haired breeds (**303**). This is often associated with a generalized greasy seborrhea (**304**). *T. mentagrophytes* typically causes more severe inflammation, alopecia, furunculosis, crusting, and granulomas of the face and feet, especially in small terrier breeds (**305, 306**)[12]. Dermatophytes are a rare cause of otitis externa[13].

DIFFERENTIAL DIAGNOSES

Because the clinical presentation can be so variable, dermatophytosis should be considered in almost any animal, but especially a cat, that presents with focal to multifocal alopecia, scaling, and crusting; diffuse alopecia, seborrhea, and scaling; nodules and draining sinus tracts; inflammation, erythema, erosions, and ulcers; and folliculitis and furunculosis.

DIAGNOSIS

Diagnosis relies on culture of hair and scale collected by scraping or plucking or by using carpet squares, grooming, or tooth brushes. These can initially be examined by microscopy for the identification of ectothrix arthroconidia spores (**307**). It is sometimes possible to identify fungal elements on tape-strip or impression smear cytology (**308**). Up to 50% of *M. canis* strains fluoresce apple green under a Wood's lamp (**309**). However, these tests are specific for infection, but poorly sensitive. Skin biopsies may be submitted, but histology is not as sensitive as culture[9].

Dermatophytes readily produce whitish colonies on dermatophyte test medium (DTM),

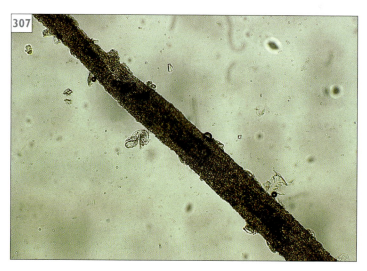

307 Dermatophytosis. Photomicrograph of a hair shaft exhibiting spores and hyphae. Note that these impart a 'dirty', thickened appearance to the hair.

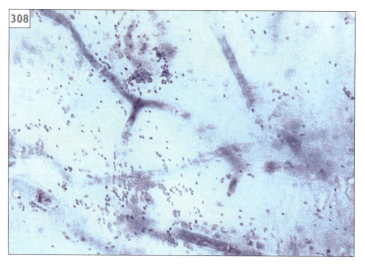

308 Hyphae seen on tape-strip cytology from a dog with dermatophytosis. (Diff-Quik stain, ×1000)

inducing a red color change that coincides with early fungal growth, usually within 7–10 days (faster if incubated above 25°C) (**310, 311**). Green or black colonies and/or color changes that coincide with late fungal growth all indicate a saprophyte. Species identification by colony and macroconidia morphology can, however, be difficult. Many dermatologists therefore prefer Sabouraud's agar, but this can take 2–3 weeks. Sabouraud's agar is more sensitive than DTM, where there can be poor fungal growth or failure to induce a color change. However, fungal isolation may simply reflect asymptomatic carriage[9].

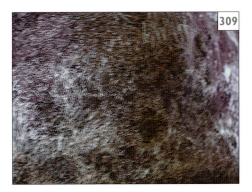

309 Fluorescing hairs and scale in a Yorkshire Terrier with dermatophytosis caused by *M. canis*.

MANAGEMENT

Clipping is not necessary in all cases, but it can facilitate topical therapy and remove infected hairs, reducing the pathogenic load and environmental contamination. This should be done with care to avoid further contamination from the clipped hair and skin trauma.

TOPICAL THERAPY

Rinses, dips, or shampoos are the preferred topical treatments, although many cats resist bathing. They should not be used alone, but they can reduce environmental contamination and the time to clinical and fungal cure[9]. Lime sulfur solutions are effective and well tolerated, although staining and pungent. Miconazole, ketoconazole, and 2% miconazole/2% chlorhexidine shampoos are also well tolerated and effective[9,14]. Enilconazole dip is highly effective and well tolerated by dogs, but idiosyncratic reactions including raised liver enzymes, muscle weakness, and death are occasionally seen in cats. Chlorhexidine is less effective[15].

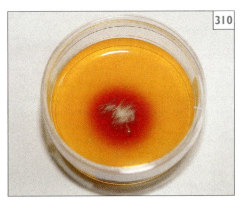

310 Positive culture on dermatophyte test medium. The critical observation is the appearance of color change at the same time as colony growth becomes apparent.

SYSTEMIC THERAPY[9,16,17]

Griseofulvin

Micronized formulation, 50–100 mg/kg q24h (dog), 25 mg/kg q24h (cat); ultramicronized/PEG formulation, 10–30 mg/kg q24h (dog), 5–10 mg/kg q24h (cat). Doses can be divided and given twice daily with a (fatty) meal until the infection has resolved. It is well tolerated, but should not be used in animals under six weeks of age. Side-effects include pruritus, anorexia, vomiting, diarrhea, liver damage, ataxia, and bone marrow suppression, which can be more severe in FIV- or FeLV-positive cats. Griseofulvin is teratogenic and may affect sperm quality.

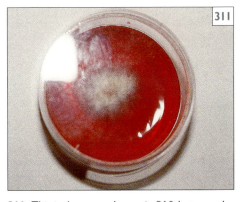

311 This is the same plate as in **310**, but a week later. The uniform red color now makes it impossible to tell if the fungal growth appeared after the color change or before.

Itraconazole

Itraconazole (5 mg/kg q24h for 7 days for 3 alternating weeks) is licensed for use in cats in Europe. It persists for 3–4 weeks after dosing. Therapeutic concentrations are maintained in the skin and hair for at least two weeks after the final dose. Itraconazole is better tolerated than ketoconazole.

Ketoconazole

Ketoconazole (5–10 mg/kg q24h) is effective and usually well tolerated, but it can cause anorexia and vomiting and is potentially terato-genic and hepatotoxic; some dermatologists recommend monitoring liver enzymes. Flucona-zole offers no advantages over itraconazole or ketoconazole, and neither fluconazole nor keto-conazole are licensed for use in animals.

Terbinafine

Terbinafine (20–30 mg/kg q24h) has been used successfully for dermatophytosis and dermato-phyte mycetomas, although it is not licensed for animals. There is a long duration of activity and this may allow relatively short courses of therapy followed by careful monitoring. Terbinafine appears to be well tolerated.

Lufenuron

A number of open studies using lufenuron at 2–3 times the standard anti-flea dose suggested that it is effective in the treatment and control of dermatophytosis in cats. Despite this, controlled studies have shown that it is ineffective in treating or controlling dermatophytosis[17,18,19].

Monitoring treatment

Clinical cure occurs before mycological cure and animals should not be regarded as cured until they have had 2–3 negative cultures at least seven days apart.

Environmental decontamination

The major source of contamination is the fungal spores on hairs. These may be removed with a combination of disposal, physical cleaning (including daily vacuuming – seal and burn the bag), and chemical agents. Effective antifungals include sodium hypochlorite (undiluted bleach is best, 1:10 dilution is effective with repeated administration), enilconazole (available as a spray or smoke generator), potassium monoperoxy-sulfate (although a recent report cast doubt on its efficacy), lime sulfur, and others (e.g. gluteralde-hyde, formaldehyde, and quaternary ammonium chlorides)[9].

Control of dermatophytosis in catteries and multi-cat households

The principles for controlling dermatophytosis in catteries and multi-cat households are:
- Isolate the cattery and suspend breeding until the outbreak is controlled.
- Separate infected and non-infected cats on the basis of culture and use barrier precautions to prevent spread of the infection. If it is impossible to isolate culture-negative cats, they should all be treated as culture positive.
- Treat infected cats.
- Eliminate environmental contamination.
- Prevent reinfection.

Pregnant queens and kittens can be isolated and treated with topical lime sulfur, miconazole/chlorhexidine, or enilconazole. Negative cats should be recultured and any that become posi-tive moved. Ideally, infected cats should not be moved until all of them are cured[9].

Prevention is better, less expensive, and less time consuming than treatment. New cats and animals that have been to shows and/or stud should be isolated and cultured; many owners can be taught to use DTM in-house. Testing, treating, and environmental monitoring using DTM have also been shown to control dermato-phytosis more cost effectively than euthanasia in rescue shelters[20–22].

KEY POINTS
- There is great potential for misdiagnosis.
- Be aware of zoonotic risk – treatment is mandatory and systemic therapy is needed in most cases.
- Good client communication is imperative.

Canine familial dermatomyositis

DEFINITION
Canine familial dermatomyositis is an hereditary inflammatory disease of skin and muscle that is characterized by symmetrical scarring alopecia about the face and limbs and atrophy of the muscles of mastication[1].

ETIOLOGY AND PATHOGENESIS
The etiopathogenesis of canine familial dermatomyositis is unknown. It is postulated that immunologic damage occurs to blood vessels, resulting in ischemic damage to the skin and muscles[2]. The condition is familial in Collies and Shetland Sheepdogs and breeding studies in Collies support an autosomal dominant mode of inheritance with variable expressivity[3,4].

CLINICAL FEATURES
The disease occurs more commonly in Collies and Shetland Sheepdogs, but it has also been reported to occur in the Welsh Corgi, Chow Chow, German Shepherd Dog, and Kuvasz, and may sporadically occur in other breeds[5]. Lesions generally develop before animals are six months of age, but they can occasionally develop in adults. The typical distribution pattern for lesions is the face (especially the bridge of the nose, around the eyes, and the tips of the ears [**312**]), carpal and tarsal areas (**313**), digits, and tip of the tail. A scarring alopecia, erythema, scaling, and mild crusting are the most common findings. Occasionally, vesicles, papules, pustules, and ulcers may be found[3]. The rate of development and progression of lesions is quite variable, as they often wax and wane and may undergo spontaneous regression. Muscle involvement occurs after the development of skin lesions and correlates with the severity of the skin lesions[3]. It is often minimal and limited to temporal and masseter atrophy. Severely affected dogs have difficulty in eating, drinking, and swallowing, and may evidence growth retardation, megaesophagus, lameness, widespread muscle atrophy, and infertility[3]. Skeletal muscle involvement may result in an abnormal gait or poor exercise intolerance. Pruritus and pain are generally not features of the disease.

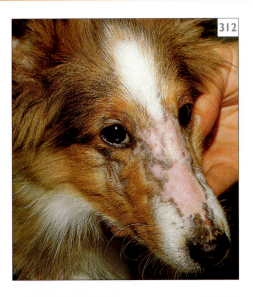

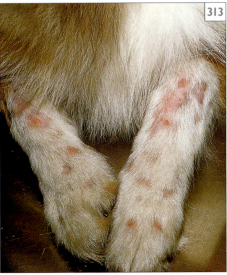

312, 313 Dermatomyositis in a Rough Collie demonstrating the alopecia and scale formation.

DIFFERENTIAL DIAGNOSES
- Cutaneous or systemic lupus erythematosus
- Dermatophytosis
- Epidermolysis bullosa
- Leishmaniasis
- Demodicosis
- Facial pyoderma
- Pemphigus foliaceus

DIAGNOSIS

Diagnosis is based on history, physical examination, compatible histologic changes in skin biopsies, and electromyography abnormalities consisting of positive sharp waves, fibrillation potentials, and bizarre high-frequency discharges of affected muscles[4].

MANAGEMENT

As the lesions of canine familial dermatomyositis can wax and wane on their own, it is difficult to determine the effectiveness of any particular treatment. No treatment may be needed for cases with minimal lesions as they may spontaneously resolve in many cases. Pentoxifylline (10–30 mg/kg p/o q12h) is felt to be the treatment of choice[6]. (**Note:** Generic forms of this drug have been less effective than the name brand Trental®[6].) Pentoxifylline improves circulation and decreases levels of inflammatory mediators such as tumor necrosis factor-alpha and collagenase. As this drug is a gastric irritant, it must be given with food. There is a lag period of 2–3 months before clinical benefits are noted. Oral vitamin E (200–800 IU/day) or marine lipid supplements may provide some improvement for skin lesions, but not the muscle lesions[3]. Prednisolone (1 mg/kg p/o q24h) can be used for the treatment of lesions when they flare. Prolonged use of prednisolone is discouraged as it may cause aggravation of the muscle atrophy. One author (PJM) has seen improvement in some dogs when they were treated with a combination of tetracycline (250 mg q8h in animals <10 kg, and 500 mg q8h in animals >10 kg) and niacinamide (250 mg q8h in animals <10 kg, and 500 mg q8h in animals >10 kg).

The various treatments suggested should not be expected to result in complete resolution of lesions, as they only minimize the development of new lesions and lessen the severity of those present. This is a heritable disease and affected dogs and their offspring should not be used for breeding.

KEY POINT

- A well-recognized disease that is not easy to diagnose or manage.

Injection site alopecia

DEFINITION

Injection site alopecia occurs at the site of subcutaneously administered drugs, including vaccines.

ETIOLOGY AND PATHOGENESIS

The etiology of this condition is not known, although a number of different mechanisms may be involved. Classic lesions are focal areas of alopecia occurring after rabies vaccination. Poodles and Bichon Frises are at increased risk, but the condition has been reported in many breeds of dogs[1]. A vasculitis has been noted in reported cases and an immune-mediated etiology proposed[2]. Inadvertent deep dermal injection may result in panniculitis and nodule formation[3]. Fibrosarcoma following feline leukemia (or rabies) vaccination has been reported in cats, although the exact mechanism of tumor induction is not known[4]. Extravascular injection of sodium thiopentone will cause a well-defined slough due to local necrosis of tissues.

CLINICAL FEATURES

Focal alopecia occurs 3–6 months after rabies injection[2]. Areas overlying the site of injection become hyperpigmented and alopecic and may measure 2–10 cm (0.8–4 in) in diameter. In rare instances animals may become depressed, lethargic, and febrile and develop alopecia over the face, limbs, margins of the pinnae, and tip of the tail. Erosions and ulcers have also been noted on the tongue, footpads, elbows, and lateral canthi. Focal decreased muscle mass has also been noticed in severe cases[1,5]. Lesions may be exacerbated upon revaccination[1]. Subcutaneous injections with progestagen suspensions may also result in focal alopecia. Reactions following progestagen injection also occur at the site of injection, although this tends to be dorsal midline in the interscapular region (**314**).

DIFFERENTIAL DIAGNOSES

- Demodicosis
- Dermatophytosis
- Dermatomyositis
- Alopecia areata
- Vasculitis
- Systemic lupus erythematosus

314 Focal alopecia and cutaneous atrophy following subcutaneous injection of progestagen.

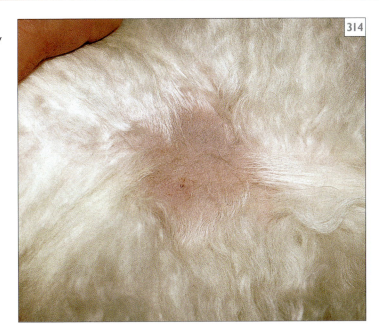

DIAGNOSIS
Clinical history and examination are normally sufficient to suggest the diagnosis. Examination of skin scrapings and fungal culture will rule out infectious causes, and histopathologic examination of biopsy samples will confirm the diagnosis.

MANAGEMENT
Pentoxifylline (25 mg/kg p/o q12h) is reported to be beneficial for lesions resulting from vaccines[5]. Hair regrowth without treatment can occur, but may take up to a year. Other treatments advocated include tacrolimus ointment 0.1% (applied q12h) and tetracycline and niacinamide (250 mg each p/o q8h if the animal is <15 kg and 500 mg each p/o q8h if the animal is >15 kg; doxycycline 10 mg/kg p/o q24h can be used instead of tetracycline)[6]. In some animals the atrophic changes are permanent. Prednisolone and/or cytotoxic drugs may be necessary to manage the vasculitis in severe, recalcitrant cases.

KEY POINT
- It may be best to avoid the dorsal midline when injecting show animals of predisposed breeds.

Alopecia areata

ETIOLOGY AND PATHOGENESIS

Alopecia areata is a rare immune-mediated condition associated with cell-mediated and humoral immune responses targeting the hair bulb[1,2].

CLINICAL FEATURES

Alopecia areata is characterized by focal to multifocal areas of well-circumscribed alopecia (**315**). These are usually irregular and asymmetric, but can appear symmetrical in some cases. The head, neck, and distal limbs are most commonly affected[2]. In some animals the disease may restrict itself to one hair color. The underlying skin appears normal, although hyperpigmentation may be present in chronic cases[2]. Rarely, it can be associated with nail disorders[3].

DIFFERENTIAL DIAGNOSES

- Post-injection alopecia
- Pseudopelade
- Dermatomyositis
- Demodicosis
- Dermatophytosis
- Follicular dysplasia
- Acquired pattern alopecia
- Leishmaniasis
- Bacterial pyoderma
- Epitheliotropic lymphoma

DIAGNOSIS

The history and clinical signs are highly suggestive. Hair plucks can reveal characteristic 'exclamation-mark' hairs – these are short and stubby with dystrophic proximal tapered portions and frayed, damaged distal portions[2]. Histopathology will usually confirm the presence of lymphocyte infiltrates targeting the hair bulb (the so-called 'swarm of bees'). Immunohistochemistry may detect immunoglobulin deposition in and around the hair bulb[1].

MANAGEMENT

There is no evidence that any therapy is beneficial. Many cases will undergo spontaneous resolution over six months to two years[2]. Glucocorticoids, imiquimod, and tacrolimus have been used with variable success in humans[2,4–6].

KEY POINT

- Definitive diagnosis is important, as some of the differentials are more serious conditions that require specific treatment.

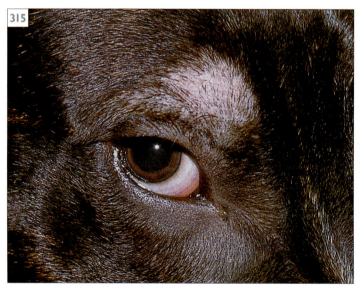

315 Focal alopecia due to alopecia areata. Note the complete absence of primary and secondary lesions apart from alopecia.

Follicular dysplasia

DEFINITION
Non-color-linked follicular dysplasia is a rare, tardive disorder in which abnormal follicular function results in either a patchy loss of hair or generalized abnormality of hair structure.

ETIOLOGY AND PATHOGENESIS
The disorder is of unknown etiology, although the fact that individuals of certain breeds appear to exhibit similar signs suggests an inherited component. The abnormalities in follicle function result in failure to cycle properly, pigment clumping, shaft abnormalities, hypotrichosis or alopecia, and follicular hyperkeratosis[1].

CLINICAL FEATURES
Although any individual animal may be affected, a number of syndromes have been recognized in various breeds. However, the face and distal extremities are areas that are seldom affected. Periodic remissions may occur in some animals, but with time the condition progresses.

Siberian Husky and Malamute
There is incomplete shedding of the juvenile coat, fracture and loss of guard hairs, and a reddish discoloration of remaining hair[1,2]. Secondary hair will appear wooly, dry, and matted. Focal areas of alopecia may occur at points of wear such as under collars and pressure points.

Doberman Pinscher and Weimaraner
There is a slowly progressive, non-pruritic symmetrical loss of hair, usually starting on the dorsal lumbosacral region[3,4]. Hair loss begins at about 12 months of age and frequently remains confined to the sublumbar fossae (**316**) and dorsal lumbosacral region. Animals are prone to secondary superficial pyoderma.

Curly Coated Retriever, Irish Water Spaniel, Portuguese Water Dog, and Chesapeake Bay Retriever
Affected individuals of these breeds exhibit loss of primary hairs and the remaining secondary hairs become dull and of a lighter shade[1,5,6]. The distribution pattern is often prominent on the ventral neck, posterior aspects of the hindlimbs, and tail (**317**). Truncal involvement may occur initially or evolve as the condition progresses. Periocular alopecia is often seen in Portuguese Water Dogs[6].

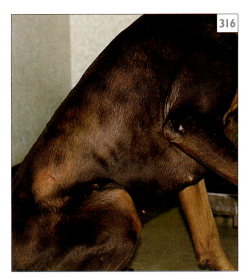

316 Follicular dysplasia in a Red Doberman Pinscher.

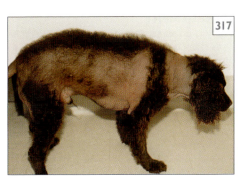

317 Alopecia of the neck, trunk, hindlimbs, and tail of an Irish Water Spaniel with follicular dysplasia.

Rottweilers
Follicular lipidosis is a rare condition seen in Rottweilers. Affected dogs start to lose hair from the brown colored areas on the face and feet. The rest of the coat is normal and there are no systemic signs. The clinical appearance is pathognomonic. Histopathology reveals follicular dysplasia of affected skin, with lipid deposition and swelling of hair bulb matrix cells. The condition can be progressive or wax and wane with periods of remission, but it largely remains a cosmetic problem.

DIFFERENTIAL DIAGNOSES

- Endocrinopathy
- Color-dilution alopecia
- Demodicosis
- Dermatophytosis
- Alopecia X
- Cyclical flank alopecia

DIAGNOSIS

Clinical history, physical examination, basic investigatory tests, and endrocrine profiles will rule out infectious causes and endocrinopathies. Hair plucks can reveal variably irregular hairs with broken shafts and dysplastic bulbs. Cytology can be useful for confirming secondary infection. Histopathology reveals variable follicular dysplasia, melanin aggregates, and follicular hyperkeratosis. Secondary infection can superimpose a perifollicular to interstitial inflammatory pattern and can mask subtle signs of dysplasia, and should therefore be controlled before biopsies are taken.

MANAGEMENT

There is no specific treatment for these conditions. Therapy is based on managing the skin to promote healthy skin turnover and normal follicular development, and control of secondary infections. Treatment measures can include:

- Avoiding further damage to coat – sun and/or cold weather protection.
- Gentle anti-scaling and moisturizing shampoos.
- Control secondary infections with topical antimicrobial shampoos and use moisturizing rinses/conditioners if the shampoo is drying.
- High-quality diets and essential fatty acid supplements can reduce scaling and promote hair growth in some dogs.
- Melatonin (5–20 mg/kg p/o q24h) and retinoids (isotretinoin [1.0 mg/kg p/o q12h] or acitretin [1.0 mg/kg p/o q24h]) may help some dogs, although neither is licensed for dogs. Retinoids are usually well tolerated, but side-effects include keratoconjunctivitis sicca, vomiting, diarrhea, joint pain and stiffness, pruritus, hyperlipidemia, and increased liver enzymes.

KEY POINTS

- The breed-associated syndromes greatly facilitate recognition of these diseases, but do not forget the differential diagnoses.
- The prognosis is generally poor for the coat, although the quality of life can be maintained for most dogs with appropriate treatment.

Black hair follicular dysplasia

DEFINITION

Black hair follicular dysplasia is a rare, tardive disorder affecting growth of black hairs, with sparing of white hairs[1].

ETIOLOGY AND PATHOGENESIS

The underlying etiology of the disorder is not understood. Abnormally large granules of melanin are present within the pigmented hair shafts, which may exhibit microscopic defects, and there are areas of epidermal pigment clumping, suggesting defects in pigment handling[1]. The dermatosis has been shown to be autosomally transmitted in one study on an affected crossbred litter[2], although the mode of inheritance was not determined[1]. Breeds reportedly affected include the Bearded Collie, Border Collie, Beagle, Basset Hound, Papillon, Saluki, Jack Russell Terrier, American Cocker Spaniel, Cavalier King Charles Spaniel, Dachshund, Gordon Setter, and Munsterlander[1,3,4]. As black hair follicular dysplasia and color-dilution alopecia share clinical and histopathologic features, it is possible that black hair follicular dysplasia is a localized form of color-dilution alopecia[5].

CLINICAL FEATURES

Only pigmented hair is affected. There is a patchy hypotrichosis associated with pigmented regions of skin (**318**). Affected areas produce short, dry, lusterless hair, although the severity varies both within and between individuals. Affected animals are normal at birth. Abnormalities may be detected both microscopically and grossly from as early as three weeks of age[2] and, rarely, they are delayed later than six weeks[1].

318 Black hair follicle
alopecia in a Jack
Russell Terrier.
(Photo courtesy
CM Knottenbelt)

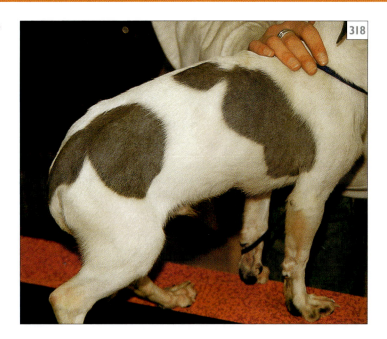

DIFFERENTIAL DIAGNOSES

- Demodicosis
- Superficial pyoderma
- Color-dilution alopecia
- Endocrinopathy
- Follicular dysplasia

DIAGNOSIS

A history of normal pups developing lesions that
are confined to the pigmented areas only is highly
suggestive of black hair follicular dysplasia. Skin
scrapes should be taken to rule out demodicosis.
Histopathologic examination of biopsy samples
is diagnostic.

MANAGEMENT

The dermatosis is not responsive to treatment.
Only the pigmented areas of the skin are affected
and there are no systemic signs. Management
should be symptomatic; mild shampoos and
systemic antibacterial therapy may be indicated if
secondary superficial pyoderma develops.

KEY POINT

- Almost pathognomonic presentation.

Color-dilution alopecia
(color-mutant alopecia, Blue Dobermann syndrome)

DEFINITION
Color-dilution alopecia is an inherited disorder of color-diluted (i.e. gray or 'blue', or red/fawn) dogs characterized by alopecia developing in the areas of the dilute-colored hair.

ETIOLOGY AND PATHOGENESIS
Color-dilution alopecia is thought to occur because of changes in genes in the D locus[1,2]. As some animals with color dilution do not develop the condition, there appear to be other alleles or factors responsible[1–3]. Affected animals have many large, irregularly shaped melanin granules in the basal keratinocytes, the hair matrix cells, and the hair shafts[1,3]. It has been suggested that hair matrix cells are affected by the cytotoxic effects of melanin precursors, which results in cessation of hair growth and, eventually, follicular dysplasia[1]. The extensive melanin clumping in the hair and associated distortion of the cuticular–cortical structure of the hair are thought to lead to fragility and breaking of hair shafts at these sites[3]. However, similar findings can be seen in normal animals with dilute-colored coats. Cats with diluted coats are only very rarely affected by color-dilution alopecia.

CLINICAL FEATURES
Color-dilution alopecia has been diagnosed mainly in Blue Doberman Pinschers, leading to the early name of Blue Doberman syndrome. However, the syndrome has also been diagnosed in other breeds with blue color dilution, including the Dachshund, Great Dane, Whippet, Italian Greyhound, Chow Chow, Standard Poodle, Yorkshire Terrier, Miniature Pinscher, Chihuahua, Bernese Mountain Dog, Shetland Sheepdog, Schipperke, Silky Terrier, Boston Terrier, Saluki, Newfoundland, German Shepherd Dog, and mixed-breed dogs[1,2,4]. The syndrome has also been diagnosed in the Fawn Doberman Pinscher, Fawn Irish Setter, and Red Doberman Pinscher[1,2,4]. The syndrome appears in approximately 93% of Blue and 83% of Fawn Doberman Pinschers[1]. Onset generally occurs in animals aged four months to three years. However, it has developed in some animals as late as six years of age[4]. Affected animals gradually develop a dull, dry, brittle, poor-quality coat with fractured hair (**319, 320**). As the condition progresses, a moth-eaten partial alopecia develops, which may continue to worsen until there is total alopecia of dilute-colored hair. Follicular papules often develop and may advance to comedo formation or secondary bacterial folliculitis. As the condition becomes chronic, the affected skin can become hyperpigmented and seborrheic. The severity of the syndrome varies, with lighter-colored animals developing the most extensive lesions. Lesions will be limited to the dilute-colored parts of the coat in multi-colored animals.

DIFFERENTIAL DIAGNOSES
- Hyperadrenocorticism
- Hypothyroidism
- Sex hormone dermatoses
- Follicular dysplasia
- Cyclical flank alopecia
- Acquired pattern alopecia
- Demodicosis
- Dermatophytosis

DIAGNOSIS
Clinical examination will raise suspicion of the disorder. Microscopic examination of affected hair may demonstrate uneven distribution and clumping of melanin (**321**) that may cause distortion of the hair shaft. Histopathologic examination of biopsy samples will confirm the diagnosis.

MANAGEMENT
There is no specific treatment that will alter the course of the syndrome. In some animals, weekly bathing with benzoyl peroxide shampoo to reduce comedo formation and seborrhea may be beneficial. Harsh, drying shampoos can accelerate coat damage, however. Gentle bathing with antimicrobial, keratolytic, and moisturizing products should be tailored to the needs of each individual case. Systemic antibiotics would be appropriate if a secondary bacterial folliculitis is present. High-quality diets and essential fatty acids may also be helpful.

KEY POINTS
- Diagnosis depends on histopathologic examination.
- There is no treatment that will alter the coat changes.

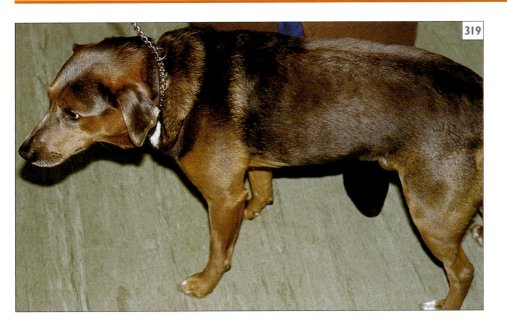

319,320 Color-dilution alopecia in a dilute-blue crossbreed (**319**) and a Red Doberman Pinscher (**320**).

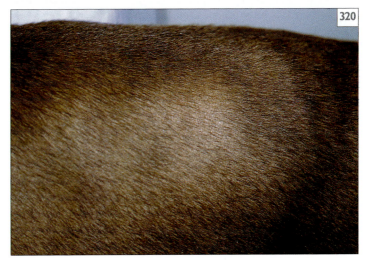

321 Photomicrograph of a hair from a color-dilute Doberman Pinscher. Note the clumping of the pigment granules.

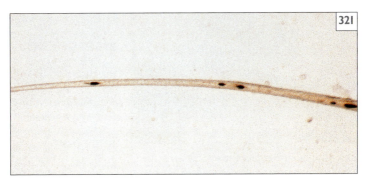

Cyclical flank alopecia
(seasonal flank alopecia, flank alopecia, recurrent flank alopecia)

DEFINITION
Cyclical flank alopecia is a follicular dysplasia of dogs resulting in alopecia and hyperpigmentation in the flank regions.

ETIOLOGY AND PATHOGENESIS
It is likely that there is some genetic predisposition to cyclical flank alopecia, as it is quite common in some breeds (e.g. Boxers, Bulldogs, Airedales, and Schnauzers) but rare in others (including German Shepherd Dogs, Spaniels, and Arctic Breeds). There is no age predisposition, although the mean age of onset is about four years[1,2]. The seasonal nature of the condition and the fact that it is more common north of 45° latitude suggest that light exposure and changing photoperiod are important. Onset in most cases is associated with short photoperiod seasons, which are opposite in the northern and southern hemispheres. Paradoxically, lesions may develop during prolonged photoperiods, with partial or complete resolution during shorter photoperiods. In other cases, lesions develop and there is no resolution with changes in photoperiod. This latter scenario is more likely to occur in areas of the world that do not have well-defined seasons[1]. Infrequently, multifocal areas of interface dermatitis affecting alopecic skin may be observed, and the etiology of this finding is unknown.

CLINICAL FEATURES
Lesions are typically manifested by the onset of well-demarcated, irregular to serpiginous areas of alopecia in the thoracolumbar areas (**322**). Occasionally, other areas such as the nose, ears, tail, back, cranial ribcage, and perineum can be affected. The underlying skin is usually hyperpigmented but otherwise normal. Airedale Terriers can have widespread involvement of the back, with lesions extending down to the trunk. Dogs with interface dermatitis may exhibit small, circular to arcuate, multifocal patches of scaling, erosions, and crusting. These lesions may be mildly painful or pruritic.

Hair regrowth usually occurs in 3–8 months as the photoperiod lengthens. However, the extent of alopecia can vary from year to year. Regrowth can be complete or partial and may be lighter or darker in color and have a different texture. Hyperpigmentation and/or alopecia may eventually become permanent.

Affected dogs have no systemic clinical signs and the rest of the skin and coat appears normal.

DIFFERENTIAL DIAGNOSES
- Demodicosis
- Dermatophytosis
- Endocrinopathies
- Injection site alopecia
- Alopecia areata
- Follicular dysplasia

DIAGNOSIS
Diagnosis is based on history, clinical findings, and ruling out other differentials. Dermatohistopathology can be supportive, with follicular atrophy, dysplastic follicles (which have infundibular hyperkeratosis extending into the secondary follicles), and sebaceous ducts giving an 'octopus'- or 'witches foot'-like appearance. Infrequently, a multifocal interface dermatitis may be seen.

MANAGEMENT
The treatment of choice is melatonin (3–12 mg/dog p/o q12h for 4–6 weeks and then as needed). As lesions are cosmetic and hair may regrow, observation only is reasonable, particularly where melatonin is unavailable.

KEY POINT
- Be aware that this is a condition that is generally controlled but not cured.

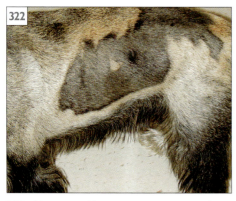

322 Alopecia and hyperpigmentation over the trunk of a Schnauzer with cyclical flank alopecia.

Acquired pattern alopecia (pattern baldness)

DEFINITION
Acquired pattern alopecia is a condition that results in thinning of hair or alopecia in specific locations over the body.

ETIOLOGY AND PATHOGENESIS
The pathogenesis of acquired pattern alopecia is unknown, although some form of genetic predisposition is suspected.

CLINICAL FEATURES
The syndrome is frequently seen in Dachshunds, but it can occur in other short-coated breeds such as the Boston Terrier, Chihuahua, Greyhound, Whippet, and Miniature Pinscher. Common features of pattern alopecia include an insidious onset and slowly progressive, symmetrical, and focal hair loss, which may result in well-demarcated patches of complete alopecia. The underlying skin is usually normal. Very short and very fine hairs may be evident, especially in the earlier stages. Affected dogs show no systemic clinical signs, and the rest of the hair coat is normal. One pattern involves gradual alopecia and hyperpigmentation of the pinnae in male and, less commonly, female Dachshunds. This usually starts at 6–12 months of age and is complete by 6–9 years of age. Another pattern is seen in young to adult Greyhounds that develop gradual hair loss of the caudal thighs. The most frequently seen pattern consists of a bilateral thinning of hair that can progress to total hair loss in one or more of the following areas: pinna and areas just caudal to the pinna, areas between ear and eye, ventral neck, chest, ventral abdomen, perianal, and caudal thighs. Of these the pinna is most frequently affected. This pattern occurs in Dachshunds, but it is also recognized in other breeds.

DIFFERENTIAL DIAGNOSES
* Endocrinopathies
* Demodicosis
* Dermatophytosis
* Follicular dysplasia
* Telogen effluvium and telogen defluxion

DIAGNOSIS
Diagnosis is based on history, clinical findings, and ruling out other differentials. Histopathology reveals normal skin with miniaturization of hair follicles and very fine hair shafts.

MANAGEMENT
Acquired pattern alopecia is a benign cosmetic disease and may not need treatment. Melatonin (3–12 mg/dog p/o q12h) may result in hair regrowth in some cases.

KEY POINT
* Be aware that this is a condition that is generally controlled but not cured.

Telogen effluvium, anagen defluxion, wave shedding, diffuse shedding, and excessive continuous shedding

ETIOLOGY AND PATHOGENESIS

These conditions result from a disruption of the normal mosaic hair replacement of dogs and cats. Normal replacement is governed primarily by photoperiod and, to a lesser extent, ambient temperature, but is largely unaffected by season under normal household conditions[1].

Telogen defluxion occurs when a condition such as whelping and lactation, pregnancy, high fever, severe illness, shock, surgery, or anesthesia results in the cessation of hair growth in many anagen follicles. This results in synchronization of these follicles to catagen and then telogen. When follicular activity begins again, typically after 1–3 months, large amounts of hair are shed[2]. The coat can also be removed by vigorous grooming and bathing.

Anagen defluxion occurs when more severe conditions such as metabolic disease, endocrine disorders, infectious diseases, or treatment with antimitotic drugs interfere with anagen, resulting in acute hair loss within days[2].

The pathogenesis of wave shedding, diffuse shedding, and excessive continuous shedding is unclear.

CLINICAL FEATURES

Telogen effluvium and anagen defluxion result in diffuse, partial to complete alopecia, especially of the trunk. Telogen effluvium may also be particularly marked in areas prone to wear and trauma. The underlying skin is usually normal (**323**).

Wave shedding can cause either a localized thinning of the coat, shedding of hair from a particular area, and a spreading difference in coat color, or differences in hair length between one region and another (**324, 325**). It is characterized by a diffuse shedding that generally starts on the dorsum of the animal and descends ventrally. The coat is almost completely shed at the edge of the wave, with new hair regrowth behind the wave. This often creates a contrast in coat length, coat color (new hair tends to be darker), coat density (new coat tends to be less dense), and coat texture (new coat has a higher ratio of primary hairs). Diffuse shedding occurs when an animal does not shed in a mosaic pattern, but sheds the majority of its coat at one time in the absence of a systemic insult, with transient diffuse, partial alopecia preceding normal regrowth. In animals with excessive continuous shedding there is no thinning of the coat or alopecia.

DIFFERENTIAL DIAGNOSES

- Systemic disease, metabolic stress, long-standing pyrexia
- Post-clipping alopecia
- Endocrine diseases
- Drug therapy

DIAGNOSIS

Diagnosis is based on history and clinical findings (**326, 327**). Appropriate diagnostics to rule in or out a particular systemic insult should be performed as indicated. Hair plucks reveal normal telogenized hairs or, with anagen defluxion, twisted and fractured dysplastic hairs that often have prominent pinch points. Histopathologic examination of biopsy samples is helpful in ruling in or out endocrinopathies.

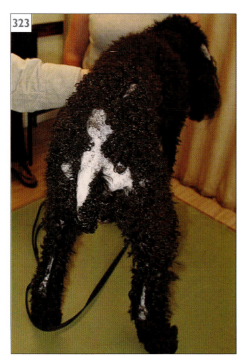

323 Anagen defluxion following azathioprine treatment in a Miniature Poodle.

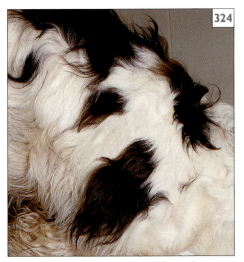
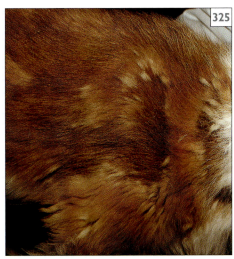

324, 325 Abnormal shedding with overlong regrowth of the black hairs (**324**) and patchy alopecia (**325**).

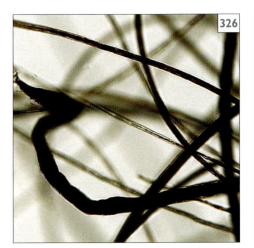
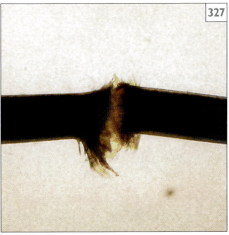

326 Hair pluck from the dog in **323** with broken and distorted hairs.

327 Trichorrhexis nodosa in a hair pluck from a cat with anagen defluxion.

MANAGEMENT

Wave and diffuse shedding usually self-cure in 3–6 months. Anagen and telogen defluxion self-cure 3–6 months after the insult has been resolved. Removal of telogen hairs with a brush or comb to prevent accumulation on household furnishings is all that can be done for excessive continuous shedding.

KEY POINTS

- Another poorly defined group of diseases.
- The prognosis is generally good.

Post-clipping alopecia

ETIOLOGY AND PATHOGENESIS

Post-clipping alopecia results from failure of hair growth after clipping. It is relatively common in dogs, but rare in cats. The exact mechanism is unknown, but one theory is that decreased perfusion of hair follicles, secondary to vasoconstriction due to cooling of the skin by removal of the hair, may lead to premature termination of the growing phase[1]. Alternatively, it may simply reflect a very long telogen period before the next hair growth cycle. In Labrador Retrievers, post-clipping regrowth takes 2.5–5 months (mean 3.7) and there is no relationship to the season in which the dogs are clipped[2]. Post-clipping alopecia can also be an early sign of an endocrinopathy or metabolic disorder (see Telogen effluvium and anagen defluxion, p. 294).

CLINICAL FEATURES

Although post-clipping alopecia may occur in any breed, it occurs primarily in long-coated breeds such as Siberian Huskies, Alaskan Malamutes, Samoyeds, Chow Chows, and Keeshonds[1]. Clinically, the hair does not regrow after clipping for venipuncture, surgery, wound management, or summer grooming (**328**). There appears to be an association with lumbar epidural anesthesia.

Occasionally, a few guard hairs will regrow in the affected area. Pyoderma is rare, but may be related to the trauma of clipping or underlying immunosuppressive conditions (**329**). Hair growth generally resumes within 6–12 months, but full regrowth can take 18–24 months.

DIFFERENTIAL DIAGNOSES

- Iatrogenic or endogenous hyperadrenocorticism
- Hypothyroidism or other endocrinopathies
- Alopecia of follicular arrest (e.g. castration responsive dermatosis, growth hormone responsive alopecia, 'alopecia X')
- Telogen effluvium and anagen defluxion

DIAGNOSIS

Diagnosis is based on history and clinical findings as well as ruling out conditions in the differential diagnosis. Histopathologic findings on biopsy samples are supportive.

MANAGEMENT

There is no treatment that benefits this condition.

KEY POINTS

- A poorly understood condition.
- With time, hair will regrow in most animals.

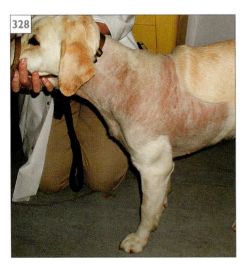

328 Post-clipping alopecia in a Labrador Retriever.

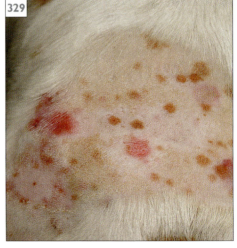

329 Post-clipping alopecia and pyoderma in an English Springer Spaniel.

Topical corticosteroid reaction

DEFINITION
Topical corticosteroid reaction is a thinning of the skin with prominent comedones associated with topical application of potent corticosteroid medications.

ETIOLOGY AND PATHOGENESIS
A wide variety of corticosteroid-containing sprays, creams, ointments, and gels might institute the lesions, but many cases are associated with products containing triamcinolone or betamethasone[1].

CLINICAL FEATURES
Lesions appear as focal areas of thin, almost translucent skin with prominent comedones (**330**). Varying degrees of erythema and hyperpigmentation may be present. Long-standing lesions may become eroded or ulcerated, or evidence scarring[1]. Other lesions include localized demodicosis and/or bacterial folliculitis, telangiectasia, and poor wound healing. Due to the difficulty of applying topical preparations to densely haired areas of the body, lesions are generally found in the glabrous skin of the ventral abdomen or axilla.

DIFFERENTIAL DIAGNOSES
Hyperadrenocorticism or prolonged use of systemic glucocorticoids may result in a thinning of the skin and comedones, but the affected area will be diffuse rather than focal.

DIAGNOSIS
Diagnosis is based on history and clinical findings.

MANAGEMENT
Discontinue application of topical corticosteroids. Return of skin to normal appearance may take several months.

KEY POINT
- Focal thinning of skin with comedones that may take several months to resolve after discontinuing topical corticosteroids.

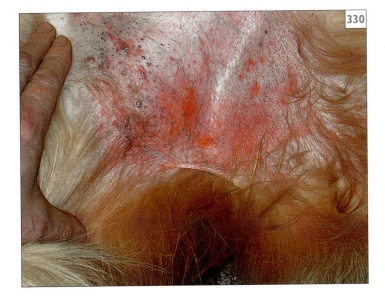

330 Thin skin, comedones, and erythema of the skin of a dog with topical corticosteroid reaction.

Feline paraneoplastic alopecia

DEFINITION

Feline paraneoplastic alopecia is a syndrome of hair loss that is a marker for underlying internal malignancy.

ETIOLOGY AND PATHOGENESIS

The condition is generally associated with a pancreatic adenocarcinoma, but in a small number of cases it has been reported in association with bile duct carcinoma[1-4].

CLINICAL FEATURES

The syndrome occurs in older cats. Alopecia first appears on the ventral abdomen, thorax, and limbs and then may generalize[1-4]. Occasionally, the pinnae and periorbital regions may also be affected. Hair adjacent to the advancing alopecia epilates easily. The alopecic skin has a characteristic smooth, shiny, glistening appearance (**331**). It is thin and inelastic, but not fragile[3]. The footpads may be affected with translucent scale often arranged in rings[3]. Excessive grooming and secondary *Malassezia* dermatitis may also develop[2,3]. Concurrent signs of underlying neoplasia include anorexia, weight loss, and lethargy.

DIFFERENTIAL DIAGNOSES

• Psychogenic alopecia
• Lymphocytic mural folliculitis
• Thymoma-associated exfoliative dermatitis
• Demodicosis
• Hyperadrenocorticism
• Telogen defluxion

DIAGNOSIS

The history and clinical findings are distinctive. Dermatohistopathology is supportive. Radiology, ultrasonography, or exploratory laparotomy will confirm neoplasia.

MANAGEMENT

Complete surgical excision of the internal malignancy is curative. However, in the majority of cases, tumor metastasis has occurred by the time a diagnosis is made and the prognosis is therefore poor[1-3]. Recurrence of the alopecia indicates metastatic disease and relapse.

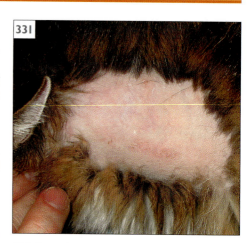

331 Smooth, shiny, glistening skin and alopecia in a cat with feline paraneoplastic alopecia.

KEY POINT

• A condition with distinctive alopecic, smooth, shiny skin that is due to internal malignancy and has a poor prognosis.

Lymphocytic mural folliculitis

Lymphocytic mural folliculitis is a recently recognized condition characterized by moderate to severe alopecia, papules and erythema, and scaling of the trunk and limbs that may resemble paraneoplastic alopecia and metabolic epidermal necrosis. Secondary *Malassezia* infection is common. The etiology is unknown; some cases spontaneously resolve or relapse, but others may be associated with epitheliotropic lymphoma, dermatophytosis, *Demodex*, and systemic illness or neoplasia.

Thymoma-associated exfoliative dermatitis is similar, but is associated with a lupus-like immune-mediated condition triggered by a thymoma. Excision of the thymoma is curative.

References

CHAPTER 1: PRURITIC DERMATOSES

Pyotraumatic dermatitis

1 Jennings S (1953) Some aspects of veterinary dermatology. *Vet Rec* **46**:809–816.

2 Reinke SI, Stannard AA, Ihrke PJ, Reinke JD (1987) Histopathological features of pyotraumatic dermatitis. *J Am Vet Med Assoc* **190**:57–60.

Canine atopic dermatitis

1 Olivry T, Hill PB (2001) The ACVD task force on canine atopic dermatitis (IX): the controversy surrounding the route of allergen challenge in canine atopic dermatitis. *Vet Immunol Immunopathol* **81**:219–225.

2 de Weck AL, Mayer P, Schiessl B *et al*. (1997) Dog allergy: a model for allergy genetics. *Int Arch Allergy Immunol* **113**:55–57.

3 DeBoer DJ, Hill PB (1999) Serum immuno-globulin E concentrations in West Highland White Terrier puppies do not predict development of atopic dermatitis. *Vet Dermatol* **10**:275–281.

4 Shaw SC, Wood N, Freeman J *et al*. (2004) Estimation of heritability of atopic dermatitis in Labrador and Golden Retrievers. *Am J Vet Res* **65**:1014–1020.

5 Scott DW, Miller WH, Reinhart GA *et al*. (1997) Effect of an omega-3/omega-6 fatty acid-containing commercial lamb and rice diet on pruritus in atopic dogs: results of a single-blinded study. *Can J Vet Res* **61**:145–153.

6 Taugbol O, Baddaky-Taugbol B, Saarem JW (1990) The fatty acid profile of subcutaneous fat and blood plasma in pruritic dogs and dogs without skin problems. *Can J Vet Res* **62**:275–278.

7 Inman AO, Olivry T, Dunston SM *et al*. (2001) Electron microscopic observations of the stratum corneum intercellular lipds in normal and atopic dogs. *Vet Pathol* **38**:720–723.

8 MacEwan NA (2000) Adherence by *Staphylo-coccus intermedius* to canine keratinocytes in atopic dermatitis. *Res Vet Sci* **68**:279–283.

9 Mason IS, Lloyd DH (1990) Factors influencing the penetration of bacterial antigens through canine skin. In *Advances in Veterinary Dermatology, Vol. I* (eds C von Tscharner, REW Halliwell). Baillière-Tindall, Philadelphia, pp. 360–366.

10 Morales CA, Schultz KT, DeBoer DJ (1994) Antistaphylococcal antibodies in dogs with recurrent pyoderma. *Vet Immunol Immunopathol* **42**:137–147.

11 Mason IS, Lloyd DH (1995) The macroscopic and microscopic effects of intradermal injection of crude and purified staphyloccal extracts on canine skin. *Vet Dermatol* **6**:197–204.

12 Nimmo-Wilkie JS, Yager JA, Wilkie BN *et al*. (1991) Abnormal cutaneous response to mitogens and a contact allergen in dogs with atopic dermatitis. *Vet Immunol Immunopathol* **28**:97–106.

13 Hendricks A, Schuberth HJ, Schueler K *et al*. (2002) Frequency of superantigen-producing *Staphylococcus intermedius* isolates from canine pyoderma and proliferation inducing potential of superantigens in dogs. *Res Vet Sci* **73**:273–277.

14 Nuttall TJ, Halliwell REW (2001) Serum antibodies to *Malassezia* yeasts in canine atopic dermatitis. *Vet Dermatol* **12**:327–332.

15 Morris DO, DeBoer DJ (2003) Evaluation of serum obtained from atopic dogs with dermatitis attributable to *Malassezia pachydermatis* for passive transfer of immediate hypersensitivity to that organism. *Am J Vet Res* **64**:262–266.

16 Belew PW, Rosenberg EW, Jennings BR (1980) Activation of the alternate pathway of complement by *Malassezia ovalis (Pityrosporum ovale)*. *Mycopathologia* **70**:187–191.

17 Lund EM, Armstrong PJ, Kirk CA *et al*. (1999) Health status and population characteristics of dogs and cats examined at private veterinary practices in the United States. *J Am Vet Med Assoc* **214**:1336–1341.

18 Griffin CE (1993) Canine atopic disease. In *Current Veterinary Dermatology* (eds CE Griffin, KW Kwochka, JM McDonald). Mosby Year Book, St. Louis, pp. 90–120.

19 Willemse T (1986) Atopic skin disease: a review and reconsideration of diagnostic criteria. *J Small Anim Pract* **27**:771–778.

20 Prèlaud P, Guarere E, Alhaidari Z *et al.* (1998) Reevaluation of diagnostic criteria of canine atopic dermatitis. *Rev Med Vet* **149**:1057–1064.

21 Plant J (1994) The reproducibility of three *in vitro* canine allergy tests: a pilot study. (Abstract) In *Proceedings of the Annual Meeting of the American Academy of Dermatology/American College of Veterinary Dermatology*, Charlston, p. 16.

22 Scott DW, Miller WH, Griffin CE (1995) Immunologic skin diseases. In *Muller and Kirk's Small Animal Dermatology*, 5th edn. WB Saunders, Philadelphia, pp. 543–666.

23 Marsella R, Olivry T (2001) The ACVD task force on canine atopic dermatits (XXII): nonsteroidal anti-inflammatory pharmacotherapy. *Vet Immunol Immunopathol* **81**:331–341.

24 Olivry, T, Steffan J, Fisch RD *et al.* (2002) Randomized controlled trial of the efficacy of cyclosporin in the treatment of atopic dermatitis in dogs. *J Am Vet Med Assoc* **221**:370–377.

25 Radowicz SN, Power HT (2003) Long-term use of cyclosporin therapy in the treatment of canine atopic dermatitis. (Abstract) *Vet Dermatol* **14**:234.

26 Olivry T, Rivierre C, Murphy KM *et al.* (2003) Maintenance treatment of canine atopic dermatitis with cyclosporin: decreasing dosages or increasing intervals? (Abstract) *Vet Dermatol* **14**:220.

27 Fontaine J, Olivry T (2001) Treatment of canine atopic dermatitis with cyclosporin: a pilot study. *Vet Rec* **148**:662–663.

28 Olivry T, Mueller RS (2003) Evidence-based veterinary dermatology: a systematic review of the pharmacology of canine atopic dermatitis. *Vet Dermatol* **14**:121–146.

29 Favrot C, Hauser B, Olivry T *et al.* (2003) Absence of detection of conventional papilloma virus DNA in cyclosporin-associated papilloma-like skin lesions in dogs. (Abstract) In *Proceedings of the Annual Meeting of the American Academy of Dermatology/American College of Veterinary Dermatology*, Monterey, p. 203.

30 Werner A (2003) Psoriasiform-lichenoid-like dermatitis in three dogs treated with microemulsified cyclosporine A. *J Am Vet Med Assoc* **223**:1013–1016.

31 Steffan J, Strehlau G, Maurer M *et al.* (2004) Cyclosporine A pharmacokinetics and efficacy in the treatment of atopic dermatitis in dogs. *J Vet Pharmacol Ther* **27**:231–238.

32 Ryffel B, Donatsch P, Madorin M *et al.* (1983) Toxicological evaluation of cyclosporin A. *Arch Toxicol* **53**:107–141.

33 Scott DW, Miller WH, Griffin CE (2001) Dermatologic therapy. In *Muller and Kirk's Small Animal Dermatology*, 6th edn. WB Saunders, Philadelphia, pp. 207–273.

34 Miller WH, Scott DW, Wellington JR *et al.* (1993) Evaluation of the performance of a serologic allergy system in atopic dogs. *J Am Anim Hosp Assoc* **29**:545–550.

Cutaneous adverse food reaction
(food or dietary allergy or intolerance)

1 Day MJ (2005) The canine model of dietary hypersensitivity. *Proceedings of the Nutrition Society* **64**:458–464.

2 Jeffers JG, Meyer EK, Sosis EJ (1996) Responses of dogs with food allergies to single ingredient dietary provocation. *J Am Vet Med Assoc* **209**:608–612.

3 Rosser EJ (1993) Diagnosis of food allergy in dogs. *J Am Vet Med Assoc* **203**:259–262.

4 White SD, Sequoia DM (1989) Food hypersensitivity in cats – 14 cases (1982–1987). *J Am Vet Med Assoc* **194**:692–695.

5 Hill PB (1999) Diagnosing cutaneous food allergies in dogs and cats – some practical considerations. *In Pract* **21**:287–294.

6 Chesney CJ (2001) Systematic review of evidence for the prevalence of food sensitivity in dogs. *Vet Rec* **148**:445–448.

7 Chesney CJ (2002) Food sensitivity in the dog: a quantitative study. *J Small Anim Pract* **43**:203–207.

8 Bourdeau P, Fer G (2004) Characteristics of the 10 most frequent feline skin disease conditions seen in the dermatology clinic at the National Veterinary School of Nantes. *Vet Dermatol* **15**:63.

9 Martin A, Sierra MP, Gonzalez JL *et al.* (2004) Identification of allergens responsible for canine cutaneous adverse food reactions to lamb, beef and cow's milk. *Vet Dermatol* **15**:349–356.

10 Paterson S (1995) Food hypersensitivity in 20 dogs with skin and gastrointestinal signs. *J Small Anim Pract* **36**:529–534.

11 Jackson HA, Jackson MW, Coblentz L *et al.* (2003) Evaluation of the clinical and allergen specific serum immunoglobulin E responses to oral challenge with cornstarch, corn, soy and a soy hydrolysate diet in dogs with spontaneous food allergy. *Vet Dermatol* **14**:181–187.

12 Bensignor E, Germain PA (2004) Canine recurrent pyoderma: a multicenter prospective study. *Vet Dermatol* **15**:42.

13 Mueller RS, Friend S, Shipstone MA *et al*. (2000) Diagnosis of canine claw disease – a prospective study of 24 dogs. *Vet Dermatol* **11**:133–141.

14 Guilford WG, Markwell PJ, Jones BR *et al*. (1998) Prevalence and causes of food sensitivity in cats with chronic pruritus, vomiting or diarrhea. *J Nutr* **128**:2790–2791.

15 Loeffler A, Lloyd DH, Bond R *et al*. (2004) Dietary trials with a commercial chicken hydrolysate diet in 63 pruritic dogs. *Vet Rec* **154**:519–522.

16 Foster AP, Knowles TG, Moore AH *et al*. (2003) Serum IgE and IgG responses to food antigens in normal and atopic dogs, and dogs with gastrointestinal disease. *Vet Immunol Immunopathol* **92**:113–124.

Allergic and irritant contact dermatitis

1 White PD (1991) Contact dermatitis in the dog and the cat. *Semin Vet Med Surg (Small Animal)* **6**:303–315.

2 Olivry T, Prelaud P, Heripret D *et al*. (1990) Allergic contact dermatitis in the dog: principles and diagnosis. *Vet Clin North Am: Small Anim Pract* **20**:1443–1456.

3 Thomsen MK, Kristensen F (1986) Contact dermatitis in the dog: a review and clinical study. *Nordisk Veterinaer Medicin* **38**:129–134.

4 Kunkle GA, Gross TL (1983) Allergic contact dermatitis to *Tradescantia fluminensis* (Wandering Jew) in a dog. *Compend Cont Educ Pract Vet* **5**:925–930.

5 Nesbitt GH, Schmitz JA (1977) Contact dermatitis in dogs: a review of 35 cases. *J Am Anim Hosp Assoc* **13**:155–163.

6 Grant DI, Thoday KL (1980) Canine allergic contact dermatitis: clinical review. *J Small Anim Pract* **21**:17–27.

7 Kimura T (2007) Contact hypersensitivity to stainless steel cages (chromium metal) in hairless descendants of Mexican hairless dogs. *Environ Toxic* **22**:176–184.

8 Nuttall TJ, Cole LK (2004) Ear cleaning: the UK and US perspective. *Vet Dermatol* **15**:127–136.

9 Bensignor E (2002) Sensitisation to the contact of prednisolone in a Golden Retriever. *Prat Med Chir Anim* **37**:141–146.

10 Thomsen MK, Thomsen HK (1989) Histopathological changes in canine allergic contact dermatitis patch test reactions: a study on spontaneously hypersensitive dogs. *Acta Vet Scand* **30**:379–386.

11 Marsella R, Kunkle GA, Lewis DT (1997) Use of pentoxifylline in the treatment of allergic contact reactions to plants of the Commelinceae family in dogs. *Vet Dermatol* **8**:121–126.

Flea bite hypersensitivity
(flea allergic dermatitis)

1 Lee SE, Johnstone IP, Lee RP *et al*. (1999) Putative salivary allergens of the cat flea, *Ctenocephalides felis felis*. *Vet Immunol Immunopathol* **69**:229–237.

2 Lewis DT, Ginn PE, Kunkle GA (1999) Clinical and histological evidence of immediate and delayed antigen intradermal skin test and flea bite sites in normal and flea allergic cats. *Vet Dermatol* **10**:29–37.

3 Scott DW, Miller WH, Griffin CE (2001) Parasitic skin diseases. In *Muller and Kirk's Small Animal Dermatology*, 6th edn. WB Saunders, Philadelphia, pp. 423–516.

4 Shaw SE, Kenny MJ, Tasker S *et al*. (2004) Pathogen carriage by the cat flea *Ctenocephalides felis* (Bouche) in the United Kingdom. *Vet Microbiol* **102**:183–188.

5 Sousa CA, Halliwell RE (2001) The ACVD task force on canine atopic dermatitis (XI): the relationship between arthropod hypersensitivity and atopic dermatitis in the dog. *Vet Immunol Immunopathol* **81**:233–237.

6 Laffort-Dassot C, Carlotti DN, Pin D *et al*. (2004) Diagnosis of flea allergy dermatitis: comparison of intradermal testing with flea allergens and a Fc epsilon RI alpha-based IgE assay in response to flea control. *Vet Dermatol* **15**:321–330.

7 Foster AP, Littlewood JD, Webb P, *et al*. (2003) Comparison of intradermal and serum testing for allergen-specific IgE using a Fc epsilon RI alpha-based assay in atopic dogs in the UK. *Vet Immunol Immunopathol* **93**:51–60.

8 Garcia E, Halpert E, Rodriguez A *et al*. (2004) Immune and histopathologic examination of flea bite-induced papular urticaria. *Ann Allergy Asthma Immunol* **92**:446–452.

9 Beugnet F, Porphyre T, Sabatier P *et al*. (2004) Use of a mathematical model to study the dynamics of *Ctenocephalides felis* populations in the home environment and the impact of various control measures. *Parasite-Journal de la Societe Francaise de Parasitologie* **11**:387–399.

10 Rust MK (2005) Advances in the control of *Ctenocephalides felis* (cat flea) on cats and dogs. *Trends in Parasitology* **21**:232–236.

11 Bossard RL, Dryden MW, Broce AB (2002) Insecticide susceptibilities of cat fleas (Siphonaptera: Pulicidae) from several regions of the United States. *J Med Entomol* **39**:742–746.

12 Endris RG, Hair JA, Anderson G *et al*. (2003) Efficacy of two 65% permethrin spot-on formulations against induced infestations of *Ctenocephalides felis* (Insecta: Siphonaptera) and *Amblyomma americanum* (Acari: Ixodidae) on beagles. *Vet Ther* **4**:47–55.

13 Cadiergues MC, Caubet C, Franc M (2001) Comparison of the activity of selamectin, imidacloprid and fipronil for the treatment of dogs infested experimentally with *Ctenocephalides canis* and *Ctenocephalides felis felis*. *Vet Rec* **149**:704–706.

14 Dryden MW, Perez HR, Ulitchny DM (1999) Control of fleas on pets and in homes by use of imidacloprid or lufenuron and a pyrethrin spray. *J Am Vet Med Assoc* **1**:36–39.

15 Dryden MW, Smith V, Payne PA *et al*. (2005) Comparative speed of kill of selamectin, imidacloprid, and fipronil-(S)-methoprene spot-on formulations against fleas on cats. *Vet Ther* **6**:228–236.

16 Young DR, Jeannin PC, Boeckh A (2004) Efficacy of fipronil/(S)-methoprene combination spot-on for dogs against shed eggs, emerging and existing adult cat fleas (*Ctenocephalides felis*, Bouche). *Vet Parasitol* **125**:397–407.

17 Rust MK, Waggoner MM, Hinkle NC *et al*. (2003) Efficacy and longevity of nitenpyram against adult cat fleas (Siphonaptera: Pulicidae). *J Med Entomol* **40**:678–681.

18 Ibrahim MA, Kainulainen P, Aflatuni A *et al*. (2001) Insecticidal, repellent, antimicrobial activity and phytotoxicity of essential oils: with special reference to limonene and its suitability for control of insect pests. *Agricultural and Food Science in Finland* **10**:243–259.

19 Cadiergues MC, Steffan J, Tinembart O *et al*. (1999) Efficacy of an adulticide used alone or in combination with an insect growth regulator for flea infestations of dogs housed in simulated home environments. *Am J Vet Res* **60(9)**:1122–1125.

20 Maynard L, Houffschmitt P, Lebreux B (2001) Field efficacy of a 10 per cent pyriproxyfen spot-on for the prevention of flea infestations on cats. *J Small Anim Pract* **42**:491–494.

Pediculosis

1 Scott DW, Miller WH , Griffin CE (2001) Skin diseases. In *Muller and Kirk's Small Animal Dermatology*, 6th edn. WB Saunders, Philadelphia, pp. 423–516.

2 Mencke N, Larsen KS, Eydal M *et al*. (2005) Dermatological and parasitological evaluation of infestations with chewing lice (*Werneckiella equi*) on horses and treatment using imidacloprid. *Parasitol Res* **97**:7–12.

3 Pollmeier M, Pengo G, Longo M *et al*. (2004) Effective treatment and control of biting lice, *Felicola subrostratus* (Nitzsch in Burmeister, 1838), on cats using fipronil formulations. *Vet Parasitol* **121**:157–165.

4 Pollmeier M, Pengo G, Jeannin P *et al*. (2002) Evaluation of the efficacy of fipronil formulations in the treatment and control of biting lice, *Trichodectes canis* (De Geer, 1778) on dogs. *Vet Parasitol* **107**:127–136.

5 Shanks DJ, Gautier R, McTier IL *et al*. (2003) Efficacy of selamectin against biting lice on dogs and cats. *Vet Rec* **152**:234.

Sarcoptic mange
(scabies, sarcoptic acariosis)

1 Bornstein S, Zakrisson G, Thebo P (1995) Clinical picture and antibody response to experimental *Sarcoptes scabiei* var *vulpes* infection in red foxes (*Vulpes vulpes*). *Acta Vet Scand* **36**:509–519.

2 Bornstein S, Zakrisson G (1993) Humoral antibody response to experimental *Sarcoptes scabiei* var. *vulpes* infection in the dog. *Vet Dermatol* **4**:107–110.

3 Mueller RS, Bettenay SV, Shipstone M (2001) Value of the pinnal-pedal reflex in the diagnosis of canine scabies. *Vet Rec* **148**:621–623.

4 Schumann RJ, Morgan MS, Glass R *et al*. (2002) Characterization of house dust mite and scabies allergens by the use of canine serum antibodies. *Am J Vet Res* **62**:1344–1348.

5 Curtis CF (2001) Evaluation of a commercially available enzyme-linked immunosorbent assay for the diagnosis of canine sarcoptic mange. *Vet Rec* **148**:238–239.

6 Curtis CF (2004) Current trends in the treatment of *Sarcoptes*, *Cheyletiella* and *Otodectes* mite infestations in dogs and cats. *Vet Dermatol* **15**:108–114.

Notoedric mange

1 Scott DW, Horn RT (1987) Zoonotic dermatoses of dogs and cats. *Vet Clin North Am: Small Anim Pract* **17**:117–144.

2 Delucchi L, Castro E (2000) Use of doramectin for treatment of notoedric mange in five cats. *J Am Vet Med Assoc* **216**:215–216.

Cheyletiella spp. infestation (cheyletiellosis)

1 Alexander MA, Ihrke PJ (1982) *Cheyletiella* dermatitis in small animal practice: a review. *Californian Vet* **36**:9–12.

2 Cohen SR (1980) *Cheyletiella* dermatitis (in rabbit, cat, dog, man). *Arch Dermatol* **116**:435–437.

3 Scott DW, Horne RT (1987) Zoonotic dermatoses of dogs and cats. *Vet Clin North Am: Small Anim Pract* **21**:535–541.

4 McKeever PJ, Allen SK (1979) Dermatitis associated with *Cheyletiella* infestation in cats. *J Am Vet Med Assoc* **174**:718–720.

5 Ottenschott TRF, Gil D (1978) Cheyletiellosis in long-haired cats. *Tijdschrift voor Diergeneeskunde* **103**:1104–1108.

6 Chadwick AJ (1997) Use of a 0.25 per cent fipronil pump spray formulation to treat canine cheyletiellosis. *J Small Anim Pract* **38**:261–262.

7 Bourdeau P, Lecanu JM (1999) Treatment of multiple infestations with *Otodectes cynotis*, *Cheyletiella yasguri* and *Trichodectes canis* with fipronil (Frontline Spot-on: Merial) in the dog. In *Proceedings of the Autumn Meeting of the British Veterinary Dermatology Study Group*, Bristol, pp. 35–36.

Harvest mite infestation

1 Greene RT, Scheidt VJ, Moncol DJ (1986) Trombiculiasis in a cat. *J Am Vet Med Assoc* **188**:1054–1055.

2 Nuttall TJ, French AT, Cheetman HC *et al*. (1998) Treatment of *Trombicula autmnalis* infestation in dogs and cats with 0.25 per cent fipronil pump spray. *J Small Anim Pract* **39**:237–239.

3 Famose F (1995) Efficacy of fipronil (Frontline) spray in the prevention of natural infestation by *Trombicula autumnalis* in dogs. In *Proceedings of the Royal Veterinary College Seminar – Ectoparasites and Their Control*, London, pp. 28–30.

Pelodera strongyloides dermatitis

1 Nesbitt GH (1983) Parasitic diseases. In *Canine and Feline Dermatology: A Systematic Approach*. Lea & Febiger, Philadelphia, p. 77.

2 Willers WB (1970) *Pelodera strongyloides* in association with canine dermatitis in Wisconsin. *J Am Vet Med Assoc* **156**:319–320.

Ancylostomiasis (hookworm dermatitis)

1 Bowman DD (1992) Hookworm parasites of dogs and cats. *Compend Cont Educ Pract Vet* **14**:585–593.

2 Scott DW, Miller WH, Griffin CE (1995) Parasitic skin diseases. In *Muller and Kirk's Small Animal Dermatology*, 5th edn. WB Saunders, Philadelphia, pp. 393–395.

3 Buelke DL (1971) Hookworm dermatitis. *J Am Vet Med Assoc* **158**:735–739.

4 Baker KP (1979) Clinical aspects of hookworm dermatitis. *Vet Dermatol* (Newsletter) **6**:69–74.

Malassezia dermatitis

1 Bond R, Ferguson EA, Curtis CF *et al*. (1996) Factors associated with elevated cutaneous *Malassezia pachydermatis* populations in dogs with pruritic skin disease. *J Small Anim Pract* **37**:103–107.

2 Akerstedt J, Vollset I (1996) *Malassezia pachydermatis* with special reference to canine skin disease. *B Vet J* **152**:269–281.

3 Nardoni S, Mancianti F, Corazza M *et al*. (2004) Occurrence of *Malassezia* species in healthy and dermatologically diseased dogs. *Mycopathologia* **157**:383–388.

4 Bensignor E, Weill FX, Couprie B (1999) Population sizes and frequency of isolation of *Malassezia* yeasts from healthy pet cats. *Journal de Mycologie Medicale* **9**:158–161.

5 Raabe P, Mayser P, Weiss R (1998) Demonstration of *Malassezia furfur* and *M. sympodialis* together with *M. pachydermatis* in veterinary specimens. *Mycoses* **41**:493–500.

6 Mason KV, Evans AG (1991) Dermatitis associated with *Malassezia pachydermatis* in 11 dogs. *J Am Anim Hosp Assoc* **27**:13–20.

7 Mauldin EA, Morris DO, Goldschmidt MH (2002) Retrospective study: the presence of *Malassezia* in feline skin biopsies. A clinicopathological study. *Vet Dermatol* **13**:7–13.

8 Bond R, Collin NS, Lloyd DH (1994) Use of contact plates for the quantitative culture of *Malassezia pachydermatis* from canine skin. *J Small Anim Pract* **35**:68–72.

9 Chen TA, Halliwell REW, Pemberton AD *et al*. (2002) Identification of major allergens of *Malassezia pachydermatis* in dogs with atopic dermatitis and *Malassezia* overgrowth. *Vet Dermatol* **13**:141–150.

10 Nuttall TJ, Halliwell REW (2001) Serum antibodies to *Malassezia* yeasts in canine atopic dermatitis. *Vet Dermatol* **12**:327–332.

11 Morris DO, DeBoer DJ (2003) Evaluation of serum obtained from atopic dogs with dermatitis attributable to *Malassezia pachydermatis* for passive transfer of immediate hypersensitivity to that organism. *Am J Vet Res* **64**:262–266.

12 Farver K, Morris DO, Shofer F *et al*. (2005) Humoral measurement of type-1 hypersensitivity reactions to a commercial *Malassezia* allergen. *Vet Dermatol* **16**:261–268.

13 Bensignor E (2001) An open trial to compare two dosages of ketoconazole in the treatment of *Malassezia* dermatitis in dogs. *Annales de Medecine Veterinaire* **145**:311–315.

14 Guillot J, Bensignor E, Jankowski F *et al*. (2003) Comparative efficacies of oral ketoconazole and terbinafine for reducing *Malassezia* population sizes on the skin of Basset Hounds. *Vet Dermatol* **14**:153–157.

15 Morris DO, O'Shea K, Shofer FS *et al*. (2005) *Malassezia pachydermatis* carriage in dog owners. *Emerg Infect Dis* **11**:83–88.

16 Fan YM, Huang WM, Li SF *et al*. (2006) Granulomatous skin infection caused by *Malassezia pachydermatis* in a dog owner. *Arch Dermatol* **142**:1181–1184.

17 Chang HJ, Miller HL, Watkins N *et al*. (1998) An epidemic of *Malassezia pachydermatis* in an intensive care nursery associated with colonization of health care workers pet dogs. *New Engl J Med* **338**:706–711.

Epitheliotropic lymphoma
(cutaneous T cell lymphoma, mycosis fungoides)

1 Baker JL, Scott DW (1989) Mycosis fungoides in two cats. *J Am Anim Hosp Assoc* **25**:97–101.

2 DeBoer DJ, Turrel JM, Moore PF (1990) Mycosis fungoides in a dog: demonstration of T cell specificity and response to radiotherapy. *J Am Anim Hosp Assoc* **26**:566–572.

3 Burg G, Dummer R, Haeffner A *et al*. (2001) From inflammation to neoplasia: mycosis fungoides evolves from reactive inflammatory conditions (lymphocytic infiltrates) transforming into neoplastic plaques and tumors. *Arch Dermatol* **137**:949–952.

4 Santoro D, Marsella R, Hernandez J (2007) Investigation on the association between atopic dermatitis and the development of mycosis fungoides in dogs: a retrospective case control study. *Vet Dermatol* **18**:101–106.

5 Moore PF, Olivry T, Naydan D (1994) Canine cutaneous epitheliotropic lymphoma (mycosis fungoides) is a proliferative disorder of CD8+ T cells. *Am J Pathol* **144**:421–429.

6 Walton DK (1986) Canine epidermotropic lymphoma. In *Current Veterinary Therapy IX* (ed RW Kirk). WB Saunders, Philadelphia, pp. 609–614.

7 Wilcock BP, Yager JA (1989) The behavior of epidermotropic lymphoma in twenty-five dogs. *Can Vet J* **30**:754–756.

8 Scott DW, Miller WH, Griffin CE (2001) Neoplastic and non-neoplastic tumors. In *Small Animal Dermatology*, 6th edn. WB Saunders, Philadelphia, pp. 1333–1338.

9 Petersen A, Wood S, Rosser E (1999) The use of safflower oil for the treatment of mycosis fungoides in two dogs. In *Proceedings of the Annual Meeting of the American Academy of Veterinary Dermatologists/American College of Veterinary Dermatology*, Maui, p. 49.

10 White SD, Rosychuk AW, Scott KV *et al*. (1993) Use of isotretinoin and etretinate for the treatment of benign cutaneous neoplasia and cutaneous lymphoma in dogs. *J Am Vet Med Assoc* **202**:387–391.

11 Kwochka KW (1989) Retinoids in dermatology. In *Current Veterinary Therapy X* (ed RW Kirk). WB Saunders, Philadelphia, pp. 553–563.

12 Williams LE, Rassnick KM, Power HT *et al*. (2006) CCNU in the treatment of canine epitheliotropic lymphoma. *J Vet Intern Med* **20**:136–143.

Acral lick dermatitis

1 Shanley K, Overall K (1992) Psychogenic dermatoses. In *Current Veterinary Therapy*, *XI* (eds RW Kirk, JD Bonagura). W B Saunders, Philadelphia, pp. 552–558.

2 Virga V (2003) Behavioral dermatology. *Vet Clin North Am: Small Anim Pract* **317**:231–251.

3 Schwartz S (1993) Naltrexone-induced pruritus in a dog with tail chasing behavior. *J Am Anim Hosp Assoc* **202**:278–280.

4 Denerolle P, White S, Taylor TS *et al*. (2007) Organic diseases mimicking acral lick dermatitis in six dogs. *J Am Anim Hosp Assoc* **43**:215–220.

5 Paterson S, Midgley D, Barclay I (2007) Canine acral lick dermatitis. *In Pract* **29**:328–332.

6 Walton DK (1986) Psychodermatoses. In *Current Veterinary Therapy IX* (ed RW Kirk). WB Saunders, Philadephia, pp. 557–559.

7 White SD (1990) Naltrexone for treatment of acral lick dermatitis in dogs. *J Am Vet Med Assoc* **196**:1073–1076.

8 Rusbridge C, Greitz D, Iskandar BJ (2006) Syringomyelia: current concepts in pathogenesis, diagnosis and treatment. *J Vet Intern Med* **20**:469–479.

9 Dodman NH, Shuster L, White SD *et al*. (1988) Use of narcotic antagonists to modify stereotypic self-licking, self-chewing, and scratching behavior in dogs. *J Am Vet Med Assoc* **193**:815–819.

10 Dodman NH, Shuster L, Nesbitt G *et al*. (2004) The use of dextromethorphan to treat repetitive self-directed scratching, biting, or chewing in dogs with allergic dermatitis. *J Vet Pharmacol Ther* **27**:99–104.

11 Gaultier E, Bonnafous L, Bougrat L *et al.* (2005) Comparison of the efficacy of a synthetic dog-appeasing pheromone with clomipramine for the treatment of separation-related disorders in dogs. *Vet Rec* **156**:533.

12 Holt TL, Mann FA (2002) Soft tissue application of lasers. *Vet Clin North Am: Small Anim Pract* **32**:535–547.

13 Rusbridge C, Jeffery ND (2008) Pathophysiology and treatment of neuropathic pain associated with syringomyelia. *Vet J* **175**:164–172.

Schnauzer comedo syndrome

1 Scott DW, Miller WH, Griffin CE (2001) Congenital and hereditary defects. In *Muller and Kirk's Small Animal Dermatology*, 6th edn. WB Saunders, Philadelphia, pp. 913–1003.

2 Hannigan MM (1997) A refractory case of schnauzer comedo syndrome. *Can Vet J* **38**:238–239.

Feline psychogenic alopecia

1 Virga V (2003) Behavioral dermatology. *Vet Clin North Am: Small Anim Pract* **317**:231–251.

2 Waisglass SE, Landsberg GM, Yager JA *et al.* (2006) Underlying medical conditions in cats with presumptive psychogenic alopecia. *J Am Vet Med Assoc* **228**:1705–1709.

CHAPTER 2: NODULAR DERMATOSES

Epidermal and follicular inclusion cysts

1 Goldschmidt MH, Hendrick MH (2007) Tumors of the skin and soft tissues. In *Tumors of Domestic Animals* (ed DE Meuten). Iowa State Press, Ames, pp. 45–117.

2 Scott DW, Miller WH, Griffin CE (2001) Neoplastic and non-neoplastic tumors. In *Muller and Kirk's Small Animal Dermatology*, 6th edn. WB Saunders, Philadelphia, pp. 1236–1414.

Infundibular keratinizing acanthoma

1 Scott DW, Miller WH, Griffin CE (1995) Neoplastic and non-neoplastic tumors. In *Muller and Kirk's Small Animal Dermatology*, 5th edn. WB Saunders, Philadelphia, pp. 999–1001.

2 Goldschmidt MH, Shofer FS (1992) Intracutaneous cornifying epithelioma. In *Skin Tumors of the Dog and Cat*. Pergamon Press, New York, pp. 109–114.

3 Gross TL, Ihrke PJ, Walder EJ (1992) Follicular tumors. In *Veterinary Dermatopathology*. Mosby Year Book, St. Louis, pp. 361–363.

4 Stannard AA, Pulley LT (1975) Intracutaneous cornifying epithelioma (keratoacanthoma) in the dog: a retrospective of 25 cases. *J Am Vet Med Assoc* **167**:385–388.

5 White SD, Rosychuk RAW, Scott KV *et al.* (1995) Sebaceous adenitis in dogs and results of treatment with isotretinoin and etretinate – 30 cases (1990–1994). *J Am Vet Med Assoc* **207**:197–200.

6 White SD, Rosychuk RAW, Scott KV *et al.* (1993) Use of isotretinoin and etretinate for the treatment of benign cutaneous neoplasia and cutaneous lymphoma in dogs. *J Am Vet Med Assoc* **202**:387–391.

7 Henfrey JI (1991) Treatment of multiple intra-cutaneous cornifying epitheliomata using isotretinoin. *J Small Anim Pract* **32**:363–365.

8 Scott DW, Miller WH, Griffin CE (1995) Dermatologic therapy. In *Muller and Kirk's Small Animal Dermatology*, 5th edn. WB Saunders, Philadelphia, pp. 238–240.

Papillomatosis

1 Goldschmidt MH, Shofer FS (1992) Cutaneous papillomas. In *Skin Tumors of the Dog and Cat*. Pergamon Press, New York, pp. 11–15.

2 Gross TL, Ihrke PJ, Walder EJ (1992) Epidermal tumors. In *Veterinary Dermatopathology*. Mosby Year Book, St. Louis, pp. 334–336.

3 Scott DW, Miller WH, Griffin CE (1995) Neoplastic and non-neoplastic tumors. In *Small Animal Dermatology*, 5th edn. WB Saunders, Philadelphia, pp. 994–997.

4 Sansom J, Barnett KC, Blunden AS *et al.* (1996) Canine conjunctival papilloma: a review of five cases. *J Small Anim Pract* **37**:84–86.

5 Nagata M, Nanko H, Moriyama A *et al.* (1995) Pigmented plaques associated with papillomavirus infection in dogs: is this epidermodysplasia verruciformis? *Vet Dermatol* **6**:179–186.

6 Watrach AM, Small E, Case MT (1970) Canine papillomas: progression of oral papilloma to carci-noma. *J Nat Cancer Inst* **45**:915–920.

7 Bergman CL, Hirth RS, Sundberg JP *et al.* (1987) Cutaneous neoplasia in dogs associated with canine papillomavirus vaccine. *Vet Pathol* **24**:477–487.

8 Foster AP (2004) Immunomodulation and immunodeficiency. *Vet Derm* **15**:115–126..

Mast cell neoplasia

1 Scott DW, Miller WH, Griffin CE (2001) Neoplastic and non-neoplastic tumors. In *Muller and Kirk's Small Animal Dermatology*, 6th edn. WB Saunders, Philadelphia, pp. 1236–1414.

2 Tyrell D, Davis RM (2001) Progressive neurological signs associated with systemic mastocytosis in a dog. *Austr Vet J* **79**:106–108.

3 Lepri E, Ricci G, Leonardi L *et al*. (2003) Diagnostic and prognostic features of feline cutaneous mast cell tumours: a retrospective analysis of 40 cases. *Vet Res Comm* **27**:707–709.

4 Elmslie R (2002) Mast cell tumours. In *The 5-minute Veterinary Consult: Small Animal Dermatology* (ed K Helton Rhodes). Lippincott Williams and Wilkins, Philadelphia, pp. 464–470.

5 Baker-Gabb M, Hunt GB, France MP (2003) Soft tissue sarcomas and mast cell tumours in dogs; clinical behaviour and response to surgery. *Austr Vet J* **81**:732–738.

6 Johnson TO, Schulman FY, Lipscomb TP *et al*. (2002) Histopathology and biologic behavior of pleomorphic cutaneous mast cell tumors in fifteen cats. *Vet Pathol* **39**:452–457.

7 Molander-McCrary H, Henry CJ, Potter K *et al*. (1998) Cutaneous mast cell tumors in cats: 32 cases (1991–1994). *J Am Anim Hosp Assoc* **34**:281–284.

8 Weisse C, Shofer FS, Sorenmo K (2002) Recurrence rates and sites for grade II canine cutaneous mast cell tumors following complete surgical excision. *J Am Anim Hosp Assoc* **38**:71–73.

9 Gerritsen RJ, Teske E, Kraus JS *et al*. (1998) Multi-agent chemotherapy for mast cell tumours in the dog. *Vet Quart* **20**:28–31.

10 LaDue T, Price GS, Dodge R *et al*. (1998) Radiation therapy for incompletely resected canine mast cell tumors. *Vet Radiol Ultrasound* **39**:57–62.

11 Misdorp W (2004) Mast cells and canine mast cell tumours. A review. *Vet Quart* **26**:156–169.

12 Moore AS (2002) Radiation therapy for the treatment of tumours in small companion animals. *Vet J* **164**:176–187.

13 Chaffin K, Thrall DE (2002) Results of radiation therapy in 19 dogs with cutaneous mast cell tumor and regional lymph node metastasis. *Vet Radiol Ultrasound* **43**:392–395.

14 Jaffe MH, Hosgood G, Kerwin SC (2000) Deionised water as an adjunct to surgery for the treatment of canine cutaneous mast cell tumours. *J Small Anim Pract* **41**:7–11.

Melanocytic neoplasia

1 Gross TH, Ihrke PJ, Walder EJ, Affolter VK (2005) Melanocytic tumors. In *Skin Diseases of the Dog and Cat: Clinical and Histopathologic Diagnosis*, 2nd edn. Blackwell Publishing, Oxford, pp. 813–833.

2 Sober AJ (1991) Biology of malignant melanoma. In *Pathophysiology of Dermatologic Diseases* (eds NA Soter, HP Baden). McGraw-Hill, New York, pp. 515–528.

3 Bostock DE (1979) Prognosis after surgical excision of canine melanomas. *Vet Pathol* **16**:32–40.

4 Aronsohn MG, Carpenter JL (1990) Distal extremity melanocytic nevi and malignant melanoma in dogs. *J Am Anim Hosp Assoc* **26**:605–612.

5 Goldschmidt MH, Liu SMS, Shofer FS (1993) Feline dermal melanoma. In *Advances in Veterinary Dermatology* (eds PJ Ihrke, IS Mason, SD White). Pergamon Press, Oxford, pp. 285–291.

6 Scott DW (1987) Lentigo simplex in orange cats. *Companion Anim Pract* **1**:23–25.

7 Conroy JD (1983) Canine skin tumors. *J Am Anim Hosp Assoc* **19**:91–114.

8 Goldschmidt MH, Shofer FS (1992) *Skin Tumors of the Dog and Cat*. Pergamon Press, Oxford, pp. 2–3, 142–151.

9 Carpenter JL, Andrew LK, Holzworth J (1987) Tumors and tumor-like lesions. In: *Diseases of the Cat* (ed J Holzworth). WB Saunders, Philadelphia, pp. 408, 579–583.

10 Richardson RC, Rebar AH, Elliott GS (1984) Common skin tumors of the dog: a clinical approach to diagnosis and treatment. *Comp Contin Ed Pract Vet* **6**:1080–1085.

Basal cell carcinoma (basal cell epithelioma)

1 Gross TH, Ihrke PJ, Walder EJ, Affolter VK (2005) Epithelial neoplasms and other tumors. In *Skin Diseases of the Dog and Cat: Clinical and Histopathologic Diagnosis*, 2nd edn. Blackwell Publishing, Oxford, pp. 589–591.

2 Miller SJ (1991) Biology of basal cell carcinoma. *J Am Acad Dermatol* **24**:161–175.

3 Miller MA, Nelson SL, Turk JR *et al*. (1991) Cutaneous neoplasia in 340 cats. *Vet Pathol* **28**:389–395.

4 Macy DW, Reynolds HA (1981) The incidence, characteristics, and clinical management of skin tumors of cats. *J Am Anim Hosp Assoc* **17**:1026–1034.

5 Goldschmidt MH, Shofer FS (1992) *Skin Tumors of the Dog and Cat*. Pergamon Press, Oxford, pp. 29–32.

6 Rothwell TLW, Howlett CR, Middleton DJ *et al.* (1987) Skin neoplasms of dogs in Sydney. *Austr Vet J* **64**:161–164.

7 Barton CL (1987) Cytological diagnosis of cutaneous neoplasia: an algorithmic approach. *Comp Cont Ed Pract Vet* **9**:20–33.

Collagenous nevi

1 Scott DW, Yager Johnson JA, Manning TO *et al.* (1984) Nevi in the dog. *J Am Anim Hosp Assoc* **20**:505–512.

2 Jones BR, Alley MR, Craig AS (1985) Cutaneous collagen nodules in a dog. *J Small Anim Pract* **26**:445–451.

3 Fox JG, Snyder SB, Campbell LH (1973) Connective tissue nevus in a dog. *Vet Pathol* **10**:65–68.

Canine eosinophilic granuloma

1 Curial da Silva JMA, Kraus KH, Brown TP *et al.* (1998) Eosinophilic granuloma of the nasal skin in a dog. *J Am Anim Hosp Assoc* **20**:603–606.

2 Gross TH, Ihrke PJ, Walder EJ, Affolter VK (2005) Canine eosinophilic granuloma. In *Skin Diseases of the Dog and Cat: Clinical and Histopathologic Diagnosis*, 2nd edn. Blackwell Publishing, Oxford, pp. 358–360.

3 Madewell BR, Stannard AA, Pulley LT *et al.* (1980) Oral eosinophilic granuloma in Siberian husky dogs. *J Am Vet Med Assoc* **177**:701–703.

4 Norris JM (1994) Cutaneous eosinophilic granuloma in a crossbred dog: a case report and literature review. *Aust Pract* **24**:74–78.

5 Potter KA, Tucker RD, Carpenter JL (1980) Oral eosinophilic granuloma of Siberian huskies. *J Am Anim Hosp Assoc* **16**:595–600.

6 Scott DW (1988) Cutaneous eosinophilic granulomas with collagen degeneration in the dog. *J Am Anim Hosp Assoc* **19**:529–532.

7 Turnwald GH, Hoskins JD, Taylor HW (1981) Cutaneous eosinophilic granuloma in a Labrador retriever. *J Am Vet Med Assoc* **179**:799–801.

8 Walsh KM (1983) Oral eosinophilic granuloma in two dogs. *J Am Vet Med Assoc* **183**:323–324.

Sterile granuloma and pyogranuloma syndrome

1 Houston DM, Clark EG, Matwichuk CL *et al.* (1993) A case of cutaneous sterile pyogranuloma/granuloma syndrome in a golden retriever. *Can Vet J* **34**:121–122.

2 Gross TH, Ihrke PJ, Walder EJ, Affolter VK (2005) Sterile granuloma and pyogranuloma syndrome. In *Skin Diseases of the Dog and Cat: Clinical and Histopathologic Diagnosis*, 2nd edn. Blackwell Publishing, Oxford, pp. 320–323.

3 Panich R, Scott DW, Miller WH (1991) Canine cutaneous sterile pyogranuloma/granuloma syndrome: a retrospective analysis of 29 cases (1976–1988). *J Am Anim Hosp Assoc* **27**:519–528.

4 Cornegliani L, Fondevla D, Vercelli A *et al.* (2005) PCR detection of *Leishmania* and *Mycobacterium* organisms in canine cutaneous sterile pyogranuloma/granuloma syndrome (SPGS). *Vet Derm* **16**:235–238.

5 Scott DW, Buerger RG, Miller WH (1990) Idiopathic sterile granulomatous and pyogranulomatous dermatitis in cats. *Vet Dermatol* **1**:129–137.

6 Rothstien E, Scott DW, Riis RC (1997) Tetracycline and niacinamide for the treatment of sterile pyogranuloma/granuloma syndrome in a dog. *J Am Anim Hosp Assoc* **33**:540–543.

7 White SA, Rosychuk RAW, Renke IS *et al.* (1992) Use of tetracycline and niacinamide for the treatment of autoimmune skin disease in 31 dogs. *J Am Vet Med Assoc* **200**:1457–1500.

Histiocytic proliferative disorders

1 Affolter VK, Moore PF (2000) Canine cutaneous and systemic histiocytosis: reactive histiocytosis of dermal dendritic cells. *Am J Dermatopathol* **22**:40–48.

2 Moore PF, Schrenzel MD, Affolter VK *et al.* (1996) Canine cutaneous histiocytoma is an epidermotropic langerhans cell histiocytosis that expresses CD1 and specific beta(2)-integrin molecules. *Am J Pathol* **148**:1699–1708.

3 Ciobotaru E, Militaru M, Soare T *et al.* (2004) Canine cutaneous histiocytoma: morphology and morphometry. *Vet Dermatol* **15**:62.

4 Affolter VK, Moore PF (2002) Localized and disseminated histiocytic sarcoma of dendritic cell origin in dogs. *Vet Pathol* **39**:74–83.

5 Moore PF, Rosin A (1986) Malignant histiocytosis of Bernese Mountain Dogs. *Vet Pathol* **23**:1–10.

6 Padgett GA, Madewell BR, Keller ET *et al.* (1995) Inheritance of histiocytosis in Bernese Mountain Dogs. *J Small Anim Pract* **36**:93–98.

7 Schmidt ML, Rutteman GR, Vanniel MHF *et al.* (1993) Clinical and radiographic manifestations of canine malignant histiocytosis. *Vet Quart* **15**:117–120.

8 Day MJ, Lopatkin I, Lucke VM *et al.* (2000) Multiple cutaneous histiocytomas in a cat. *Vet Dermatol* **11**:305–310.

Panniculitis

1 Scott DW, Anderson WI (1988) Panniculitis in dogs and cats: a retrospective analysis of 78 cases. *J Am Anim Hosp Assoc* **24:**551–559.

2 Shanley KJ, Miller WH (1985) Panniculitis in the dog: a report of five cases. *J Am Anim Hosp Assoc* **21:**545–550.

3 Hendrick MJ, Dunagan CA (1991) Focal necrotizing granulomatous panniculitis associated with subcutaneous injection of rabies vaccine in cats and dogs: 10 cases (1988–1989). *J Am Vet Med Assoc* **198:**304–305.

4 Gross TL, Ihrke PJ, Walder EJ (1992) Diseases of the panniculus. In *Veterinary Dermatopathology*. Mosby Year Book, St. Louis, pp. 316–326.

5 Hagiwara MK, Guerra JL, Maeoka MRM (1986) Pansteatitis (yellow fat disease) in a cat. *Feline Pract* **16:**25–27.

6 Edgar TP, Furrow RD (1984) Idiopathic nodular panniculitis in a German Shepherd Dog. *J Am Anim Hosp Assoc* **20:**603–606.

7 Kunkle GA, White SD, Calderwood-Mays M *et al.* (1993) Focal metatarsal fistulas in five dogs. *J Am Vet Med Assoc* **202:**756–757.

8 Paterson S (1995) Sterile idiopathic pedal panniculitis in the German Shepherd Dog – clinical presentation and response to treatment of four cases. *J Small Anim Pract* **36:**498–501.

Cryptococcosis

1 Wolf AM, Troy GC (1995) Deep mycotic diseases. In *Textbook of Veterinary Internal Medicine* (eds SJ Ettinger, EC Feldman). WB Saunders, Philadelphia, pp. 439–462.

2 Ackerman L (1988) Feline cryptococcosis. *Comp Cont Ed Pract Vet* **10:**1049–1055.

3 Medleau L, Barsanti JA (1990) Cryptococcosis. In *Infectious Diseases of Dogs and Cats* (ed CE Green). WB Saunders, Philadelphia, pp. 687–695.

4 Medleau L, Hall EJ, Goldschmidt MH, Irby N (1995) Cutaneous cryptococcosis in three cats. *J Am Vet Med Assoc* **187:**169–170.

5 Legendre AM (1995) Antimycotic drug therapy. In *Current Veterinary Therapy XII* (ed JD Bonagura). WB Saunders, Philadelphia, pp. 327–331.

6 Medleau L, Jacobs GJ, Marks MA (1995) Itraconazole for the treatment of cryptococcosis in cats. *J Vet Int Med* **9:**39–42.

Phaeohyphomycosis

1 Odds FC, Arai T, Disalvo AF *et al.* (1992) Nomenclature of fungal diseases: a report and recommendations from a sub-committee of the International Society for Human and Animal Mycology (ISHAM). *J Med Vet Mycology* **30:**1–10.

2 Dhein CR, Leathers CW, Padhye AA *et al.* (1988) Phaeomycosis caused by *Alternaria alternata* in a cat. *J Am Vet Med Assoc* **193:**1101–1103.

3 Beale KM, Pinson D (1990) Phaeomycosis caused by two different species of *Curvularia* in two animals from the same household. *J Am Anim Hosp Assoc* **26:**67–70.

4 Attleburger MH (1980) Mycoses and mycosis-like diseases. In *Current Veterinary Therapy VII* (ed RW Kirk). WB Saunders, Philadelphia, pp. 1177–1180.

5 Fadok VA (1987) Granulomatous dermatitis in dogs and cats. *Semin Vet Med Surg (Small Anim)* **2:**186–194.

6 Kettlewell P, McGinnis MR, Wilkinson GT (1989) Phaeomycosis caused by *Exophiala spinifera* in two cats. *J Med Vet Mycology* **27:**257–264.

7 Abramo F, Bastelli F, Nardoni S *et al.* (2003) Case report: feline cutaneous phaeohyphomycosis due to *Cladophyalophora bantiana*. *J Feline Med Surg* **4:**157–163.

Cuterebra spp. infestation

1 Bowman DD, Lynn RC (1995) Arthropods. In *Georgis' Parasitology for Veterinarians*. WB Saunders, Philadelphia, pp. 29–31.

2 Hatziolos BC (1966) *Cuterebra* larva in the brain of a cat. *J Am Vet Med Assoc* **148:**787–792.

3 Hendrix CM, Cox NR, Clemans-Chevis CL *et al.* (1989) Aberrant intracranial myiasis caused by larval *Cuterebra* infection. *Comp Cont Ed Pract Vet* **11:**550–562.

4 Kazocos KR, Bright RM, Johnson KE *et al.* (1980) *Cuterebra* species as a cause of pharyngeal myiasis in cats. *J Am Anim Hosp Assoc* **16:**773–776.

Dracunculiasis

1 Giovengo SL (1993) Canine dracunculiasis. *Comp Cont Ed Pract Vet* **15:**726–729.

2 Scott DW, Miller WH, Griffin CE (1995) Parasitic skin diseases. In *Muller and Kirk's Small Animal Dermatology*, 5th edn. WB Saunders, Philadelphia, pp. 400–401.

Calcinosis circumscripta

1 Gross TH, Ihrke PJ, Walder EJ, Affolter VK (2005) Calcinosis circumscripta. In *Skin Diseases of the Dog and Cat: Clinical and Histopathologic Diagnosis*, 2nd edn. Blackwell Publishing, Oxford, pp. 378–380.

2 Scott DW, Buerger RG (1988) Idiopathic calcinosis circumscripta in the dog: a retrospective analysis of 130 cases. *J Am Anim Hosp Assoc* **24:**187–189.

3 Stampley A, Bellah JR (1990) Calcinosis circumscripta of the metacarpal pad in a dog. *J Am Vet Med Assoc* **196:**113–114.

CHAPTER 3: ULCERATIVE DERMATOSES

German Shepherd Dog pyoderma

1 Wisselink MA, Willemse A, Koeman JP (1985) Deep pyoderma in the German Shepherd dog. *J Am Anim Hosp Assoc* **21:**773–776.

2 Wisselink MA, Bouw J, Drweduwen SA *et al*. (1989) German Shepherd Dog pyoderma: a genetic disorder. *Vet Quart* **11:**161–164.

3 Rosser EJ (2006) German shepherd dog pyoderma. *Vet Clin North Am: Small Anim Pract* **36:**203–214.

4 Rosser EJ (1998) German shepherd pyoderma. *Compend Cont Educ Pract Vet* **20:**831–839.

5 Wisselink MA, Koeman JP, van den Ingh TSGA *et al*. (1990) Investigations on the role of flea antigen in the pathogenesis of German Shepherd dog pyoderma (GSP). *Vet Quart* **12:**21–28.

6 Wisselink MA, Koeman JP, van den Ingh TSGA *et al*. (1990) Investigations on the role of staphylococci in the pathogenesis of German Shepherd dog pyoderma (GSP). *Vet Quart* **12:**29–34.

7 Day MJ (1994) An immunopathological study of deep pyoderma in the dog. *Res Vet Sci* **56:**18–23.

8 Day MJ, Mazza G (1995) Tissue immunoglobulin G subclasses observed in immune mediated dermatopathy, pyoderma and hypersensitivity dermatitis in dogs. *Res Vet Sci* **58:**82–89.

9 Denerolle P, Bourdoiseau G, Magnol JP *et al*. (1998) German Shepherd dog pyoderma: a prospective study of 23 cases. *Vet Dermatol* **9:**243–248.

10 Wisselink MA, Bernadina WE, Willemse A *et al*. (1988) Immunological aspects of German Shepherd Dog pyoderma (GSP). *Vet Immunol Immunopathol* **19:**67–77.

11 Chabanne L, Marchal T, Denerolle P *et al*. (995) Lymphocyte subset abnormalities in German Shepherd dog pyoderma (GSP). *Vet Immunol Immunopathol* **49:**189–198.

12 Koch HJ, Peters S (1996) Antimicrobial therapy in German Shepherd dog pyoderma (GSP). An open clinical study. *Vet Dermatol* **7:**177–181.

13 Bell A (1995) Prophylaxis of German Shepherd dog recurrent furunculosis (German Shepherd dog pyoderma) using cephalexin pulse therapy. *Austr Vet Pract* **25:**30–36.

14 Carlotti DN, Jasmin P, Gardey L *et al*. (2004) Evaluation of cephalexin intermittent therapy (weekend therapy) in the control of recurrent idiopathic pyoderma in dogs: a randomized, double-blinded, placebo-controlled study. *Vet Dermatol* **15:**8–9.

Feline idiopathic ulcerative dermatosis

1 Medleau L, Hnilica KA (2006) Feline idiopathic ulcerative dermatosis. In *Small Animal Dermatology: a Color Atlas and Therapeutic Guide*. WB Saunders, Philadelphia, pp. 352–353.

2 Gross TH, Ihrke PJ, Walder EJ, Affolter VK (2005) Feline idiopathic ulcerative dermatosis. In *Skin Diseases of the Dog and Cat: Clinical and Histopathologic Diagnosis*, 2nd edn. Blackwell Publishing, Oxford, pp. 130–132.

3 Mason K, Robson DC (2002) Clinical pearls of wisdom: practice tips for skin cases. In *Advances in Veterinary Dermatology, Vol 3* (eds KL Thoday, CS Foil, R Bond). Blackwell Publishing, Oxford, pp. 254–265.

Feline eosinophilic granuloma complex

1 Scott DW, Miller WH, Griffin C (2001) Skin immune system and allergic skin disease. In: *Muller and Kirk's Small Animal Dermatology*, 6th edn. WB Saunders, Philadelphia, pp. 543–666.

2 Foster A (2003) Clinical approach to feline eosinophilic granuloma complex. *In Pract* **25:**2–10.

3 Bardagi M, Fondati A, Fondevila D *et al*. (2003) Ultrastructural study of cutaneous lesions in feline eosinophilic granuloma complex. *Vet Dermatol* **14:**297–303.

4 Wilkinson GT, Bate MJ (1984) A possible further clinical manifestation of the feline eosinophilic granuloma complex. *J Am Anim Hosp Assoc* **20:**325–331.

5 Leistra WHG, van Oost BA, Willemse T (2005) Non-pruritic granuloma in Norwegian Forest cats. *Vet Rec* **56:**575–577.

6 Mason KV, Evans AG (1991) Mosquito bite-caused eosinophilic dermatitis in cats. *J Am Vet Med Assoc* **198:**2086–2088.

7 Nagata M, Ishida T (1997) Cutaneous reactivity to mosquito bites and its antigens in cats. *Vet Dermatol* **8:**19–26.

8 Noli C, Scarampella F (2006) Prospective open pilot study on the use of ciclosporin for feline allergic skin disease. *J Small Anim Pract* **47**:434–438.

9 Last RD, Suzuki Y, Manning T *et al.* (2004) A case of fatal systemic toxoplasmosis in a cat being treated with cyclosporin A for feline atopy. *Vet Dermatol* **15**:194–198.

Drug eruptions

1 Mason KV (1990) Cutaneous drug eruptions. *Vet Clin North Am: Small Anim Pract* **20**:1633–1653.

2 Medleau L, Shanley KJ, Rakich PM *et al.* (1999) Trimethoprim sulfonamide associated drug eruptions in dogs. *J Am Anim Hosp Assoc* **26**:305–311.

3 Trepanier LA (1999) Delayed hypersensitivity reactions to sulphonamides: syndromes, pathogenesis and management. *Vet Dermatol* **10**:241–248.

4 Trepanier LA, Danhof R, Toll J *et al.* (2003) Clinical findings in 40 dogs with hypersensitivity associated with administration of potentiated sulfonamides. *J Vet Int Med* **17**:647–652.

5 Papadogiannakis EI (2000) Cutaneous adverse drug reactions in the dog and cat. *Eur J Companion Anim Pract* **10**:71–77.

6 Hinn AC, Olivry T, Luther PB *et al.* (1998) Erythema multiforme, Stevens–Johnson syndrome and toxic epidermal necrolysis in the dog: classification, drug exposure and histopathological correlations. *J Vet Allergy Clin Immunol* **6**:13–20.

7 Nuttall TJ, Burrow R, Fraser I *et al.* (2004) Thrombovascular pinnal necrosis in a dog caused by fenbendazole administration. *J Small Anim Pract* **46**:243–246.

8 Nuttall TJ, Mallam T (2004) Successful intravenous human immunoglobulin treatment of drug-induced Stevens–Johnson syndrome in a dog. *J Small Anim Pract* **45**:357–361.

9 Mellor PJ, Roulois AJA, Day MJ *et al.* (2005) Neutrophilic dermatitis and immune-mediated haematological disorders in a dog: suspected adverse reaction to carprofen. *J Small Anim Pract* **46**:237–242.

10 Vasilopulos RJ, Mackin A, Lavergne SN *et al.* (2005) Nephrotic syndrome associated with administration of sulfadimethoxine/ormetoprim in a Dobermann. *J Small Anim Pract* **46**:232–236.

11 Scott DW, Miller WH, Griffin CE (2001) Immune-mediated disorders. In *Muller and Kirk's Small Animal Dermatology*, 6th edn. WB Saunders, Philadelphia, pp. 667–779.

Cutaneous lupus erythematosus
(discoid lupus erythematosus)

1 Norris DA (1993) Pathomechanisms of photosensitive lupus erythematosus. *J Invest Dermatol* **100**:58S–68S.

2 Walton DK, Scott DW, Smith CS *et al.* (1981) Canine discoid lupus erythematosus. *J Am Anim Hosp Assoc* **17**:851–858.

3 Scott DW, Walton DK, Manning TO *et al.* (1983) Canine lupus erythematosus. Part 2. Discoid lupus erythematosus. *J Am Anim Hosp Assoc* **19**:481–486.

4 Scott DW, Walton DK, Slater MR *et al.* (1987) Immune-mediated dermatoses in domestic animals: ten years after. Part 2. *Comp Cont Ed Pract Vet* **9**:539–551.

5 Willemse T and Koeman JP (1989) Discoid lupus erythematosus in cats. *Vet Dermatol* **1**:19–24.

6 White SD, Rosychuk RAW, Reinke SI *et al.* (1992) Use of tetracycline and niacinamide for treatment of autoimmune skin disease in 31 dogs. *J Am Vet Med Assoc* **200**:1497–1500.

7 Griffies JD, Mendelson CL, Rosenkrantz WS *et al.* (2004) Topical 0.1% tacrolimus for the treatment of discoid lupus erythematosus and pemphigus erythematosus in dogs. *J Am Anim Hosp Assoc* **40**:29–41.

Systemic lupus erythematosus

1 Chabanne L, Fournel C, Monestier M *et al.* (1999) Canine systemic lupus erythematosus. Part I. Clinical and biologic aspects. *Compend Cont Educ Pract Vet* **21**:135–141.

2 Chabanne L, Fournel C, Rigal D *et al.* (1999) Canine systemic lupus erythematosus. Part II. Diagnosis and treatment. *Compend Cont Educ Pract Vet* **21**:402–409.

3 Clercx C, McEntee K, Gilbert S *et al.* (1999) Nonresponsive generalized bacterial infection associated with systemic lupus erythematosus in a Beauceron. *J Am Anim Hosp Assoc* **35**:220–223.

4 Foster AP, Sturgess CP, Gould DJ *et al.* (2000) Pemphigus foliaceus in association with systemic lupus erythematosus and subsequent lymphoma in a cocker spaniel. *J Small Anim Pract* **41**:266–270.

5 Scott DW, Miller WH (1995) Squamous cell carcinoma arising in chronic discoid lupus erythematosus nasal lesions in two German Shepherd Dogs. *Vet Dermatol* **6**:99–104.

6 Chabanne L, Fournel C, Caux C *et al.* (1995) Abnormalities of lymphocyte subsets in canine systemic lupus erythematosus. *Autoimmunity* **22**:1–8.

7 Fournel C, Chabanne L, Caux C *et al*. (1992) Canine systemic lupus erythematosus. I: A study of 75 cases. *Lupus* **1**:133–139.

8 Goudswaard J, Schell WER, van Toor AJ *et al*. (1993) SLE (systemic lupus erythematosus): related clinical features in the dog. *Tijdschrift Diergeneesk* **118**:185–189.

9 Person JM, Person P, Pellerin JL (1998) Systemic lupus erythematosus in a cat. *Rev Med Vet-Toulouse* **149**:1125–1129.

10 Vitale CB, Ihrke PJ, Gross TL *et al*. (1997) Systemic lupus erythematosus in a cat: fulfillment of the American Rheumatism Association criteria with supportive skill histopathology. *Compend Cont Educ Pract Vet* **8**:133–138.

11 Hansson-Hamlin H, Lilliehook I, Trowald-Wigh G (2006) Subgroups of canine antinuclear antibodies in relation to laboratory and clinical findings in immune-mediated disease. *Vet Clin Pathol* **35**:397–404.

12 Henriksson EW, Hansson H, Karlsson-Parra A *et al*. (1998) Autoantibody profiles in canine ANA-positive sera investigated by immunoblot and ELISA. *Vet Immunol Immunopathol* **61**:157–170.

13 Monier JC, Ritter J, Caux C *et al*. (1992) Canine systemic lupus erythematosus. II: Antinuclear antibodies. *Lupus* **1**:287–293.

14 Choi EW, Shin IS, Youn HY *et al*. (2005) Gene therapy using non-viral peptide vector in a canine systemic lupus erythematosus model. *Vet Immunol Immunopathol* **103**:223–233.

Vesicular cutaneous lupus erythematosus of the Shetland Sheepdog and Collie

1 Gross TH, Ihrke PJ, Walder EJ, Affolter VK (2005) Vesicular cutaneous lupus erythematosus of the Shetland sheepdog and collie. In *Skin Diseases of the Dog and Cat: Clinical and Histopathologic Diagnosis*, 2nd edn. Blackwell Publishing, Oxford, pp. 61–63.

2 Jackson HA, Olivry T, Berget F *et al*. (2004) Immunopathology of vesicular cutaneous lupus erythematosus in the Rough Collie and Shetland Sheepdog: a canine homologue of subacute cutaneous lupus erythematosus in humans. *Vet Dermatol* **15**:230–239.

3 Jackson HA, Olivry T (2001) Ulcerative dermatosis of the Shetland Sheepdog and Rough Collie dog may represent a novel vesicular variant of cutaneous lupus erythematosus. *Vet Dermatol* **12**:19–27.

4 Jackson HA (2004) Eleven cases of vesicular cutaneous lupus erythematosus in Shetland Sheepdogs and Rough Collies: clinical management and prognosis. *Vet Dermatol* **15**:37–41.

5 Jackson HA (2006) Vesicular cutaneous lupus. *Vet Clin North Am: Small Anim Pract* **36**:251–255.

6 Font A, Bardagi M, Mascort J *et al*. (2006) Treatment with oral cyclosporin A of a case of vesicular cutaneous lupus erythematous in a Rough Collie. *Vet Dermatol* **17**:440–442.

Pemphigus vulgaris

1 Olivry T, Joubeh S, Dunston SM *et al*. (2003) Desmoglein-3 is a target autoantigen in spontaneous canine pemphigus vulgaris. *Exp Dermatol* **12**:198–203.

2 Olivry T, Alhaidari Z, Ghohestani RF (2000) Anti-plakin and desmoglein autoantibodies in a dog with pemphigus vulgaris. *Vet Pathol* **37**:496–499.

3 Carlotti DN, Terrier S, Bensignor E *et al*. (2000) Pemphigus vulgaris in the dog: a report of 8 cases. *Prat Med Chir Anim* **35**:301–307.

4 Foster AP, Olivry T (2001) Nasal dermatitis as a manifestation of canine pemphigus vulgaris. *Vet Rec* **148**:450–451.

5 Marsella R (2000) Canine pemphigus complex: diagnosis and therapy. *Compend Cont Educ Pract Vet* **22**:680–689.

6 Mimouni D, Anhalt GJ, Cummins DL *et al*. (2003) Treatment of pemphigus vulgaris and pemphigus foliaceus with mycophenolate mofetil. *Arch Dermatol* **139**:739–742.

7 Gomez SM, Morris DO, Rosenbaum MR *et al*. (2004) Outcome and complications associated with treatment of pemphigus foliaceus in dogs: 43 cases (1994–2000). *J Am Vet Med Assoc* **224**:1312–1316.

Bullous pemphigoid

1 Olivry T, Dunston SM, Schachter M *et al*. (2001) A spontaneous canine model of mucous membrane (cicatricial) pemphigoid, an autoimmune blistering disease affecting mucosae and mucocutaneous junctions. *J Autoimmun* **16**:411–421.

2 Peng J, Hernandez C, Chen M *et al*. (1997) Molecular cloning of a cDNA encoding the canine bullous pemphigoid antigen 2 (BP180, type XVII collagen). *J Investig Dermatol* **108**:462.

3 Mason KV (1987) Subepidermal bullous drug eruption resembling bullous pemphigoid in a dog. *J Am Vet Med Assoc* **190**:881–883.

4 Kunkle GA, Goldschmidt MH, Halliwell REW (1978) Bullous pemphigoid in a dog – case report with immunofluorescent findings. *J Am Anim Hosp Assoc* **14**:52–57.

5 Olivry T, Chan LS, Xu L *et al*. (1999) Novel feline autoimmune blistering disease resembling bullous pemphigoid in humans: IgG autoantibodies target the NC16A ectodomain of type XVII collagen (BP180/BPAG2). *Vet Pathol* **36**:328–335.

6 Carlotti DN, Terrier S, Bensignor E *et al*. (2000) Pemphigus vulgaris in the dog: a report of 8 cases. *Prat Med Chir Anim* **35**:301–307.

7 White SD, Rosychuk RAW, Reinke SI *et al*. (1992) Use of tetracycline and niacinamide for the treatment of autoimmune skin disease in 31 dogs. *J Am Vet Med Assoc* **200**:1497–1500.

8 Marsella R (2000) Canine pemphigus complex: diagnosis and therapy. *Compend Contin Educ Pract Vet* **22**:680–686.

9 Mimouni D, Anhalt GJ, Cummins DL *et al*. (2003) Treatment of pemphigus vulgaris and pemphigus foliaceus with mycophenolate mofetil. *Arch Dermatol* **139**:739–742.

Epidermis bullosa acquisita

1 Olivry T, Fine JD, Dunston SM *et al*. (1998) Canine epidermolysis bullosa acquisita: autoantibodies target the aminoterminal (NC1) domain of collagen VII in anchoring fibrils. *Vet Dermatol* **9**:19–31.

2 Olivry T (2003) Spontaneous canine model of epidermolysis bullosa acquista. In: *Animal Models of Immune Dermatoses* (ed LS Chan). CRC Press, Boca Raton, pp. 227–237.

3 Olivry T, Chan LS (2001) Autoimmune blistering dermatosis in domestic animals. *Clin Dermatol* **19**:750–760.

Plasma cell pododermatitis of cats

1 Gruffyd-Jones TJ, Orr CM, Lucke VM (1980) Foot pad swelling and ulceration in cats: a report of five cases. *J Small Anim Pract* **21**:381–389.

2 Taylor JE, Schmeitzel LP (1990) Plasma cell pododermatitis with chronic footpad ulceration in two cats. *J Am Vet Med Assoc* **197**:375–377.

3 Medleau L, Kaswan RL, Lorenz MD *et al*. (1982) Ulcerative pododermatitis in a cat: immunofluorescent findings and response to chrysotherapy. *J Am Anim Hosp Assoc* **18**:449–451.

4 Guaguere E, Declercq J (2000) Viral dermatoses. In *A Practical Guide to Feline Dermatology* (eds E Guaguere, P Prelaud). Blackwell Science, Oxford, pp. 7.1–7.11.

5 Bettenay SV, Mueller RS, Dow K *et al*. (2003) Prospective study of the treatment of feline plasmacytic pododermatitis with doxycycline. *Vet Rec* **152**:564–566.

Idiopathic ear margin vasculitis
(proliferative thrombovascular necrosis of the pinna)

1 Gross TL, Ihrke PJ, Walder EJ (1992) Vascular diseases of the dermis. In *Veterinary Dermatopathology*. Mosby Year Book, St. Louis, pp. 135–140.

2 Griffin CE (1985) Pinnal diseases. In *The Complete Manual of Ear Care, Solvay Animal Health*. Veterinary Learning Systems, Trenton, pp. 21–35.

3 Manning TO, Scott DW (1980) Cutaneous vasculitis in a dog. *J Am Anim Hosp Assoc* **16**:61–67.

Proliferative arteritis of the nasal philtrum

1 Torres SM, Brien TO, Scott DW (2002) Dermal arteritis of the nasal philtrum in a Giant Schnauzer and three Saint Bernard dogs. *Vet Dermatol* **13**:275–281.

2 Gross TH, Ihrke PJ, Walder EJ, Affolter VK (2005) Proliferative arteritis of the nasal philtrum. In *Skin Diseases of the Dog and Cat: Clinical and Histopathologic Diagnosis*, 2nd edn. Blackwell Publishing, Oxford, pp. 255–256.

Vasculopathy of Greyhounds

1 Cowan LA, Hertzke DM, Fenwick BW *et al*. (1997) Clinical and clinicopathologic abnormalities in Greyhounds with cutaneous and renal glomerular vasculopathy: 18 cases (1992–1994). *J Am Vet Med Assoc* **210**:789–793.

2 Rotermund A, Peters M, Hewicker-Trautwein M *et al*. (2002) Cutaneous and renal glomerular vasculopathy in a Great Dane resembling 'Alabama rot' of Greyhounds. *Vet Rec* **151**:510–512.

Feline cowpox infection

1 Bennett M, Gaskell CJ, Gaskell RM *et al*. (1986) Poxvirus infection in the domestic cat: some clinical and epidemiologic observations. *Vet Rec* **118**:387–390.

2 Gaskell RM, Gaskell CJ, Evans RJ (1983) Natural and experimental poxvirus infection in the domestic cat. *Vet Rec* **112**:164–170.

3 Godfrey DR, Blundell CJ, Essbauer S *et al*. (2004) Unusual presentations of cowpox infections in cats. *J Small Anim Pract* **45**:202–205.

4 Thomsett LR (1989) Cowpox in cats. *J Small Anim Pract* **30**:236–241.

5 Brown A, Bennett M, Gaskell CJ (1989) Fatal poxvirus infection in association with FIV infection. *Vet Rec* **124**:19–20.

6   Hinrichs U, van de Poel H, van den Ingh TSGA (1999) Necrotizing pneumonia in a cat caused by an orthopox virus. *J Comp Pathol* **121**:191–196.

7   Bennett M, Baxby D, Gaskell RM *et al.* (1985) The laboratory diagnosis of orthopoxvirus infection in the domestic cat. *J Small Anim Pract* **26**:653–661.

8   Czerny CP, Wagner K, Gessler K *et al.* (1996) A monoclonal blocking-ELISA for detection of orthopoxvirus antibodies in feline sera. *Vet Microbiol* **52**:185–200.

9   Hawranek T, Tritscher M, Muss WH *et al.* (2003) Feline orthopoxvirus infection transmitted from cat to human. *J Am Acad Dermatol* **49**:513–518.

Feline cutaneous herpesvirus and calicivirus infections

1   Gaskell R, Dawson S, Radford A *et al.* (2007) Feline herpesvirus. *Vet Res* **38**:337–354.

2   Rong S, Slade D, Floyd-Hawkins K *et al.* (2006) Characterization of a highly virulent feline calicivirus and attenuation of this virus. *Virus Res* **122**:95–108.

3   Holland JL, Outerbridge CA, Affolter VK *et al.* (2006) Detection of feline herpesvirus 1 DNA in skin biopsy specimens from cats with or without dermatitis. *J Am Vet Med Assoc* **229**:1442–1446.

4   Pesavento PA, MacLachlan NJ, Dillard-Telm L *et al.* (2004) Pathologic, immunohistochemical, and electron microscopic findings in naturally occurring virulent systemic feline calicivirus infection in cats. *Vet Pathol* **41**:257–263.

5   Suchy A, Bauder B, Gelbmann W *et al.* (2000) Diagnosis of feline herpesvirus infection by immunohistochemistry, polymerase chain reaction, and *in situ* hybridization. *J Vet Diagn Invest* **12**:186–191.

6   Hargis AM, Ginn PE, Mansell JEKL *et al.* (1999) Ulcerative facial and nasal dermatitis and stomatitis in cats associated with feline herpesvirus 1. *Vet Dermatol* **10**:267–274.

7   Maggs DJ (2005) Update on pathogenesis, diagnosis, and treatment of feline herpesvirus type 1. *Clin Tech Small Anim Pract* **20**:94–101.

8   Gutzwiller MER, Brachelente C, Taglinger K *et al.* (2007) Feline herpes dermatitis treated with interferon omega. *Vet Dermatol* **18**:50–54.

Mucocutaneous pyoderma

1   Ihrke PJ, Gross TL (1964) Canine mucocutaneous pyoderma. In *Current Veterinary Therapy XII* (ed JD Bonagura). WB Saunders, Philadelphia, pp. 618–619.

2   Gross TH, Ihrke PJ, Walder EJ, Affolter VK (2005) Mucocutaneous pyoderma. In *Skin Diseases of the Dog and Cat: Clinical and Histopathologic Diagnosis*, 2nd edn. Blackwell Publishing, Oxford, pp. 261–263.

Nocardiosis

1   Hardie EM (1990) Actinomycosis and nocardiosis. In *Infectious Diseases of Dogs and Cats* (ed CE Green). WB Saunders, Philadelphia, pp. 585–591.

2   Kirpensteijn J, Fingland RB (1992) Cutaneous actinomycosis and nocardiosis in dogs: 48 cases (1980–1990). *J Am Vet Med Assoc* **201**:917–920.

Blastomycosis

1   Attleberger MH (1980) Subcutaneous and opportunistic mycoses. In *Current Veterinary Therapy VII* (ed RW Kirk). WB Saunders, Philadelphia, pp. 1177–1180.

2   Fadok VA (1987) Granulomatous dermatitis in dogs and cats. *Seminars in Vet Med and Surg (Small Animal)* **2**:186–194.

3   Rudmann DG, Coolman BR, Perez CM *et al.* (1992) Evaluation of risk factors for blastomycosis in dogs: 857 cases (1980–1990). *J Am Vet Med Assoc* **201**:1754–1759.

4   Taboada J, Grooters AM (2005) Systemic mycoses. In *Textbook of Veterinary Internal Medicine* (eds SJ Ettinger, EC Feldman). Elsevier Saunders, St. Louis, pp. 671–690.

5   Spector AM, Legendre AM, Wheat J *et al.* (2008) Antigen and antibody testing for the diagnosis of blastomycosis in dogs. *J Vet Intern Med* **22**:839–843.

6   Legendre AM (1995) Antimycotic drug therapy. In *Current Veterinary Therapy XII* (ed JD Bonagura). WB Saunders, Philadelphia, pp. 327–331.

Sporotrichosis

1   Wolf AM, Troy GC (1995) Deep mycotic diseases. In *Textbook of Veterinary Internal Medicine* (eds SJ Ettinger, EC Feldman). WB Saunders, Philadelphia, pp. 453–455.

2   Gross TL, Ihrke PJ, Walder EJ (1992) Infectious nodular and diffuse granulomatous and pyogranulomatous diseases of the dermis. In *Veterinary Dermatopathology*. Mosby Year Book, St. Louis, pp. 181–184.

3 Dunston R, Lanham RF, Reimann KA *et al*. (1996) Feline sporotrichosis. A report of five cases with transmission to humans. *J Am Acad Derm* **15**:37–45.

4 Sykes JE, Torres SM, Armstrong J *et al*. (2001) Itraconazole for treatment of sporotrichosis in a dog residing on a Christmas tree farm. *J Am Vet Med Assoc* **218**:1440–1442.

Calcinosis cutis

1 Scott DW (1982) Histopathological findings in endocrine skin disorders. *J Am Anim Hosp Assoc* **18**:173–183.

2 Zerbe CA, MacDonald JM (1994) Canine and feline Cushing's syndrome. In *Current Veterinary Dermatology* (eds CE Griffin, KW Kwochka, JM McDonald). Mosby Year Book, St. Louis, pp. 273–287.

3 White SD, Ceragioli KL, Bullock LP *et al*. (1989) Cutaneous markers of canine hyperadrenocorticism. *Compend Contin Educ Pract Vet* **11**:446–464.

4 Scott DW (1979) Hyperadrenocorticism. *Vet Clin North Am: Small Anim Pract* **9**:3–28.

Squamous cell carcinoma

1 Scott DW, Miller WH (1995) Squamous cell carcinoma arising in chronic discoid lupus erythematosus nasal lesions in two German Shepherd Dogs. *Vet Dermatol* **6**:99–104.

2 Calmon JP (2002) Solar dermatosis. Part 2. Tumours induced by UV rays. *Prat Med Chir Anim* **37**:269–279.

3 Lana SE, Ogilvie GK, Withrow SJ *et al*. (1997) Feline cutaneous squamous cell carcinoma of the nasal planum and the pinnae: 61 cases. *J Am Anim Hosp Assoc* **33**:329–332.

4 Rogers KS (1994) Feline cutaneous squamous cell carcinoma. *Feline Pract* **22**:7–9.

5 Scott DW, Teixeira EAC (1995) Multiple squamous cell carcinomas arising from multiple cutaneous follicular cysts in a dog. *Vet Dermatol* **6**:27–31.

6 Callan MB, Preziosi D, Mauldin E (2005) Multiple papillomavirus-associated epidermal hamartomas and squamous cell carcinomas in situ in a dog following chronic treatment with prednisone and cyclosporine. *Vet Dermatol* **16**:338–345.

7 Guaguere E, Olivry T, Delverdier-Poujade A *et al*. (1999) *Demodex cati* infestation in association with feline cutaneous squamous cell carcinoma in situ: a report of five cases. *Vet Dermatol* **10**:61–67.

8 O'Brien MG, Berg J, Engler SJ (1992) Treatment by digital amputation of subungual squamous cell carcinoma in dogs: 21 cases (1987–1988). *J Am Vet Med Assoc* **201**:759–761.

9 Barton CL (1987) Cytological diagnosis of cutaneous neoplasia – an algorithmic approach. *Compend Cont Educ Pract Vet* **9**:20–33.

10 Lascelles BDX, Parry AT, Stidworthy MF *et al*. (2000) Squamous cell carcinoma of the nasal planum in 17 dogs. *Vet Rec* **147**:473–476.

11 Schmidt K, Bertani C, Martano M *et al*. (2005) Reconstruction of the lower eyelid by third eyelid lateral advancement and local transposition cutaneous flap after en bloc resection of squamous cell carcinoma in 5 cats. *Vet Surg* **34**:78–82.

12 Stell AJ, Dobson JM, Langmack K (2001) Photodynamic therapy of feline superficial squamous cell carcinoma using topical 5-aminolaevulinic acid. *J Small Anim Pract* **42**:164–169.

13 Peaston AE, Leach MW, Higgins RJ (1993) Photodynamic therapy for nasal and aural squamous cell carcinoma in cats. *J Am Vet Med Assoc* **202**:1261–1265.

14 Kinzel S, Hein S, Stopinski T *et al*. (2003) The hypofractionated radiation therapy for the treatment of melanoma and squamous cell carcinoma in dogs and cats. *Berl Munch Tierarztl Wochenschr* **116**:134–138.

15 Goodfellow M, Hayes A, Murphy S *et al*. (2006) A retrospective study of (90)Strontium plesiotherapy for feline squamous cell carcinoma of the nasal planum. *J Feline Med Surg* **8**:169–176.

Metabolic epidermal necrosis

1 Cellio LM, Dennis J (2005) Canine superficial necrolytic dermatitis. *Compend Cont Educ Pract Vet* **27**:820–824.

2 Allenspach K, Arnold P, Glaus T *et al*. (2000) Glucagon producing neuroendocrine tumour associated with hypoaminoacidaemia and skin lesions. *J Small Anim Pract* **41**:402–406.

3 Peikes H, Morris DO, Hess RS (2001) Dermatologic disorders in dogs with diabetes mellitus: 45 cases (1986–2000). *J Am Vet Med Assoc* **219**:203–208.

4 Turek MM (2003) Cutaneous paraneoplastic syndromes in dogs and cats: a review of the literature. *Vet Dermatol* **14**:279–296.

5 Kimmel SE, Christiansen W, Byrne KP (2003) Clinicopathological, ultrasonographic, and histopathological findings of superficial necrolytic dermatitis with hepatopathy in a cat. *J Am Anim Hosp Assoc* **39**:23–27.

6 Torres SMF, Caywood DD, O'Brien TD *et al*. (1997) Resolution of superficial necrolytic dermatitis following excision of a glucagon-secreting pancreatic neoplasm in a dog. *J Am Anim Hosp Assoc* **33**:313–319.

7 March PA, Hillier A, Weisbrode SE *et al*. (2004) Superficial necrolytic dermatitis in 11 dogs with a history of phenobarbital administration (1995–2002). *J Vet Int Med* **18**:65–74.

8 Outerbridge CA, Marks SL, Rogers QR (2002) Plasma amino acid concentrations in 36 dogs with histologically confirmed superficial necrolytic dermatitis. *Vet Dermatol* **13**:177–186.

9 Hill PB, Auxilia ST, Munro EAC *et al*. (2000) Resolution of skin lesions and long-term survivial in a dog with superficial necrolytic dermatitis and liver cirrhosis. *J Small Anim Pract* **41**:519–523.

Decubital ulcers (pressure sores)

1 Fadok VA (1983) Necrotizing skin diseases. In *Current Veterinary Therapy VIII* (ed RW Kirk). WB Saunders, Philadelphia, pp. 473–480.

2 Waldron DR, Trevor P (1993) Management of superficial skin wounds. In *Textbook of Small Animal Surgery* (ed D Slatter). WB Saunders, Philadelphia, pp. 276–279.

Ehlers–Danlos syndrome
(cutaneous asthenia, dermatosparaxis)

1 Hegreberg GA, Counts DF (1979) Ehlers–Danlos syndrome. In *Spontaneous Animal Models of Human Disease, Vol. II* (eds ED Andrews, BC Ward, NH Altman). Academic Press, New York, pp. 36–39.

2 Patterson DF, Minor RR (1977) Hereditary fragility and hyperextensibility of the skin of cats. A defect in collagen fibrillogenesis. *Lab Invest* **37**:170–179.

3 Counts DF, Byers PH, Holbrook KA *et al*. (1980) Dermatosparaxis in a Himalayan cat: I. Biochemical studies of dermal collagen. *J Invest Dermatol* **74**:96–99.

4 Scott DW, Miller WH, Griffin CE (2001) Ehlers–Danlos syndrome. In *Muller and Kirk's Small Animal Dermatology*, 6th edn. WB Saunders, Philadelphia, pp. 979–984.

5 Fernandez CJ, Scott DW, Erb HN *et al*. (1998) Staining abnormalities of dermal collagen in cats with cutaneous asthenia or acquired skin fragility as demonstrated with Masson's trichrome stain. *Vet Dermatol* **9**:49–54.

CHAPTER 4: PAPULAR AND PUSTULAR DERMATOSES

Superficial pyoderma

1 Mason IS, Mason KV, Lloyd DH (1996) A review of the biology of canine skin with respect to the commensals *Staphylococcus intermedius*, *Demodex canis* and *Malassezia pachydermatis*. *Vet Dermatol* **7**:119–132.

2 Hillier A, Alcorn JR, Cole LK *et al*. (2006) Pyoderma caused by *Pseudomonas aeruginosa* infection in dogs: 20 cases. *Vet Dermatol* **17**:432–439.

3 Bensignor E, Germain PA, Daix B *et al*. (2005) Aetiologic study of recurrent pyoderma in dogs. *Rev Med Vet* **156**:183–189.

4 Hendricks A, Schuberth H-J, Schueler K *et al*. (2002) Frequency of superantigen-producing *Staphylococcus intermedius* isolates from canine pyoderma and proliferation inducing potential of superantigens in dogs. *Res Vet Sci* **73**:273–277.

5 Mason IS, Lloyd DH (1995) The macroscopic and microscopic effects of intradermal injection of crude and purified staphylococcal extracts on canine skin. *Vet Dermatol* **6**:197–204.

6 Frank LA, Kania SA, Hnilica KA *et al*. (2003) Isolation of *Staphylococcus schleiferi* from dogs with pyoderma. *J Am Vet Med Assoc* **222**:451–454.

7 Medleau L, Long RE, Brown J *et al*. (1986) Frequency and antimicrobial susceptibility of *Staphylococcus* species isolated from canine pyodermas. *Am J Vet Res* **47**:229–231.

8 Rich M (2005) Staphylococci in animals: prevalence, identification and antimicrobial susceptibility, with an emphasis on methicillin-resistant *Staphylococcus aureus*. *Br J Biomed Sci* **62**:98–105.

9 Patel A, Lloyd DH, Lamport AI (1999) Antimicrobial resistance of feline staphylococci in southeastern England. *Vet Dermatol* **10**:257–261.

10 Kania SA, Williamson NL, Frank LA *et al*. (2004) Methicillin resistance of staphylococci isolated from the skin of dogs with pyoderma. *Am J Vet Res* **65**:1265–1268.

11 Duquette RA, Nuttall TJ (2004) Methicillin-resistant *Staphylococcus aureus* in dogs and cats: an emerging problem? *J Small Anim Pract* **45**:591–597.

12 Weese JS (2005) Methicillin-resistant *Staphylococcus aureus*: an emerging pathogen in small animals. *J Am Anim Hosp Assoc* **41**:150–157.

13 Morris DO, Rook KA, Shofer FS *et al*. (2006) Screening of *Staphylococcus aureus*, *Staphylococcus intermedius*, and *Staphylococcus schleiferi* isolates obtained from small companion animals for antimicrobial resistance: a retrospective review of 749 isolates (2003–2004). *Vet Dermatol* **17**:332–337.

14 Wildermuth BE, Griffin CE, Rosenkrantz WS (2006) Feline pyoderma therapy. *Clin Tech Small Anim Pract* **21**:150–156.

15 Terauchi R, Sato H, Hasegawa T *et al*. (2003) Isolation of exfoliative toxin from *Staphylococcus intermedius* and its local toxicity in dogs. *Vet Microbiol* **94**:19–29.

16 Authier S, Paquette D, Labrecque O *et al*. (2006) Comparison of susceptibility to antimicrobials of bacterial isolates from companion animals in a veterinary diagnostic laboratory in Canada between two time points 10 years apart. *Can Vet J* **47**:774–778.

17 Rosenkrantz W (2006) Practical applications of topical therapy for allergic, infectious, and seborrheic disorders. *Clin Tech Small Anim Pract* **21**:106–116.

18 de Jaham C (2003) Effects of an ethyl lactate shampoo in conjunction with a systemic antibiotic in the treatment of canine superficial bacterial pyoderma in an open-label, non-placebo controlled study. *Vet Ther* **4**:94–100.

19 Carlotti DN, Jasmin P, Gardey L *et al*. (2004) Evaluation of cephalexin intermittent therapy (weekend therapy) in the control of recurrent idiopathic pyoderma in dogs: a randomized, double-blinded, placebo-controlled study. *Vet Dermatol* **15**:8–9.

20 Curtis CF, Lamport AI, Lloyd DH (2006) Masked, controlled study to investigate the efficacy of a *Staphylococcus intermedius* autogenous bacterin for the control of canine idiopathic recurrent superficial pyoderma. *Vet Dermatol* **17**:163–168.

21 Simou C, Hill PB, Forsythe PJ *et al*. (2005) Species specificity in the adherence of staphylococci to canine and human corneocytes: a preliminary study. *Vet Dermatol* **16**:156–161.

22 Guardabassi L, Loeber ME, Jacobson A (2004) Transmission of multiple antimicrobial-resistant *Staphylococcus intermedius* between dogs affected by deep pyoderma and their owners. *Vet Microbiol* **98**:23–27.

23 Hanselman BA, Kruth SA, Rousseau J *et al*. (2006) Methicillin-resistant *Staphylococcus aureus* colonization in veterinary personnel. *Emerg Infect Dis* **12**:1933–1938.

24 Hanselman B, Kruth SA, Weese JS (2007) Evaluation of coagulase-positive staphylococcal carriage in people and their household pets. *J Vet Intern Med* **21**:627.

Pemphigus foliaceus

1 Iwasaki T, Shimizu M, Obata H *et al*. (1997) Detection of canine pemphigus foliaceus autoantigen by immunoblotting. *Vet Immunol Immunopathol* **59**:1–10.

2 White SD, Carlotti DN, Pin D *et al*. (2002) Putative drug-related pemphigus foliaceus in four dogs. *Vet Dermatol* **13**:195–202.

3 Gross TH, Ihrke PJ, Walder EJ, Affolter VK (2005) Pustular diseases of the epidermis. In *Skin Diseases of the Dog and Cat: Clinical and Histopathologic Diagnosis*, 2nd edn. Blackwell Publishing, Oxford, pp. 13–18.

4 Angarano DW (1987) Autoimmune dermatoses. In *Contemporary Issues in Small Animal Practice* . (ed GH Nesbitt). Churchill Livingstone, New York, pp. 79–94.

5 Halliwell REW, Gorman NT (1989) (eds) *Veterinary Clinical Immunology*. WB Saunders, Philadelphia, pp. 285–307.

6 Serra DA, White SD (1989) Oral chrysotherapy with auranofin in dogs. *J Am Vet Med Assoc* **194**:1327–1330.

7 Kristensen F, Mehl NB (1989) The use of gold in the treatment of autoimmune disease in the dog and cat. *Dansk Veterinäer Tidskrift* **15**:883–887.

8 McEwan NA, McNeil PE, Kirkham D (1986) Pemphigus foliaceus: a report of two cases in the dog. *J Small Anim Pract* **27**:567–575.

9 Norman NJ (1990) Pemphigus. *Dermatol Clinics* **84**:689–700.

10 August JR, Chickering WR (1985) Pemphigus foliaceus causing lameness in four dogs. *Compend Cont Educ Pract Vet* **7**:894–902.

11 Guaguere E, Degorce-Rubiales F (2004) Pemphigus foliaceus confined to the nails in a Hungarian short-haired pointer. *Vet Dermatol* **15**:56.

12 Manning TO, Scott DW, Smith CA *et al*. (1982) Pemphigus diseases in the feline: seven case reports. *J Am Anim Hosp Assoc* **18**:433–443.

13 Beale KM (1988) Azathioprine for treatment of immune-mediated disease of dogs and cats. *J Am Vet Med Assoc* **192**:1316–1318.

14 Rosenkrantz WS (2004) Pemphigus: current therapy. *Vet Dermatol* **15**:90–98.

15 Marsella R (2000) Canine pemphigus complex: diagnosis and therapy. *Compend Cont Educ Pract Vet* **22**:680–689.

16 Mimouni D, Anhalt GJ, Cummins D *et al*. (2003) Treatment of pemphigus vulgaris and pemphigus foliaceus with mycophenolate mofetil. *Arch Dermatol* **139**:739–745.

17 Gomez SM, Morris DO, Rosenbaum MR *et al.* (2004) Outcome and complications associated with treatment of pemphigus foliaceus in dogs: 443 cases (1994–2000). *J Am Vet Med Assoc* **224:**1312–1316.

Canine juvenile cellulitis
(juvenile sterile granulomatous dermatitis and lymphadenitis, juvenile pyoderma, puppy strangles)

1 Mason IS, Jones J (1989) Juvenile cellulitis in Gordon Setters. *Vet Rec* **124:**642.

2 White SD, Rosychuk RAW, Stewart LJ *et al.* (1989) Juvenile cellulitis in dogs: 15 cases (1979–1988). *J Am Vet Med Assoc* **195:**1609–1611.

3 Moriello KA, Mason IS (1995) Nodular lesions, non-healing wounds and common skin tumours. In *Handbook of Small Animal Dermatology.* Elsevier Science Ltd, Oxford, p. 146.

4 Scott DW, Miller WH, Griffin CE (1995) Miscellaneous skin diseases. In *Muller and Kirk's Small Animal Dermatology*, 5th edn. WB Saunders, Philadelphia, pp. 938–941.

CHAPTER 5: DISEASES CHARACTERIZED BY SINUS FORMATION

Bite wounds

1 Davidson EB (1998) Managing bite wounds in dogs and cats. Part II. *Compend Cont Educ Pract Vet* **20:**974–983.

2 Griffin GM, Holt DE (2001) Dog-bite wounds: bacteriology and treatment outcome in 37 cases. *J Am Anim Hosp Assoc* **37:**453–460.

3 Davidson EB (1998) Managing bite wounds in dogs and cats. Part I. *Compend Cont Educ Pract Vet* **20:**811–819.

4 Pavletic MM, Trout NJ (2006) Bullet, bite, and burn wounds in dogs and cats. *Vet Clin North Am: Small Anim Pract* **36:**873–885.

Foreign body sinus

1 Fadok VA (1987) Granulomatous dermatitis in dogs and cats. *Semin Vet Med Surg (Small Anim)* **2:**186–194.

2 Gross TL, Ihrke PJ, Walder EJ, Affolter VK (2005) Noninfectious nodular and diffuse granulomatous and pyogranulomatous diseases of the dermis. In *Skin Diseases of the Dog and Cat: Clinical and Histopathologic Diagnosis*, 2nd edn. Blackwell Publishing, Oxford, pp. 334–337.

Deep pyoderma

1 Bensignor E, Germain PA, Daix B *et al.* (2005) Aetiologic study of recurrent pyoderma in dogs. *Rev Med Vet-Toulouse* **156:**183–189.

2 Bensignor E, Germain PA (2004) Canine recurrent pyoderma: a multicenter prospective study. *Vet Dermatol* **15:**42.

3 Scott DW, Miller WH, Griffin CE (2001) Bacterial skin diseases. In *Muller and Kirk's Small Animal Dermatology*, 6th edn. WB Saunders, Philadelphia, pp. 274–335.

4 Frank LA, Kania SA, Hnilica KA *et al.* (2003) Isolation of *Staphylococcus schleiferi* from dogs with pyoderma. *J Am Vet Med Assoc* **222:**451–454.

5 Jones RD, Kania SA, Rohrbach BW *et al.* (2007) Prevalence of oxacillin- and multidrug-resistant staphylococci in clinical samples from dogs: 1,772 samples (2001–2005). *J Am Vet Med Assoc* **230:**221–227.

6 Kania SA, Williamson NL, Frank LA *et al.* (2004) Methicillin resistance of staphylococci isolated from the skin of dogs with pyoderma. *Am J Vet Res* **65:**1265–1268.

7 Hillier A, Alcorn JR, Cole LK *et al.* (2006) Pyoderma caused by *Pseudomonas aeruginosa* infection in dogs: 20 cases. *Vet Dermatol* **17:**432–439.

8 Rantala M, Lahti E, Kuhalampi J *et al.* (2004) Antimicrobial resistance in *Staphylococcus* spp., *Escherichia coli* and *Enterococcus* spp. in dogs given antibiotics for chronic dermatological disorders, compared with non-treated control dogs. *Acta Vet Scand* **45:**37–45.

9 Breathnach RM, Fanning S, Mulcahy G *et al.* (2006) Evaluation of Th-1-like and Th-2-like and immunomodulatory cytokine mRNA expression in the skin of dogs with immunomodulatory-responsive lymphocytic-plasmacytic pododermatitis. *Vet Dermatol* **17:**313–321.

10 Breathnach RM, Baker KP, Quinn PJ *et al.* (2005) Clinical, immunological and histopathological findings in a subpopulation of dogs with pododermatitis. *Vet Dermatol* **16:**364–372.

Opportunistic (atypical) mycobacterial infections

1 Malik R, Hunt GB, Goldsmid SE *et al.* (1994) Diagnosis and treatment of pyogranulmatous panniculitis due to *Mycobacterium smegmatis* in cats. *J Small Anim Pract* **35:**524–530.

2 Henderson SM, Baker J, Williams R *et al.* (2003) Opportunistic mycobacterial granuloma in a cat associated with a member of the *Mycobacterium terrae* complex. *J Feline Med Surg* **5:**37–41.

3 Jang SS, Hirsh DC (2002) Rapidly growing members of the genus *Mycobacterium* affecting dogs and cats. *J Am Anim Hosp Assoc* **38**:217–220.

4 Davies JL, Sibley JA, Myers S *et al*. (2006) Histological and genotypical characterization of feline cutaneous mycobacteriosis: a retrospective study of formalin-fixed paraffin-embedded tissues. *Vet Dermatol* **17**:155–162.

5 Appleyard GD, Clark EG (2002) Histologic and genotypic characterization of a novel *Mycobacterium* species found in three cats. *J Clin Microbiol* **40**:2425–2430.

6 Malik R, Shaw SE, Griffin C *et al*. (2004) Infections of the subcutis and skin of dogs caused by rapidly growing mycobacteria. *J Small Anim Pract* **45**:485–494.

7 Rossmeisl JH, Manning TO (2004) The clinical signs and diagnosis of feline atypical mycobacterial panniculitis. *Vet Med* **99**:694–704.

8 Manning TO, Rossmeisl JH, Lanz OI (2004) Feline atypical mycobacterial panniculitis: Treatment, monitoring, and prognosis. *Vet Med* **99**:705–715.

9 Cai H, Archambault M, Prescott JF (2003) 16S ribosomal RNA sequence-based identification of veterinary clinical bacteria. *J Vet Diag Invest* **15**:465–469.

10 Calfee T, Manning TO (2002) Non-healing subcutaneous wounds in the cat and proposed surgical management techniques. *Clin Tech Small Anim Pract* **17**:162–167.

Feline leprosy

1 Malik R, Hughes MS, James G *et al*. (2003) Feline leprosy: two different syndromes. *J Feline Med Surg* **4**:43–59.

2 Appleyard GD, Clark EG (2002) Histologic and genotypic characterization of a novel *Mycobacterium* species found in three cats. *J Clin Microbiol* **40**:2425–2430.

3 Davies JL, Sibley J, Clark EG *et al*. (2003) Feline leprosy syndrome is associated with several mycobacterial species: a histologic and genotypic retrospective study on formalin-fixed and paraffin embedded tissues. *Vet Pathol* **40**:613.

4 Gross TH, Ihrke PJ, Walder EJ, Affolter VK (2005) Infectious nodular and diffuse granulomatous and pyogranulomatous diseases of the dermis. In *Skin Diseases of the Dog and Cat: Clinical and Histopathologic Diagnosis*, 2nd edn. Blackwell Publishing, Oxford, pp. 272–317.

5 Hughes MS, Ball NW, Beck LA *et al*. (1997) Determination of the etiology of presumptive feline leprosy by 16S rRNA gene analysis. *J Clin Microbiol* **35**:2464–2471.

6 McIntosh DW (1982) Feline leprosy: a review of forty-four cases from Western Canada. *Can Vet J* **23**:291–295.

7 Schieffer HB, Middleton DM (1983) Experimental transmission of a feline mycobacterial skin disease (feline leprosy). *Vet Pathol* **20**:460–471.

8 Hartmann K, Greene CGC (2005) Diseases caused by systemic bacterial infections. In *Textbook of Veterinary Internal Medicine* (eds SJ Ettinger, EC Feldman). WB Saunders, Philadelphia, pp. 616–631.

9 Mundell AC (1989) The use of clofazimine in the treatment of three cases of feline leprosy. In *Advances in Veterinary Dermatology, Vol. 1* (eds C von Tscharner, REW Halliwell). Baillière Tindall, London, p. 451.

Dermoid sinus

1 Salmon Hillbertz NHC, Andersson G (2006) Autosomal dominant mutation causing the dorsal ridge predisposes for dermoid sinus in Rhodesian Ridgeback dogs. *J Small Anim Pract* **47**:184–188.

2 Burrow RD (2004) A nasal dermoid sinus in an English bull terrier. *J Small Anim Pract* **45**:572–574.

3 Salmon Hillbertz NHC (2005) Inheritance of dermoid sinus in the Rhodesian Ridgeback. *J Small Anim Pract* **46**:71–74.

4 Cornegliani L, Ghibaudo G (1999) A dermoid sinus in a Siberian Husky. *Vet Dermatol* **10**:47–49.

5 Cornegliani L, Jommi E, Vercelli A (2001) Dermoid sinus in a golden retriever. *J Small Anim Pract* **42**:514–516.

6 Pratt JNJ, Knottenbelt CM, Welsh EM (2000) Dermoid sinus at the lumbosacral junction in an English springer spaniel. *J Small Anim Pract* **41**:24–26.

Anal furunculosis (perianal fistulas)

1 Harvey CE (1972) Perianal fistula in the dog. *Vet Rec* **91**:25–32.

2 Day MJ (1993) Immunopathology of anal furunculosis in the dog. *J Small Anim Pract* **34**:381–389.

3 Christie TR (1975) Perianal fistulas in the dog. *Vet Clin North Am: Small Anim Pract* **5**:353–362.

4 Patricelli AJP, Hardie RJ, McAnulty JF (2002) Cyclosporine and ketoconazole for the treatment of perianal fistulas in dogs. *J Am Vet Med Assoc* **220**:1009–1016.

5 Van Ee RT (1993) Perianal fistulas. In *Disease Mechanisms in Small Animal Surgery*, 2nd edn (ed. MJ Bojrab). Lea & Febiger, Philadelphia, pp. 285–286.

6 Mathews KA, Ayres SA, Tano CA *et al*. (1977) Cyclosporine treatment of perianal fistulas in dogs. *Can Vet J* **38**:39–41.

7 Mathews KA, Sukhiani HR (1997) Randomized controlled trial of cyclosporine for treatment of perianal fistulas in dogs. *J Am Vet Med Assoc* **211**:1249–1253.

8 Doust R, Griffiths LG, Sullivan M (2003) Evaluation of once daily treatment with cyclosporine for anal furunculosis in dogs. *Vet Rec* **152**:225–229.

9 Griffiths LG, Sullivan M, Bortland WW (1999) Cyclosporine as the sole treatment for anal furunculosis: preliminary results. *J Small Anim Pract* **40**:569–572.

10 Mouatt JG (2002) Cyclosporine and ketoconazole interaction for treatment of perianal fistulas in the dog. *Aust Vet J* **80**:207–211.

Metatarsal fistulation of the German Shepherd Dog

1 Scott DW, Miller WH, Griffin CE (1995) Focal metatarsal fistulation of German Shepherd Dogs. In *Muller and Kirk's Small Animal Dermatology*, 5th edn. WB Saunders, Philadelphia, pp. 985–986.

2 Gross TL, Ihrke PJ, Walder EJ, Affolter VK (2005) Metatarsal fistulation of German Shepherd Dogs. In *Skin Diseases of the Dog and Cat: Clinical and Histopathologic Diagnosis*, 2nd edn. Blackwell Publishing, Oxford, pp. 553–555.

CHAPTER 6: DISEASES CHARACTERIZED BY CRUST AND SCALE

Actinic dermatosis

1 Bensignor E (1999) The sun and the skin in dogs and cats. 2. Photo-induced or photo-aggravated conditions. *Point Vet* **30**:49–56.

2 Frank LA, Calderwood Mays MB (1994) Solar dermatitis in dogs. *Compend Cont Educ Pract Vet* **16**:465–469.

3 Frank LA, Calderwood Mays MB *et al*. (1996) Distribution and appearance of elastic fibers in the dermis of clinically normal dogs and dogs with solar dermatitis and other dermatoses. *Am J Vet Res* **57**:178–181.

4 Ruslander D, KaserHotz B, Sardinas JC (1997) Cutaneous squamous cell carcinoma in cats. *Compend Cont Educ Pract Vet* **19**:1119–1124.

5 Friberg C (2006) Feline facial dermatoses. *Vet Clin North Am: Small Anim Pract* **36**:115–123.

6 Hadley G, Derry S, Moore RA (2006) Imiquimod for actinic keratosis: systematic review and meta-analysis. *J Invest Dermatol* **126**:1251–1255.

Sebaceous adenitis

1 Scarff DH (2000) Sebaceous adenitis in standard poodles. *Vet Rec* **146**:476.

2 Sousa CA (2006) Sebaceous adenitis. *Vet Clin North Am: Small Anim Pract* **36**:243–249.

3 Reichler IM, Hauser B, Schiller I *et al*. (2001) Sebaceous adenitis in the Akita: clinical observations, histopathology and heredity. *Vet Dermatol* **12**:243–253.

4 Vercelli A, Cornegliani L, Tronca L (2004) Sebaceous adenitis in three related Hovawart dogs. *Vet Dermatol* **15**:52.

5 Noli C, Toma S (2006) Three cases of immune-mediated adnexal skin disease treated with cyclosporin. *Vet Dermatol* **17**:85–92.

6 White SD, Linder KE, Schultheiss P *et al*. (2000) Sebaceous adenitis in four domestic rabbits (*Oryctatagus cuniculus*). *Vet Dermatol* **11**:53–60.

7 Jazic E, Coyner KS, Loeffler DG *et al*. (2006) An evaluation of the clinical, cytological, infectious and histopathological features of feline acne. *Vet Dermatol* **17**:134–140.

8 Linek M, Boss C, Haemmerling R *et al*. (2005) Effects of cyclosporine A on clinical and histologic abnormalities in dogs with sebaceous adenitis. *J Am Vet Med Assoc* **226**:59–64.

9 Mueller RS, Bettenay SV, Vogelnest LJ (2001) Sebaceous adenitis in three German Shepherd Dogs. *Aust Vet Pract* **31**:110–114.

10 Paterson S (2004) Successful therapy of sebaceous adenitis with topical cyclosporine in 20 dogs. *Vet Dermatol* **15**:64.

Vitamin A responsive dermatosis

1 Ihrke PJ, Goldschmidt MH (1983) Vitamin A responsive dermatosis in the dog. *J Am Vet Med Assoc* **182**:687–690.

2 Scott DW (1986) Vitamin A responsive dermatosis in the Cocker Spaniel. *J Am Anim Hosp Assoc* **22**:125–129.

3 Parker W, Yager Johnson JA, Hardy MH (1983) Vitamin A responsive seborrheic dermatosis in the dog – case report. *J Am Anim Hosp Assoc* **19**:548–553.

4 Schweigert FJ, Zucker H (1991) Novel aspects of vitamin A metabolism in the order Carnivora: a review. *Berl Munch Tierarztl Wochenschr* **104**:89–90, 95–98.

Feline acne

1 Rosenkrantz WS (1991) The pathogenesis, diagnosis, and management of feline acne. *Vet Med* **86**:504–512.

2 Gross TL, Ihrke PJ, Walder EJ (1992) Pustular and nodular diseases with follicular destruction. In *Veterinary Dermatopathology*. Mosby Year Book, St. Louis, pp. 258–259.

Idiopathic (primary) keratinization defect (seborrhea)

1 Kwochka KW, Rademakers AM (1989) Cell proliferation of epidermis, hair follicles and sebaceous glands of Beagles and Cocker Spaniels with healthy skin. *Am J Vet Res* **50**:587–591.

2 Kwochka KW, Rademakers AM (1989) Cell proliferation kinetics of epidermis, hair follicles and sebaceous glands of Cocker Spaniels with idiopathic seborrhea. *Am J Vet Res* **50**:1918–1922.

3 Kwochka KW (1990) Cell proliferation kinetics in the hair root matrix of dogs with healthy skin and dogs with idiopathic seborrhoea. *Am J Vet Res* **51**:1570–1573.

4 Scott DW, Miller WH (1996) Primary seborrhoea in English springer spaniels: a retrospective study of 14 cases. *J Small Anim Pract* **37**:173–178.

5 Fadok VA (1986) Treatment of canine idiopathic seborrhea with isotretinoin. *Am J Vet Res* **47**:1730–1733.

6 Power HT, Ihrke PJ, Stannard AA *et al.* (1992) Use of etretinate for treatment of primary keratinization disorders (idiopathic seborrhea) in Cocker Spaniels, West Highland White Terriers, and Bassett Hounds. *J Am Vet Med Assoc* **201**:419–429.

7 Rosenkrantz W (2006) Practical applications of topical therapy for allergic, infectious, and seborrheic disorders. *Clin Tech Small Anim Pract* **21**:106–116.

Nasal and digital hyperkeratosis

1 Paradis M (1992) Footpad hyperkeratosis in a family of Dogues de Bordeaux. *Vet Dermatol* **3**:75–78.

2 August JR, Chickering WR (1985) Pemphigus foliaceus causing lameness in four dogs. *Compend Cont Educ Pract Vet* **11**:894–902.

3 Ihrke PJ (1980) Topical therapy – uses, principles, and vehicles in dermatologic therapy. Part 1. *Compend Cont Educ Pract Vet* **11**:28–35.

4 Kwochka KW (1993) Primary keratinization disorders of dogs. In *Current Veterinary Dermatology* (eds CE Griffin, KW Kwochka, JM McDonald). Mosby Year Book, St Louis, pp. 176–190.

Erythema multiforme complex

1 Hinn AC, Olivry T, Luther PB *et al.* (1998) Erythema multiforme, Stevens–Johnson syndrome and toxic epidermal necrolysis in the dog: classification, drug exposure and histopathological correlations. *J Vet Allergy Clin Immunol* **6**:13–20.

2 Noli C, von Tscharner C, Suter MM (1998) Apoptosis in selected skin diseases. *Vet Dermatol* **9**:221–229.

3 Affolter VK, von Tscharner C (1993) Cutaneous drug reactions: a retrospective study of histopathological changes and their correlation with the clinical disease. *Vet Dermatol* **4**:79–86.

4 Scott DW, Miller WH (1999) Erythema multiforme in dogs and cats: literature review and case material from the Cornell University College of Veterinary Medicine (1988–96). *Vet Dermatol* **10**:297–309.

5 Scott DW, Miller WH, Griffin CE (2001) Immune-mediated disorders. In *Muller and Kirk's Small Animal Dermatology*, 6th edn. WB Saunders, Philadelphia, pp. 667–779.

6 Byrne KP, Giger U (2002) Use of human immunoglobulin for treatment of severe erythema multiforme in a cat. *J Am Vet Med Assoc* **220**:197–201.

7 Nuttall TJ, Mallam T (2004) Successful intravenous human immunoglobulin treatment of drug-induced Stevens–Johnson Syndrome in a dog. *J Small Anim Pract* **45**:357–361.

Canine ear margin seborrhea

1 Gross TL, Ihrke PJ, Walder EJ, Affolter VK (2005) Canine ear margin seborrhea. In *Skin Diseases of the Dog and Cat: Clinical and Histopathologic Diagnosis*, 2nd edn. Blackwell Publishing, Oxford, pp. 167–169.

Exfoliative cutaneous lupus erythematosus of the German Shorthaired Pointer

1 Ihrke PJ, Gross TL (1964) Hereditary lupoid dermatosis of the German Shorthaired Pointer. In *Current Veterinary Therapy XII* (ed JD Bonagura). WB Saunders, Philadelphia, pp. 605–606.

2 Gross TL, Ihrke PJ, Walder EJ, Affolter VK (2005) Exfoliative cutaneous lupus erythematosus of the German Shorthaired Pointer. In *Skin Diseases of the Dog and Cat: Clinical and Histopathologic Diagnosis*, 2nd edn. Blackwell Publishing, Oxford, pp. 59–61.

3 Vroom MW, Theaker MJ, Rest J *et al.* (1995) Lupoid dermatosis in five German Shorthaired Pointers. *Vet Dermatol* **6**:93–98.

4 Bryden SL, White SD, Dunston SM *et al*. (2005) Clinical, histopathological and immunological characteristics of exfoliative cutaneous lupus erythematosus in 25 German Shorthaired Pointers. *Vet Derm* **16**:239–252.

Leishmaniasis

1 Paradies P, Capelli G, Cafarchia C *et al*. (2006) Incidences of canine leishmaniasis in an endemic area of southern Italy. *J Vet Med B* **53**:295–298.

2 Solano-Gallego L, Rodriguez-Cortes A, Iniesta L *et al*. (2007) Cross-sectional serosurvey of feline leishmaniasis in ecoregions around the North-western Mediterranean. *Am J Trop Med Hyg* **76**:676–680.

3 Duprey ZH, Steurer FJ, Rooney JA *et al*. (2006) Canine visceral leishmaniasis, United States and Canada, 2000–2003. *Emerg Infect Dis* **12**:440–446.

4 Franca-Silva JC, da Costa RT, Siqueira AM *et al*. (2003) Epidemiology of canine visceral leishmaniosis in the endemic area of Montes Claros Municipality, Minas Gerais State, Brazil. *Vet Parasitol* **111**:161–173.

5 Lainson R, Rangel EF (2005) *Lutzomyia longipalpis* and the eco-epidemiology of American visceral leishmaniasis, with particular reference to Brazil: a review. *Mem I Oswaldo Cruz* **100**:811–827.

6 Grosjean NL, Vrable RA, Murphy AJ *et al*. (2003) Seroprevalence of antibodies against *Leishmania* spp. among dogs in the United States. *J Am Vet Med Assoc* **222**:603–606.

7 Manna L, Reale S, Viola E *et al*. (2006) *Leishmania* DNA load and cytokine expression levels in asymptomatic naturally infected dogs. *Vet Parasitol* **142**:271–280.

8 Oliva G, Scalone A, Manzillo VF *et al*. (2006) Incidence and time course of *Leishmania infantum* infections examined by parasitological, serologic, and nested-PCR techniques in a cohort of naive dogs exposed to three consecutive transmission seasons. *J Clin Microbiol* **44**:1318–1322.

9 Reis AB, Teixeira-Carvalho A, Vale AM *et al*. (2006) Isotype patterns of immunoglobulins: Hallmarks for clinical status and tissue parasite density in Brazilian dogs naturally infected by *Leishmania chagasi*. *Vet Immunol Immunopath* **112**:102–116.

10 Barbieri CL (2006) Immunology of canine leishmaniasis. *Parasite Immunol* **28**:329–337.

11 Quinnell RJ, Courtenay O, Garcez LM *et al*. (2003) IgG subclass responses in a longitudinal study of canine visceral leishmaniasis. *Vet Immunol Immunopathol* **91**:161–168.

12 Rodriguez-Cortes A, Fernandez-Bellon H, Ramis A *et al*. (2007) *Leishmania*-specific isotype levels and their relationship with specific cell-mediated immunity parameters in canine leishmaniasis. *Vet Immunol Immunopathol* **116**:190–198.

13 Solano-Gallego L, Llull J, Ramos G *et al*. (2000) The Ibizian hound presents a predominantly cellular immune response against natural *Leishmania* infection. *Vet Parasitol* **90**:37–45.

14 Giunchetti RC, Mayrink W, Genaro O *et al*. (2006) Relationship between canine visceral leishmaniosis and the *Leishmania chagasi* burden in dermal inflammatory foci. *J Comp Path* **135**:100–107.

15 Maroli M, Pennisi MG, Di Muccio T *et al*. (2007) Infection of sandflies by a cat naturally infected with *Leishmania infantum*. *Vet Parasitol* **145**: 357–360.

16 Lasri S, Sahibi H, Natami A *et al*. (2003) Western blot analysis of *Leishmania infantum* antigens using sera from pentamidine-treated dogs. *Vet Immunol Immunopathol* **91**:13–18.

17 Ikonomopoulos J, Kokotas S, Gazouli M *et al*. (2003) Molecular diagnosis of leishmaniosis in dogs. Comparative application of traditional diagnostic methods and the proposed assay on clinical samples. *Vet Parasitol* **113**:99–113.

18 Joao A, Pereira MA, Cortes S *et al*. (2006) Canine leishmaniasis chemotherapy: dog's clinical condition and risk of *Leishmania* transmission. *J Vet Med A* **53**:540–545.

19 Noli C, Auxilia ST (2005) Treatment of canine Old World visceral leishmaniasis: a systematic review. *Vet Dermatol* **16**:213–232.

20 Lamothe J (2001) Activity of amphotericin B in lipid emulsion in the initial treatment of canine leishmaniasis. *J Small Anim Pract* **42**:170–175.

21 Miro G, Galvez R, Mateo M *et al*. (2007) Evaluation of the efficacy of a topically administered combination of imidacloprid and permethrin against *Phlebotomus perniciosus* in dogs. *Vet Parasitol* **143**:375–379.

22 Molina R, Miró G, Gálvez R *et al*. (2006) Evaluation of a spray of permethrin and pyriproxyfen for the protection of dogs against *Phlebotomus perniciosus*. *Vet Rec* **159**:206–209.

23 Dantas-Torres F (2006) Leishmune® vaccine: the newest tool for prevention and control of canine visceral leishmaniosis and its potential as a transmission-blocking vaccine. *Vet Parasitol* **141**:1–8.

24 Saraiva EM, Barbosa AD, Santos FN *et al*. (2006) The FML-vaccine (Leishmune®) against canine visceral leishmaniasis: a transmission blocking vaccine. *Vaccine* **24**:2423–2431.

Cutaneous horn

1 Gross TH, Ihrke PJ, Walder EJ, Affolter VK (2005) Cutaneous horn of feline pawpad. *Skin Diseases of the Dog and Cat; Clinical and Histopathological Diagnosis*, 2nd edn. Blackwell Publishing, Oxford, p. 562.

2 Scott DW (1984) Feline dermatology, 1979–1982: introspective retrospections. *J Am Anim Hosp Assoc* **20**:537.

3 Center SA, Scott DW, Scott FW (1982) Multiple cutaneous horns on the footpads of a cat. *Feline Pract* **12**:26–30.

Zinc responsive dermatosis

1 Colombini S (1999) Canine zinc-responsive dermatosis. *Vet Clin North Am: Small Anim Pract* **29**:1373–1381.

2 White SD, Bourdeau P, Rosychuk RAW *et al.* (2001) Zinc-responsive dermatosis in dogs: 41 cases and literature review. *Vet Dermatol* **12**:101–109.

3 Colombini S, Dunstan RW (1997) Zinc-responsive dermatosis in northern-breed dogs: 17 cases (1990–1996). *J Am Vet Med Assoc* **211**:451–457.

4 McEwan NA, McNeil PE, Thompson H *et al.* (2000) Diagnostic features, confirmation and disease progression in 28 cases of lethal acrodermatitis of Bull Terriers. *J Small Anim Pract* **41**:507–513.

5 McEwan NA (2001) *Malassezia* and *Candida* infections in Bull Terriers with lethal acrodermatitis. *J Small Anim Pract* **42**:291–297.

6 Bensignor E, Germain PA (2004) Canine recurrent pyoderma: a multicenter prospective study. *Vet Dermatol* **15**:42.

7 van den Broek AHM, Stafford WL (1988) Diagnostic value of zinc concentrations in serum, leukocytes and hair of dogs with zinc-responsive dermatosis. *Res Vet Sci* **44**:41–44.

8 Burton G, Mason KV (1998) The possible role of prednisolone in 'zinc-responsive dermatosis' in the Siberian Husky. *Aust Vet Pract* **28**:20–24.

Lethal acrodermatitis of Bull Terriers

1 Jezyk PF, Haskins ME, MacKay-Smith WE *et al.* (1986) Lethal acrodermatitis in Bull Terriers. *J Am Vet Med Assoc* **188**:833–839.

2 Uchida Y, Moon-Fanelli AA, Dodman NH *et al.* (1997) Serum concentrations of zinc and copper in Bull Terriers with lethal acrodermatitis and tail-chasing behavior. *Am J Vet Res* **58**:808–810.

3 McEwan NA, McNeil PE, Thompson H *et al.* (2000) Diagnostic features, confirmation and disease progression in 28 cases of lethal acrodermatitis in Bull Terriers. *J Small Anim Pract* **41**:501–507.

Facial dermatitis of Persian and Himalayan cats

1 Bond R, Curtis CF, Ferguson EA *et al.* (2000) An idiopathic facial dermatitis of Persian cats. *Vet Dermatol* **11**:35–41.

Spiculosis

1 McKeever PJ, Torres SM, O'Brien TD (1992) Spiculosis. *J Am Anim Hosp Assoc* **28**:257–262.

CHAPTER 7: PIGMENTARY ABNORMALITIES

Vitiligo

1 Naughton GK, Mahaffey M, Bystryn JC (1986) Antibodies to surface antigens of pigmented cells in animals with vitiligo. *Proceedings of the Society for Experimental Biology and Medicine* **181**:423–426.

2 Mosher DB, Fitzpatrick TB, Ortonne JP *et al.* (1987) Disorders of pigmentation. In *Dermatology in General Medicine* (eds TB Fitzpatrick, AZ Eisen, K Wolff, I Freedberg, KF Austen). McGraw-Hill Inc., New York, pp. 794–876.

3 Gross TL, Ihrke PJ, Walder EJ (1992) Vitiligo. In *Veterinary Dermatopathology*. Mosby Year Book, St. Louis, pp. 150–153.

4 Guagure E, Alhaidari Z (1989) Disorders of melanin pigmentation in the skin of dogs and cats. In *Current Veterinary Therapy X* (ed RW Kirk). WB Saunders, Philadelphia, pp. 628–632.

Canine uveodermatologic syndrome
(Vogt–Koyanagi–Harada-like [VKH] syndrome)

1 Gross TH, Ihrke PJ, Walder EJ, Affolter VK (2005) Vogt–Koyanagi–Harada-like syndrome. In *Skin Diseases of the Dog and Cat: Clinical and Histopathologic Diagnosis*, 2nd edn. Blackwell Publishing, Oxford, pp. 266–268.

2 Kern TJ, Walton DK, Riis RC *et al.* (1985) Uveitis associated with poliosis and vitiligo in six dogs. *J Am Vet Med Assoc* **187**:408–414.

3 Morgan RV (1989) Vogt–Koyanagi–Harada syndrome in humans and dogs. *Compend Cont Educ Pract Vet* **11**:1211–1218.

4 Murphy C, Belhorn R, Thirkill C (1991) Anti-retinal antibodies associated with Vogt–Koyanagi–Harada-like syndrome in a dog. *J Am Anim Hosp Assoc* **27**:399–402.

5 Vercelli A, Taraglio S (1990) Canine Vogt–Koyanagi–Harada-like syndrome in two Siberian Husky dogs. *Vet Dermatol* **1**:151–158.

6 Sigle KJ, McLellan GJ, Haynes JS *et al.* (2006) Unilateral uveitis in a dog with uveodermatologic syndrome. *J Am Vet Med Assoc* **228**:543–548.

Lentigo and lentiginosis profusa

1 Briggs OM (1985) Lentiginosis profusa in the Pug: 3 case reports. *J Small Anim Pract* **26**:675–680.

2 Scott DW (1987) Lentigo simplex in orange cats. *Companion Anim Pract* **1**:23–25.

3 van Rensburg IBJ, Briggs OM (1986) Pathology of canine lentiginosis profusa. *J South African Vet Assoc* **57**:159–161.

4 Le Net JL, Orth G, Sundberg JP *et al.* (1997) Multiple pigmented cutaneous papules associated with a novel canine papillomavirus in an immunosuppressed dog. *Vet Pathol* **34**:8–14.

5 Nagata M, Nanko H, Moriyama A *et al.* (1995) Pigmented plaques associated with papillomavirus infection in dogs. Is this epidermodysplasia verruciformis? *Vet Dermatol* **6**:179–186.

6 Stokking LB, Ehrhart EJ, Lichtensteiger CA *et al.* (2004) Pigmented epidermal plaques in three dogs. *J Am Anim Hosp Assoc* **40**:411–417.

7 Nash S, Paulsen D (1990) Generalized lentigenes in a silver cat. *J Am Vet Med Assoc* **196**:1500–1501.

CHAPTER 8: ENVIRONMENTAL DERMATOSES

Tick infestation

1 Dryden MW (2006) Challenges and solutions to tick control. *Compend Cont Educ Pract Vet* **28**:10–13.

2 Blagburn BL (2006) Control of tick-borne diseases: a complete review. *Compend Cont Educ Pract Vet* **28**:14–22.

3 Dryden MW, Payne PA (2004) Biology and control of ticks infesting dogs and cats in North America. *Vet Ther* **5**:139–154.

4 Trotz-Williams LA, Trees AJ (2003) Systematic review of the distribution of the major vector-borne parasitic infections in dogs and cats in Europe. *Vet Rec* **152**:97–105.

5 Shaw SE, Day MJ, Birtles RJ *et al.* (2001) Tick-borne infectious diseases of dogs. *Trends Parasitol* **17**:74–80.

6 Kidd L, Breitschwerdt EB (2003) Transmission times and prevention of tick-borne diseases in dogs. *Compend Cont Educ Pract Vet* **25**:742–747.

7 Raghavan M, Glickman N, Moore G *et al.* (2007) Prevalence of and risk factors for canine tick infestation in the United States, 2002–2004. *Vector Borne Zoonotic Dis* **7**:65–75.

8 Parker A (2005) Risk factors for canine tick paralysis: a case control study. *Aust Vet Pract* **35**:132–136.

9 Zenner L, Drevon-Gaillot E, Callait-Cardinal MP (2006) Evaluation of four manual tick-removal devices for dogs and cats. *Vet Rec* **159**:526–529.

10 Dautel H, Cranna R (2006) Assessment of repellency and mortality of an imidacloprid plus permethrin spot-on solution against *Ixodes holocyclus* using a moving object bioassay. *Aust Vet Pract* **36**:138–141.

11 Dryden MW, Payne PA, Smith V *et al.* (2006) Evaluation of an imidacloprid (8.8% w/w)-permethrin (44.0% w/w) topical spot-on and a fipronil (9.8% w/w)-(S)-methoprene (8.8% w/w) topical spot-on to repel, prevent attachment, and kill adult *Ixodes scapularis* and *Amblyomma americanum* ticks on dogs. *Vet Ther* **7**:173–186.

12 Dryden MW, Payne PA, Smith V *et al.* (2006) Evaluation of an imidacloprid (8.8% w/w)-permethrin (44.0% w/w) topical spot-on and a fipronil (9.8% w/w)-(S)-methoprene (8.8% w/w) topical spot-on to repel, prevent attachment, and kill adult *Rhipicephalus sanguineus* and *Dermacentor variabilis* ticks. *Vet Ther* **7**:187–198.

Bee stings and spider bites

1 Fitzgerald KT, Flood AA (2006) Hymenoptera stings. *Clin Tech Small Anim Pract* **21**:194–204.

2 Conceicao LG, Haddad V, Loures FH (2006) Pustular dermatosis caused by fire ant (*Solenopsis invicta*) stings in a dog. *Vet Dermatol* **17**:453–455.

3 Peterson ME (2006) Black widow spider envenomation. *Clin Tech Small Anim Pract* **21**:187–190.

4 Peterson ME (2006) Brown spider envenomation. *Clin Tech Small Anim Pract* **21**:191–193.

5 Antin IP (1963) Fatal anaphylactic reaction of dog to bee sting. *J Am Vet Med Assoc* **142**:775.

6 Walker T, Tidwell AS, Rozanski EA *et al.* (2005) Imaging diagnosis: acute lung injury following massive bee envenomation in a dog. *Vet Radiol Ultrasound* **46**:300–303.

7 Curtis CF, Bond R, Blunden AS *et al.* (1995) Canine eosinophilic folliculitis and furunculosis in three cases. *J Small Anim Pract* **36**:119–123.

8 Guaguere E, Prelaud P, Peyronnet L *et al.* (1996) Eosinophilic furunculosis. A study of 12 dogs. *Prat Med Chir Anim* **31**:413–419.

9 Walder EJ, Howard EB (1981) Persistent insect bite granuloma in a dog. *Vet Pathol* **18**:839–841.

10 Isbister GK, Seymour JE, Gray MR *et al.* (2003) Bites by spiders of the family Theraphosidae in humans and canines. *Toxicon* **41**:519–524.

11 Sousa CA, Halliwell RE (2001) The ACVD task force on canine atopic dermatitis (XI): the relationship between arthropod hypersensitivity and atopic dermatitis in the dog. *Vet Immunol Immunopathol* **81**:233–237.

Fly and mosquito bite dermatosis

1 Mason KV, Evans AG (1991) Mosquito bite-caused eosinophilic dermatitis in cats. *J Am Vet Med Assoc* **198**:2086–2088.

2 Wilkinson GT, Bates MJ (1984) A possible further clinical manifestation of the feline eosinophilic granuloma complex. *J Am Anim Hosp Assoc* **20**:325–331.

Myiasis

1 Hendrix CM (1991) Facultative myiasis in dogs and cats. *Compend Cont Educ Pract Vet* **13**:86–93.

Burns

1 McKeever PJ (1980) Thermal injury. In *Current Veterinary Therapy VII* (ed RW Kirk). WB Saunders, Philadelphia, pp. 191–194.

2 Saxon WD, Kirby R (1992) Treatment of acute burn injury and smoke inhalation. In *Current Veterinary Therapy XI* (eds RW Kirk, JD Bonagura). WB Saunders, Philadelphia, pp. 146–152.

3 Rudowski W, Nasitowski W, Zietkiewiez W *et al.* (1976) *Burn Therapy and Research*. Johns Hopkins University Press, Baltimore.

4 Stamp GL, Crow DT (1992) Triage and resuscitation of the catastrophic trauma patient. In *Current Veterinary Therapy XI* (eds RW Kirk, JD Bonagura). WB Saunders, Philadelphia, pp. 75–82.

5 Ofeigsson OJ (1995) Water cooling: first aid treatment for scalds and burns. *Surgery* **57**:391–400.

Frostbite

1 Dietrich RA (1983) Cold injury (hypothermia, frostbite, freezing). In *Current Veterinary Therapy VIII* (ed RW Kirk). WB Saunders, Philadelphia, pp. 187–189.

CHAPTER 9: ENDOCRINE DERMATOSES

Hypothyroidism

1 Frank LA (2006) Comparative dermatology: canine endocrine dermatoses. *Clin Dermatol* **24**:317–325.

2 Panciera DL (2001) Conditions associated with canine hypothyroidism. *Vet Clin North Am: Small Anim Pract* **31**:935–942.

3 Gulikers KP, Panciera DL (2002) Influence of various medications on canine thyroid function. *Compend Cont Educ Pract Vet* **24**:511–523.

4 Frank LA, Hnilica KA, May ER *et al.* (2005) Effects of sulfamethoxazole-trimethoprim on thyroid function in dogs. *Am J Vet Res* **66**:256–259.

5 Shiel RE, Acke E, Puggioni A *et al.* (2007) Tertiary hypothyroidism in a dog. *Irish Vet J* **60**:88–93.

6 Dixon RM, Reid SJ, Mooney CT (1999) Epidemiological, clinical, haematological and biochemical characteristics of canine hypothyroidism. *Vet Rec* **145**:481–487.

7 Kennedy LJ, Quarmby S, Happ GM *et al.* (2006) Association of canine hypothyroidism with a common major histocompatibility complex DLA class II allele. *Tissue Antigens* **68**:82–86.

8 Fyfe JC, Kampschmidt K, Dang V *et al.* (2003) Congenital hypothyroidism with goiter in toy fox terriers. *J Vet Int Med* **17**:50–57.

9 Greco DS (2006) Diagnosis of congenital and adult-onset hypothyroidism in cats. *Clin Tech Small Anim Pract* **21**:40–44.

10 Dixon RM, Mooney CT (1999) Evaluation of serum-free thyroxine and thyrotropin concentrations in the diagnosis of canine hypothyroidism. *J Small Anim Pract* **40**:72–78.

11 Kemppainen RJ, Behrend EN (2001) Diagnosis of canine hypothyroidism – perspectives from a testing laboratory. *Vet Clin North Am: Small Anim Pract* **31**:951–967.

12 Schachter S, Nelson RW, Scott-Moncrieff C *et al.* (2004) Comparison of serum-free thyroxine concentrations determined by standard equilibrium dialysis, modified equilibrium dialysis, and 5 radioimmunoassays in dogs. *J Vet Int Med* **18**:259–264.

13 Iversen L, Jensen AL, Hoier R *et al.* (1999) Biological variation of canine serum thyrotropin (TSH) concentration. *Vet Clin Pathol* **28**:16–19.

14 Dixon RM, Reid SWJ, Mooney CT (2002) Treatment and therapeutic monitoring of canine hypothyroidism. *J Small Anim Pract* **43**:334–340.

15 Boretti FS, Sieber-Ruckstuhl NS, Favrot C et al. (2006) Evaluation of recombinant human thyroid-stimulating hormone to test thyroid function in dogs suspected of having hypothyroidism. *Am J Vet Res* **67**:2012–2016.

16 Dixon RM, Mooney CT (1999) Canine serum thyroglobulin autoantibodies in health, hypothyroidism and non-thyroidal illness. *Res Vet Sci* **66**:243–246.

17 Taeymans O, Daminet S, Duchateau L et al. (2007) Pre- and post-treatment ultrasonography in hypothyroid dogs. *Vet Radiol Ultrasound* **48**:262–269.

18 Espineira MMD, Mol JA, Peeters ME et al. (2007) Assessment of thyroid function in dogs with low plasma thyroxine concentration. *J Vet Int Med* **21**:25–32.

Hyperadrenocorticism

1 Merchant SR, Taboada J (1997) Endocrinopathies: thyroid and adrenal disorders. *Vet Clin North Am: Small Anim Pract* **27**:1285–1297.

2 Mooney C (1998) Unusual endocrine disorders in the cat. *In Pract* **20**:345–351.

3 Rosychuk RAW (1998) Cutaneous manifestations of endocrine disease in dogs. *Compend Cont Educ Pract Vet* **20**:287–392.

4 Watson PJ, Herrtage ME (1998) Hyperadrenocorticism in six cats. *J Small Anim Pract* **39**:175–184.

5 Hoenig M (2002) Feline hyperadrenocorticism – where are we now? *J Feline Med Surg* **4**:171–174.

6 Behrend EN, Kemppainen RJ (2001) Diagnosis of canine hyperadrenocorticism. *Vet Clin North Am: Small Anim Pract* **31**:985–997.

7 Gould SM, Baines EA, Mannion PA et al. (2001) Use of endogenous ACTH concentration and adrenal ultrasonography to distinguish the cause of canine hyperadrenocorticism. *J Small Anim Pract* **42**:113–121.

8 van der Vlugt-Meijer R, Meij BP et al. (2003) Dynamic computed tomography of the pituitary gland in dogs with pituitary-dependent hyperadrenocorticism. *J Vet Int Med* **17**:773–780.

9 Benitah NM, Feldman EC, Kass PH et al. (2005) Evaluation of serum 17-hydroxyprogesterone concentration after administration of ACTH in dogs with hyperadrenocorticism. *J Am Vet Med Assoc* **227**:1095–1101.

10 Bruyette DS (2000) An approach to diagnosing and treating feline hyperadrenocorticism. *Vet Med* **95**:142–148.

11 Schoeman JP, Evans HJ, Childs D et al. (2000) Cortisol response to two different doses of intravenous synthetic ACTH (tetracosactrin) in overweight cats. *J Small Anim Pract* **41**:552–557.

12 Ruckstuhl NS, Nett CS, Reusch CE (2002) Results of clinical examinations, laboratory tests, and ultrasonography in dogs with pituitary-dependent hyperadrenocorticism treated with trilostane. *Am J Vet Res* **63**:506–512.

13 Bell R, Neiger R, McGrotty Y et al. (2006) Study of the effects of once daily doses of trilostane on cortisol concentrations and responsiveness to adrenocorticotrophic hormone in hyperadrenocorticoid dogs. *Vet Rec* **159**:277–281.

14 Alenza DP, Arenas C, Lopez ML et al. (2006) Long-term efficacy of trilostane administered twice daily in dogs with pituitary-dependent hyperadrenocorticism. *J Am Anim Hosp Assoc* **42**:269–276.

15 Chapman PS, Kelly DF, Archer J et al. (2004) Adrenal necrosis in a dog receiving trilostane for the treatment of hyperadrenocorticism. *J Small Anim Pract* **45**:307–310.

16 Barker EN, Campbell S, Tebb AJ et al. (2005) A comparison of the survival times of dogs treated with mitotane or trilostane for pituitary-dependent hyperadrenocorticism. *J Vet Int Med* **19**:810–815.

17 den Hertog E, Braakman JCA, Teske E et al. (1999) Results of non-selective adrenocorticolysis by o,p'-DDD in 129 dogs with pituitary-dependent hyperadrenocorticism. *Vet Rec* **144**:12–17.

18 Anderson CR, Birchard SJ, Powers BE et al. Surgical treatment of adrenocortical tumors: 21 cases (1990–1996). *J Am Anim Hosp Assoc* **37**:93-97.

19 van Sluijs FJ, Sjollema BE, Voorhout G et al. (1995) Results of adrenalectomy in 36 dogs with hyperadrenocorticism caused by adrenocortical tumor. *Vet Quart* **17**:113–116.

20 Meij B, Voorhout G, Rijnberk A (2002) Progress in transsphenoidal hypophysectomy for treatment of pituitary-dependent hyperadrenocorticism in dogs and cats. *Mol Cell Endocrinol* **197**:89–96.

21 Bruyette DS, Ruehl WW, Entriken TL et al. (1997) Treating canine pituitary-dependent hyperadrenocorticism with L-deprenyl. *Vet Med* **92**:711–727.

22 Braddock JA, Church DB, Robertson ID et al. (2004) Inefficacy of selegiline in treatment of canine pituitary-dependent hyperadrenocorticism. *Aust Vet J* **82**:272–277.

23 Mayer MN, Greco DS, LaRue SM (2006) Outcomes of pituitary tumor irradiation in cats. *J Vet Int Med* **20**:1151–1154.

24 Mayer-Stankeova S, Bley CR, Wergin M et al. (2004) Efficacy of radiotherapy in 13 dogs treated for pituitary tumors. *Tierarztl Prax K H* **32**:232–237.

25 Boag AK, Neiger R, Church DB (2004) Trilostane treatment of bilateral adrenal enlargement and excessive sex steroid production in a cat. *J Small Anim Pract* **45**:263–266.

26 Neiger R, Witt AL, Noble A et al. (2004) Trilostane therapy for treatment of pituitary-dependent hyperadrenocorticism in 5 cats. *J Vet Int Med* **18**:160–164.

27 Skelly BJ, Petrus D, Nicholls PK (2003) Use of trilostane for the treatment of pituitary-dependent hyperadrenocorticism in a cat. *J Small Anim Pract* **44**:269–272.

28 Moore LE, Biller DS, Olsen DE (2000) Hyperadrenocorticism treated with metyrapone followed by bilateral adrenalectomy in a cat. *J Am Vet Med Assoc* **217**:691–696.

29 Duesberg CA, Nelson RW, Feldman EC et al. (1995) Adrenalectomy for the treatment of hyperadrenocorticism in cats – 10 cases (1988–1992). *J Am Vet Med Assoc* **207**:1066–1070.

30 Dunn K (1997) Complications associated with the diagnosis and management of canine hyperadrenocorticism. *In Pract* **19**:246–251.

Hyperandrogenism

1 Rosychuk RAW (1998) Cutaneous manifestations of endocrine disease in dogs. *Compend Cont Educ Pract Vet* **20**:287–296.

2 Frank LA (2006) Comparative dermatology – canine endocrine dermatoses. *Clin Dermatol* **24**:317–325.

3 Dow SW, Olson PN, Rosychuk RAW et al. (1988) Perianal adenomas and hypertestosteronemia in a spayed bitch with pituitary-dependent hyperadrenocorticism. *J Am Vet Med Assoc* **192**:1439–1441.

4 Hill KE, Scott-Moncrieff JCR, Koshko MA et al. (2005) Secretion of sex hormones in dogs with adrenal dysfunction. *J Am Vet Med Assoc* **226**:556–561.

Sertoli cell and other testicular neoplasia

1 Rosychuk RAW (1998) Cutaneous manifestations of endocrine disease in dogs. *Compend Cont Educ Pract Vet* **20**:287–292.

2 Turek MM (2003) Cutaneous paraneoplastic syndromes in dogs and cats: a review of the literature. *Vet Dermatol* **14**:279–296.

3 Doxsee AL, Yager JA, Best SJ et al. (2006) Extra-testicular interstitial and Sertoli cell tumors in previously neutered dogs and cats: a report of 17 cases. *Can Vet J* **47**:763–766.

4 Peters MAJ, de Jong FH, Teerds KJ et al. (2000) Ageing, testicular tumours and the pituitary-testis axis in dogs. *J Endocrinol* **166**:153–161.

5 Kim O, Kim KS (2005) Seminoma with hyperesterogenemia in a Yorkshire Terrier. *J Vet Med Sci* **67**:121–123.

6 Mischke R, Meurer D, Hoppen HO et al. (2002) Blood plasma concentrations of oestradiol-17 beta, testosterone and testosterone/oestradiol ratio in dogs with neoplastic and degenerative testicular diseases. *Res Vet Sci* **73**:267–272.

7 Brazzell JL, Weiss DJ (2006) A retrospective study of aplastic pancytopenia in the dog: 9 cases (1996–2003). *Vet Clin Pathol* **35**:413–417.

8 Pugh CR, Konde LJ (1991) Sonographic evaluation of canine testicular and scrotal abnormalities – a review of 26 case histories. *Vet Radiol* **32**:243–250.

9 Masserdotti C, Bonfanti U, De Lorenzi D et al. (2005) Cytologic features of testicular tumours in dog. *J Vet Med A* **52**:339–346.

Pituitary dwarfism

1 Scott DW, Miller WH, Griffin CE (1995) Endocrine and metabolic diseases. In *Small Animal Dermatology*, 5th edn. WB Saunders, Philadelphia, pp. 628–719.

2 Lund-Larson TR, Grondalen J (1976) Aetiolitic dwarfism in the German Shepherd Dog. Low somatomedin activity associated with apparently normal pituitary function (two cases) and with panadenopituitary dysfunction (one case). *Acta Vet Scand* **17**:293–306.

3 Chastain CB, Ganjam VK (1986) The endocrine brain. In *Clinical Endocrinology of Companion Animals*. Lea & Febiger, Philadelphia, pp. 37–96.

4 Eigenmann JE (1986) Growth hormone-deficient disorders associated with alopecia in the dog. In *Current Veterinary Therapy IX* (ed RW Kirk). WB Saunders, Philadelphia, pp. 1006–1014.

5 DeBowes LJ (1987) Pituitary dwarfism in a German Shepherd dog puppy. *Compend Cont Educ Pract Vet* **9**:931–937.

6 Feldman EC, Nelson RW (1987) Growth hormone. In *Canine and Feline Endrocrinology and Reproduction*. WB Saunders, Philadelphia, pp. 29–54.

7 Bell AG (1993) Growth hormone responsive dermatosis in three dogs. *N Z Vet J* **41**:195–199.

8 Kooistra HS, Voorhout G, Carlotti DN, et al. (1998) Progestin induced growth hormone (GH) production in treatment of dogs with congenital GH deficiency. *Domest Anim Endocrinol* **15**:93–102.

Alopecia X
(adrenal sex hormone imbalance, follicular dysfunction of plush-coated breeds, adrenal hyperplasia-like syndrome, growth hormone/castration responsive dermatoses, adult-onset hyposomatotropism, pseudo-Cushing's disease, alopecia of follicular arrest)

1 Schmeitzel LP, Parker W (1992) Growth hormone and sex hormone alopecia. In *Advances in Veterinary Dermatology, Vol.* 2 (eds PJ Ihrke, IS Mason, SD White). Pergamon Press, Oxford, pp. 451–454.

2 Schmeitzel LP, Lothrop CD (1990) Hormonal abnormalities in Pomeranians with normal coat and in Pomeranians with growth hormone-responsive dermatosis. *J Am Vet Med Assoc* **107**:1333–1341.

3 Schmeitzel LP, Lothrop CD, Rosenkrantz WS (1995) Congenital adrenal hyperplasia-like syndrome. In *Current Veterinary Therapy XII* (ed JD Bonagura). WB Saunders, Philadelphia, pp. 600–604.

4 Frank LA, Hnilica KA, Rohrbach BW *et al.* (2003) Retrospective evaluation of sex hormone and steroid hormone intermediates in dogs with alopecia. *Vet Dermatol* **14**:91–97.

5 Paradis M (2004) Miscellaneous hormone-responsive alopecias. In *Small Animal Dermatology Secrets* (ed KL Campbell). Hanley & Belfus, Philadelphia, pp. 288–296.

6 Cerundolo R, Lloyd DH, Persechino A *et al.* (2004) Treatment of canine alopecia X with trilostane. *Vet Dermatol* **15**:285–293.

CHAPTER 10: OTITIS EXTERNA

1 August JR (1988) Otitis externa: a disease of multifactorial etiology. *Vet Clin North Am: Small Anim Pract* **18**:731–742.

2 McKeever PJ (1995) Canine otitis externa. *Current Veterinary Therapy XII* (ed JD Bonagura). WB Saunders, Philadelphia, pp. 647–655.

3 McArthy G, Kelly WR (1982) Microbial species associated with canine ear disease and their antibacterial sensitivity patterns. *Irish Vet J* **36**:53–56.

4 Mansfield PD, Boosinger TR, Attleburger MH (1990) Infectivity of *Malassezia pachydermatis* in the external ear canal of dogs. *J Am Anim Hosp Assoc* **26**:97–100.

5 Stout-Graham MS, Kainer RA, Whalen LR *et al.* (1990) Morphological measurements of the horizontal ear canal of dogs. *Am J Vet Res* **51**:990–994.

6 Hendricks A, Brooks H, Pocknell A *et al.* (2002) Ulcerative otitis externa responsive to immunosuppressive therapy in two dogs. *J Small Anim Pract* **43**:350–354.

7 Van der Gaag I (1986) The pathology of the external ear canal in dogs and cats. *Vet Quart* **8**:307–317.

8 Mansfield PD (1990) Ototoxicity in dogs and cats. *Compend Cont Educ Pract Vet* **12**:331–337.

9 Neer MT, Howard PE (1982) Otitis media. *Compend Cont Educ Pract Vet* **4**:410–417.

10 Sanchez-Leal J, Mayos I, Homedes J *et al.* (2006) *In vitro* investigation of ceruminolytic activity of various otic cleansers for veterinary use. *Vet Dermatol* **17**:121–127.

11 Nielloud F, Reme CA, Fortune R *et al.* (2004) Development of an *in vitro* test to evaluate the cerumen dissolving properties of several veterinary ear cleansing solutions. *J Drug Deliv Sci Tech* **14**:235–238.

12 Swinney A, Fazakerley J, McEwan NA *et al.* (2008) Comparative *in vitro* antimicrobial efficacy of commercial ear cleaners. *Vet Dermatol* **19**:373–379.

13 Lloyd DH, Bond R, Lamport I (1998) Antimicrobial activity *in vitro* and *in vivo* of a canine ear cleanser. *Vet Rec* **143**:111–112.

14 Cole LK, Kwochka KW, Kowalski JJ *et al.* (2003) Evaluation of an ear cleanser for the treatment of infectious otitis externa in dogs. *Vet Ther* **4**:12–23.

15 Reme CA, Pin D, Collinot C *et al.* (2006) The efficacy of an antiseptic and microbial anti-adhesive ear cleanser in dogs with otitis externa. *Vet Ther* **7**:15–26.

16 Strauss TB, McKeever TM, McKeever PJ (2005) The efficacy of an acidified sodium chlorite solution to treat canine *Pseudomonas aeruginosa* otitis externa. *Vet Med* **100**:55–63.

17 Bassett RJ, Burton GG, Robson DC *et al.* (2004) Efficacy of an acetic acid/boric acid ear cleaning solution for treatment and prophylaxis of *Malassezia* sp. otitis externa. *Aust Vet Pract* **34**:79–82.

18 Cole LK, Luu DH, Rajala-Schultz PJ *et al.* (2006) *In vitro* activity of an ear rinse containing tromethamine, EDTA, and benzyl alcohol on bacterial pathogens from dogs with otitis. *Am J Vet Res* **67**:1040–1044.

19 McEwan NA, Reme CA, Gatto H (2005) Sugar inhibition of adherence by *Pseudomonas* to canine corneocytes. *Vet Dermatol* **16**:204–205.

20 McEwan NA, Reme CA, Gatto H *et al.* (2006) Sugar inhibition of adherence by *Staphylococcus intermedius* to canine corneocytes. *Vet Dermatol* **17**:358.

21 McEwan NA, Kelly R, Woolley K *et al.* (2007) Sugar inhibition of *Malassezia pachydermatis* to canine corneocytes. *Vet Dermatol* **18**:187–188.

22 Morrielo KA, Fehrer-Sawyer SL, Meyer DJ *et al.* (1988) Adrenocortical suppression associated with topical otic administration of glucocorticoids in dogs. *J Am Vet Med Assoc* **193:**329–331.

23 Paradis M (1989) Ivermectin in small animal dermatology. *Current Veterinary Therapy X* (ed RW Kirk). WB Saunders, Philadelphia, pp. 560–563.

CHAPTER 11: DISORDERS OF THE NAILS

1 Scott DW, Miller WH (1992) Disorders of the claw and clawbed in dogs. *Compend Cont Educ Pract Vet* **14:**1448–1458.

2 Rosychuck RAW (1995) Diseases of the claw and claw fold. In *Current Veterinary Therapy XII* (ed JD Bonagura). WB Saunders, Philadelphia, pp. 641–647.

3 Foil CS (1987) Disorders of the feet and claws. *Proceedings of Annual Kal Kan Symposium* **11:**23–32.

4 Muller RS, Friend S, Shipstone MA *et al.* (2000) Diagnosis of canine claw disease – a prospective study of 24 dogs. *Vet Dermatol* **11:**133–141.

5 McKeever PJ (1972–96) Unpublished observations.

6 Scott DW, Rousselle S, Miller WH (1995) Symmetrical lupoid onychodystrophy in dogs: a retrospective analysis of 18 cases (1989–1993). *J Am Anim Hosp Assoc* **31:**194–201.

CHAPTER 12: DERMATOSES CHARACTERIZED BY PATCHY ALOPECIA

Canine demodicosis (red mange, demodectic mange, demodicosis, demodectic acariosis, follicular mange)

1 Chesney CJ (1999) Short form of *Demodex* species mite in the dog: occurrence and measurements. *J Small Anim Pract* **40:**58–61.

2 Desch CE, Hillier A (2003) *Demodex injai*: a new species of hair follicle mite (Acari : Demodecidae) from the domestic dog (Canidae). *J Med Entomol* **40:**146–149.

3 Scott DW, Farrow BRH, Schulz RD (1974) Studies on the therapeutic and immunological aspects of generalized demodectic mange in the dog. *J Am Anim Hosp Assoc* **10:**233–244.

4 Barta O, Waltman C, Oyekan PP *et al.* (1983) Lymphocyte-transformation suppression caused by pyoderma: failure to demonstrate it in uncomplicated demodectic mange. *Comp Immunol Microbiol Infect Dis* **6:**9–18.

5 Barriga OO, Alkhalidi NW, Martin S *et al.* (1992) Evidence of immunosuppression by *Demodex canis*. *Vet Immunol Immunopathol* **32:**37–46.

6 Scott DW, Miller WH, Griffin CE (2001) Parasitic skin diseases. In: *Muller and Kirk's Small Animal Dermatology*, 6th edn. WB Saunders, Philadelphia, pp. 423–516.

7 Lemarie SL, Hosgood G, Foil CS (1996) A retrospective study of juvenile- and adult-onset generalized demodicosis in dogs (1986–91). *Vet Dermatol* **7:**3–10.

8 Bensignor E (2003) Comparaison of three diagnostic techniques of *Demodex canis* demodicosis in the dog. *Prat Med Chir Anim* **38:**167–171.

9 Saridomichelakis MN, Koutinas AF, Farmaki R *et al.* (2004) Sensitivity of deep skin scrapings, hair pluckings and exudate microscopy in the diagnosis of canine demodicosis. *Vet Dermatol* **15:**48.

10 Mueller RS (2004) Treatment protocols for demodicosis: an evidence-based review. *Vet Dermatol* **15:**75–89.

11 Medleau L, Willemse T (1995) Efficacy of daily amitraz therapy for refractory, generalized demodicosis in dogs – two independent studies. *J Am Anim Hosp Assoc* **31:**246–249.

12 Holm BR (2003) Efficacy of milbemycin oxime in the treatment of canine generalized demodicosis: a retrospective study of 99 dogs (1995–2000). *Vet Dermatol* **14:**189–195.

13 Ristic Z, Medleau L, Paradis M *et al.* (1995) Ivermectin for the treatment of generalized demodicosis in dogs. *J Am Vet Med Assoc* **207:**1308–1311.

14 Paradis M, Page N (1998) Topical (pour-on) ivermectin in the treatment of chronic generalized demodicosis in dogs. *Vet Dermatol* **9:**55–59.

Feline demodicosis

1 Desch CE, Stewart TB (1999) *Demodex gatoi*: new species of hair follicle mite (Acari: Demodecidae) from the domestic cat (Carnivora: Felidae). *J Med Entomol* **36:**167–170.

2 Morris DO (1996) Contagious demodicosis in three cats residing in a common household. *J Am Anim Hosp Assoc* **32:**350–352.

3 Guaguere E, Olivry T, Delverdier-Poujade A *et al.* (1999) *Demodex cati* infestation in association with feline cutaneous squamous cell carcinoma in situ: a report of five cases. *Vet Dermatol* **10:**61–67.

4 Vogelnest LJ (2001) Cutaneous xanthomas with concurrent demodicosis and dermatophytosis in a cat. *Aust Vet J* **79:**470–475.

5 Guaguere E, Muller A, Degorce-Rubiales F (2004) Feline demodicosis: a retrospective study of 12 cases. *Vet Dermatol* **15:**34.

6 van Poucke S (2001) Ceruminous otitis externa due to *Demodex cati* in a cat. *Vet Rec* **149:**651–652.

7 Mueller RS (2004) Treatment protocols for demodicosis: an evidence-based review. *Vet Dermatol* **15**:75–89.

8 Johnstone IP (2002) Doramectin as a treatment for canine and feline demodicosis. *Aust Vet Pract* **32**:98–103.

Dermatophytosis

1 Lewis DT, Foil CS, Hopgood G (1991) Epidemiology and clinical features of dermatophytosis in dogs and cats at Louisiana State University: 1981–1990. *Vet Dermatol* **2**:53–58.

2 Sparkes AH, Gruffydd Jones TJ, Shaw SE *et al.* (1993) Epidemiological and diagnostic features of canine and feline dermatophytosis in the United Kingdom from 1956–1991. *Vet Rec* **133**:57–61.

3 Cabanes FJ, Abarca ML, Bragulat MR (1997) Dermatophytes isolated from domestic animals in Barcelona, Spain. *Mycopathologia* **137**:107–113.

4 Cafarchia C, Romito D, Sasanelli M *et al.* (2004) The epidemiology of canine and feline dermatophytoses in southern Italy. *Mycoses* **47**:508–513.

5 Moriello KA, DeBoer DJ (1991) Fungal flora of the haircoat of cats with and without dermatophytosis. *J Med Vet Mycol* **29**:285–292.

6 Moriello KA, DeBoer DJ (1991) Fungal flora of the coat of pet cats. *Am J Vet Res* **52**:602–606.

7 Moriello KA, Kunkle GA, DeBoer DJ (1994) Isolation of dermatophytes from the haircoats of stray cats from selected animal shelters in two different geographic regions in the United States. *Vet Dermatol* **5**:57–62.

8 Sparkes AH, Werrett G, Stokes CR *et al.* (1994) *Microsporum canis* – inapparent carriage by cats and the viability of arthrospores. *J Small Anim Pract* **35**:397–401.

9 Moriello KA, DeBoer DJ (1995) Feline dermatophytosis. *Vet Clin North Am: Small Anim Pract* **25**:901–921.

10 DeBoer DJ, Moriello KA (1995) Investigations of a killed dermatophyte cell-wall vaccine against infection with *Microsporum canis* in cats. *Res Vet Sci* **59**:110–113.

11 Mancianti F, Nardoni S, Corazza M *et al.* (2003) Environmental detection of *Microsporum canis* arthrospores in the households of infected cats and dogs. *J Feline Med Surg* **5**:323–328.

12 Bergman RL, Medleau L, Hnilica K *et al.* (2002) Dermatophyte granulomas caused by *Trichophyton mentagrophytes* in a dog. *Vet Dermatol* **13**:49–52.

13 Godfrey DR (2001) *Microsporum canis* associated with otitis externa in a Persian cat. *Vet Rec* **147**:50–51.

14 Paterson S (1999) Miconazole/chlorhexidine shampoo as an adjunct to systemic therapy in controlling dermatophytosis in cats. *J Small Anim Pract* **40**:163–166.

15 DeBoer DJ, Moriello KA (1995) Inability of two topical treatments to influence the course of experimentally induced dermatophytosis in cats. *J Am Vet Med Assoc* **207**:52–57.

16 Hill PB, Moriello KA, Shaw SE (1995) A review of systemic antifungal agents. *Vet Dermatol* **6**:59–66.

17 Moriello KA (2004) Treatment of dermatophytosis in dogs and cats: review of published studies. *Vet Dermatol* **15**:99–107.

18 Moriello KA, DeBoer DJ, Schenker R *et al.* (2004) Efficacy of pretreatment with lufenuron for the prevention of *Microsporum canis* infection in a feline direct topical challenge model. *Vet Dermatol* **15**:357–362.

19 DeBoer DJ, Moriello KA, Blum JL *et al.* (2003) Effects of lufenuron treatment in cats on the establishment and course of *Microsporum canis* infection following exposure to infected cats. *J Am Vet Med Assoc* **222**:1216–1220.

20 Newbury S, Verbrugge M, Steffen T *et al.* (2005) Management of naturally occurring dermatophytosis in an open shelter. Part 1: Development of a cost effective screening and monitoring program. *Vet Dermatol* **16**:205.

21 Newbury S, Verbrugge M, Steffen T *et al.* (2005) Management of naturally occurring dermatophytosis in an open shelter. Part 2: Treatment of cats in an off-site facility. *Vet Dermatol* **16**:206.

22 Heinrich K, Newbury S, Verbrugge M *et al.* (2005) Detection of environmental contamination with *Microsporum canis* arthrospores in exposed homes and efficacy of the triple cleaning decontamination technique. *Vet Dermatol* **16**:205–206.

Canine familial dermatomyositis

1 Hargis AM, Haupt KH (1990) Review of familial canine dermatomyositis. *Vet Ann* **30**:227–282.

2 Gross TH, Ihrke PJ, Walder EJ, Affolter VK (2005) Cell-poor vasculitis. In *Skin Diseases of the Dog and Cat: Clinical and Histopathologic Diagnosis*, 2nd edn. Blackwell Publishing, Oxford, pp. 247–250.

3 Hargis AM, Mundell AC (1992) Familial canine dermatomyositis. *Compend Cont Educ Pract Vet* **14**:855–864.

4 Haupt KH, Prieur DJ, Moore MP *et al.* (1985) Familial canine dermatomyositis: clinical, electrodiagnostic, and genetic studies. *Am J Vet Res* **46**:1861–1869.

5 Gross TH, Ihrke PJ, Walder EJ, Affolter VK
   (2005) Ischemic dermatopathy/canine dermatomyositis. In *Skin Diseases of the Dog and Cat:
   Clinical and Histopathologic Diagnosis*, 2nd edn.
   Blackwell Publishing, Oxford, pp. 49–52.

6 Rees CA (2004) Inherited vesiculobullous
   disorders. *Small Animal Dermatology Secrets*
   (ed KL Campbell). Hanley & Belfus,
   Philadelphia, pp. 112–119.

Injection site alopecia

1 Gross TH, Ihrke PJ, Walder EJ, Affolter VK
   (2005) Post rabies vaccination panniculitis. In
   *Skin Diseases of the Dog and Cat: Clinical and
   Histopathologic Diagnosis*, 2nd edn. Blackwell
   Publishing, Oxford, pp. 538–541.

2 Wilcock BP, Yager JA (1986) Focal cutaneous
   vasculitis and alopecia at sites of rabies vaccination
   in dogs. *J Am Vet Med Assoc* **188:**1174–1177.

3 Gross TL, Ihrke PJ, Walder EJ (1992) Atrophic
   diseases of the hair follicle. In *Veterinary Dermatopathology*. Mosby Yearbook, St. Louis,
   pp. 287–298.

4 Lester S, Clemett T, Burt A (1996) Vaccine site-
   associated sarcomas in cats: clinical experience and
   a laboratory review (1982–1993). *J Am Anim
   Hosp Assoc* **32:**91–95.

5 Vitale CB, Gross TL, Margro CM (1999) Case
   report: vaccine-induced ischemic dermatopathy in
   the dog. *Vet Dermatol* **10:**131–142.

6 Medleau L, Hnilica KA (2006) Injection reaction
   and post-rabies vaccination alopecias. In *Small
   Animal Dermatology: A Color Atlas and Therapeutic Guide*. Elsevier, St. Louis, p. 267.

Alopecia areata

1 Olivry T, Moore PF, Naydan DK *et al.* (1996)
   Antifollicular cell-mediated and humoral immunity in canine alopecia areata. *Vet Dermatol*
   7:67–79.

2 Tobin DJ, Gardner SH, Luther PB *et al.* (2003)
   A natural canine homologue of alopecia areata in
   humans. *Br J Dermatol* **149:**938–950.

3 De Jonghe SR, Ducatelle RV, Mattheeuws DR
   (1999) Trachyonychia associated with alopecia
   areata in a Rhodesian Ridgeback. *Vet Dermatol*
   10:123–126.

4 Letada PR, Sparling JD, Norwood C (2007)
   Imiquimod in the treatment of alopecia univer-
   salis. *Cutis* **79:**138–140.

5 Letko E, Bhol K, Pinar V *et al.* (1999) Tacrolimus
   (FK 506). *Ann Allergy Asthma Immun*
   83:179–189.

6 Price VH (2003) Therapy of alopecia areata: on
   the cusp and in the future. *J Invest Dermatol*
   8:207–211.

Follicular dysplasia

1 Gross TH, Ihrke PJ, Walder EJ, Affolter VK
   (2005) Cell-poor vasculitis. In *Skin Diseases of
   the Dog and Cat: Clinical and Histopathologic
   Diagnosis*, 2nd edn. Blackwell Publishing, Oxford,
   pp. 247–250.

2 Post K, Dignean MA, Clark E (1988) Hair follicle
   dysplasia of Siberian Huskies. *J Am Anim Hosp
   Assoc* **24:**659–662.

3 Miller WH (1990) Follicular dysplasia in adult black
   and red Doberman Pinschers. *Vet Dermatol*
   1:181–187.

4 Laffort-Dassot C, Beco L, Carlotti DN (2003)
   Follicular dysplasia in five Weimaraners. *Vet
   Dermatol* **13:**253–260.

5 Cerundolo R, Lloyd DH, McNeil PE *et al.* (2000)
   An analysis of factors underlying hypotrichosis and
   alopecia in Irish Water Spaniels in the United
   Kingdom. *Vet Dermatol* **11:**107–122.

6 Miller WH, Scott DW (1995) Follicular dysplasia
   of the Portuguese Water Dog. *Vet Dermatol*
   6:67–74.

Black hair follicular dysplasia

1 Hargis AM, Brignac MM, Al-Bagdadi FAK *et al.*
   (1991) Black hair follicular dysplasia in black and
   white Saluki dogs: differentiation from color-
   mutant alopecia in the Doberman Pinscher by
   microscopic examination of hairs. *Vet Dermatol*
   2:69–83.

2 Selmanowitz VJ, Markofsky F, Orentreich N
   (1977) Black hair follicular dysplasia in dogs.
   J Am Vet Med Assoc **171:**1079–1081.

3 Harper RC (1978) Congenital black hair
   follicle dysplasia in Bearded Collie pups. *Vet Rec*
   102:87.

4 Scott DW, Miller WH, Griffin CE (2001) Black
   hair follicular dysplasia. In *Muller and Kirk's Small
   Animal Dermatology*, 6th edn. WB Saunders,
   Philadelphia, pp. 959–970.

5 Gross TH, Ihrke PJ, Walder EJ, Affolter VK
   (2005) Color-dilution alopecia and black hair
   follicular dysplasia. In *Skin Diseases of the Dog
   and Cat: Clinical and Histopathologic Diagnosis*,
   2nd edn. Blackwell Publishing, Oxford,
   pp. 518–522.

Color-dilution alopecia
(color-mutant alopecia, Blue Dobermann syndrome)

1 Miller WH (1990) Color-dilution alopecia in Doberman Pinschers with blue or fawn coat colors: a study of the incidence and histopathology of this disorder. *Vet Dermatol* **1**:113–121.

2 Miller WH (1991) Alopecia associated with coat color dilution in two Yorkshire Terriers, one Saluki, and one mix-breed. *J Am Anim Hosp Assoc* **27**:39–43.

3 Brignac MM, Foil CS, Al-Bagdadi FAK *et al*. (1990) Microscopy of color-mutant alopecia. In *Advances in Veterinary Dermatology, Vol. 1* (eds C von Tscharner, REW Halliwell). Baillière Tindall, London, p. 448.

4 Gross TH, Ihrke PJ, Walder EJ, Affolter VK (2005) Color-dilution alopecia and black hair follicular dysplasia. *Skin Diseases of the Dog and Cat: Clinical and Histopathologic Diagnosis*, 2nd edn. Blackwell Publishing, Oxford, pp. 518–522.

Cyclical flank alopecia
(seasonal flank alopecia, flank alopecia, recurrent flank alopecia)

1 Gross TL, Ihrke PJ, Walder EJ, Affolter VK (2005) Cyclical flank alopecia. In *Skin Diseases of the Dog and Cat: Clinical and Histopathologic Diagnosis*, 2nd edn. Blackwell Publishing, Oxford, pp. 525–528.

2 Miller MA, Dunstan RW (1993) Seasonal flank alopecia in Boxers and Airedale Terriers: 24 cases (1985–1992). *J Am Vet Med Assoc* **203**:1567–1572.

Telogen effluvium, anagen defluxion, wave shedding, diffuse shedding, and excessive continuous shedding

1 Diaz SF, Torres SMF, Dunstan RW *et al*. (2004) An analysis of canine hair re-growth after clipping for a surgical procedure. *Vet Dermatol* **15**:25–30.

2 Scott DW, Miller WH, Griffin CE (2001) Acquired alopecias. In *Muller and Kirk's Small Animal Dermatology*, 6th edn. WB Saunders, Philadelphia, pp. 887–912.

Post-clipping alopecia

1 Gross TL, Irhke PJ, Walder EJ (1992) Post-clipping alopecia. In *Veterinary Dermatopathology*. Mosby Year Book, St. Louis, pp. 285–286.

2 Diaz SF, Torres SMF, Dunstan RW *et al*. (2004) An analysis of canine hair re-growth after clipping for a surgical procedure. *Vet Dermatol* **15**:25–30.

Topical corticosteroid reaction

1 Gross TL, Ihrke PJ, Walder EJ, Affolter VK (2005) Topical corticosteroid reaction. In *Skin Diseases of the Dog and Cat: Clinical and Histopathologic Diagnosis*, 2nd edn. Blackwell Publishing, Oxford, pp. 392–394.

Feline paraneoplastic alopecia

1 Brooks DG, Campbell KL, Dennis JS *et al*. (1994) Pancreatic paraneoplastic alopecia in three cats. *J Am Anim Hosp Assoc* **30**:557–563.

2 Godfrey DR (1998) A case of feline paraneoplastic alopecia with secondary *Malassezia*-associated dermatitis. *J Small Anim Pract* **39**:394–396.

3 Pascal A, Olivry T, Gross TL *et al*. (1997) Paraneoplastic alopecia associated with internal malignancies in the cat. *Vet Dermatol* **8**:47–52.

4 Tasker S, Griffon DJ, Nuttall TJ *et al*. (1999) Resolution of paraneoplastic alopecia following surgical removal of a pancreatic carcinoma in a cat. *J Small Anim Pract* **40**:16–19.

Index